Molecular Orbital Studies in Chemical Pharmacology

Molecular Orbital Studies In Chemical Pharmacology

Edited by

Lemont B. Kier

SPRINGER-VERLAG BERLIN • HEIDELBERG • NEW YORK 1970

Molecular Orbital Studies in Chemical Pharmacology

a symposium held at

Battelle Seattle Research Center
4000 N.E. 41st Street
Seattle, Washington

October 20-22, 1969

Chairman:

Lemont B. Kier
Associate Fellow in Medicinal Chemistry
Columbus Laboratories
Battelle Memorial Institute
Columbus, Ohio

Participants:

Arthur Cammarata
Jack Peter Green
James R. Hoyland
Lemont B. Kier
W. Brock Neely
Bernard Pullman
William P. Purcell
Robert Rein
Solomon H. Snyder
Arnold J. Wohl

ISBN 978-3-540-04972-2 ISBN 978-3-642-87536-6 (eBook)
DOI 10.1007/978-3-642-87536-6

Library of Congress Catalog Card Number 77-120374

Title Number 1690

Preface

A symposium on molecular orbital studies in chemical pharmacology was held at the Battelle Seattle Research Center of Battelle Memorial Institute in Seattle, Washington, U.S.A, on October 20-22, 1969. This volume is a collection of the lectures presented at that symposium.

The use of quantum mechanics to study the actions of molecules of biological importance is being developed by a number of scientists concerned with these phenomena. The advent of high speed computers has made possible the application of this technique to large molecules, of the kind important in living systems. One result of this expanded computational ability has been the utilization of molecular orbital theory by a group of scientists of diverse backgrounds. The lecturers at this symposium, all interested in molecular orbital theory, have backgrounds in pharmacology, physical chemistry, theoretical chemistry, biochemistry and medicinal chemistry. The common denominator among these scientists has been the realization that they must search at the primary level of chemical events for explanations of biological phenomena. Since these events are governed to a large extent by the properties of the valence electrons of molecules, molecular orbital theory offers great promise in explaining and predicting biological phenomena.

October, 1969 Lemont B. Kier

Table of Contents

ELECTRONS IN NUCLEIC ACIDS AND THEIR CONSTITUENTS*

by

Bernard Pullman**

I. INTRODUCTION

To choose the problem of the electronic structure of the nucleic acids and of their constituents as the subject of an introductory lecture to a symposium on Quantum Biology certainly does not require any justification. The central role played by these substances in modern Molecular Biology is in itself the most evident reason for such a choice. In our case, however, there are two complementary reasons for this selection.

The first of them lies in the central role played by these same compounds in the historical and technical development of quantitative quantum biochemistry, the designation referring to the application of the concepts and methods of wave-mechanics, as developed previously, e.g., in the field of quantum chemistry, to the investigation of the electronic structure of biological molecules in relation to their behavior as substrates of life and to their involvement in the biochemical and biophysical processes characteristic of living matter [1]. Although isolated attempts have been made occasionally earlier in this field, they have been very scarce and generally of a qualitative and speculative nature. It was the sudden understanding by quantum chemists of the central role played in the phenomena of life by the purines and pyrimidines of the nucleic acids, i.e., by molecules very similar to those that they have been familiar with for a long time (conjugated heterocycles), which more than anything else pointed to the possibility of applying

* This work was supported by grant number 66 236 of the Institut National de la Santé et de la Recherche Médicale (Intergroupe Cancer et Leucémie).

** University of Paris, Institut de Biologie Physico-Chimique, 13, rue P. et M. Curie Paris 5e, France.

the ideas and procedures of quantum chemistry to the problems of molecular biology. The historical discovery by Watson and Crick of the main features of the molecular structure of DNA dates back to 1953. The first theoretical calculation on the fundamental purines and pyrimidines has been carried out in 1956 [2] and the first theoretical calculation on the purine-pyrimidine complementary base pairs in 1959 [3]. Quantum biology is a direct outcome of the DNA revolution.

The second reason for the selection of the outlined subject for our talk resides in the fact that not only were these compounds the first studied but that they are also the most studied and this, moreover, not only in the numerical but also in the technical sense of the word. Because of the obvious importance of these molecules and of the problems involved, the calculations on purines and pyrimidines, although carried out always within the general frame of the molecular orbital method, have been constantly refined.

For a number of approximations of the method they represent the biggest molecules to have been studied. The history of the calculations on the electronic structure of purines and pyrimidines reflects, in fact, the recent rapid evolution of the methods of quantum chemistry as applied or applicable to large molecules, whether conjugated, saturated, or of a mixed nature.

II. THE DEVELOPMENT OF CALCULATIONS

Thus, in spite of the limited period (approximately fifteen years) of their elaboration, five stages may be distinguished in the development of the calculations on the electronic structure of the purine and pyrimidine bases:

1) The first period, starting with the publications mentioned above and embracing a large number of subsequent papers [4-13], corresponds to calculations carried out within the classical Hückel approximation of the molecular orbital method (HMO) and is limited to the π-electronic system of the compounds studied. In spite of the well-known shortcomings of the Hückel approximation, these calculations yielded a great mass of extremely useful information concerning the structure and the properties of purines and pyrimidines which enabled a general interpretation of a large body of

experimental data concerning the chemical, physicochemical, and biochemical properties of these molecules and of the nucleic acids themselves and led to a number of predictions which have since been largely substantiated by more refined treatments and, what is more important, by subsequent experimentation. The success of the procedure was due mainly to the careful manipulation of the method, which was used essentially for the comparative study of the electronic characteristics of the compounds investigated, in other words for the classification on a relative scale of compounds or molecular regions or their constituent atoms with respect to the electronic properties under investigation. The results of this work are summarized in [1].

2) The second stage corresponds to the advent of more refined calculations going beyond the HMO procedure. The first step in these refinements consisted of adopting the self-consistent field molecular orbital procedure (SCF-MO), generally in one of its semi-empirical versions, (in particular the so-called Pariser-Parr-Pople approximation, PPP-SCF-MO), where some of the calculations included a further refinement in the form of allowing configurational interaction or mixing (SCF-CI-MO). The calculations were still limited to the π-electronic system of the compounds studied.

The first calculation utilizing the PPP-SCF-MO method is due to Veillard and Pullman [14,15]. It was followed by a number of other similar publications [16-33]. As is well known, the self-consistent field methods yield, in principle, more reliable absolute values for a number of indices of electronic structure and should therefore be suitable for a direct comparison of theoretical and experimental results. In practice, although the whole scheme of these procedures is more satisfactory than that of the HMO method, they nevertheless suffer in calculations concerning heteromolecules from many of the same drawbacks. Generally, they do introduce in one way or another some semi-empirical parameters into their scheme, in particular in connection with the different integrals related to heteroatoms. As a consequence of this situation the absolute values of the quantities which they evaluate may be appreciably in error. A very careful scrutinization of the choice of the integrals appearing in the method, their optimization on reference compounds, is indispensable for a successful calculation. This, unfortunately, has not always been done, leading in some cases to drastic mistakes.

3) Calculations referred to above were limited, as stated, to the π-electronic system of the molecules considered. This is, as is well known, a very classical and usual way of dealing when studying quantum-mechanically the electronic structure of conjugated molecules, especially in connection with their chemical properties. It cannot, of course, be considered as completely satisfactory, especially when investigating certain physicochemical properties of molecules (e.g., their dipole moments) in which the distribution of the σ electrons must also play an important role.

For these reasons, concomitantly with the late period of stage 1 and with stage 2, calculations have been performed, essentially by Berthod and Pullman [34,35], (see also [36]) on the characteristics of the underlying σ skeleton of the purine and pyrimidine bases. These calculations have been carried out by a refinement, due to these authors, of the method of Del Re [37,38] for studying σ bonds which may be considered as the counterpart for σ electrons of the Hückel method for π electrons. The results of this type of calculations (DRBP) for the σ electrons have then been combined with the results of the calculations carried out for the π electrons, whether by the HMO or the SCF-MO method, leading thus to a general picture of the electronic distribution.

4) This way of calculating separately and then adding together the distribution of the σ and π electrons suffers from the obvious drawback of neglecting the fine aspects of their mutual interactions. To remedy for this defect, all-valence electrons calculations, dealing simultaneously with the σ and π systems, have been carried out recently for the purines and pyrimidines [39-42] by three procedures developed in recent years. These are the extended Hückel theory (EHT), the iterative extended Hückel theory (IEHT), and the CNDO method (the abbreviation standing for "complete neglect of differential overlap"). While the first two of these procedures are extensions

to all valence electrons of the basic Hückel procedure for π systems, the CNDO method is based on the SCF-MO scheme. A general comparison of the results obtained by the three procedures is given in [43 and 44].

5) Finally, the last of the five stages in the computational refinements of purines and pyrimidines is represented by *ab initio* all electrons (and not only all-valence electrons) calculations. This work utilizes the approach developed primarily by Clementi and his associates [45, 46] and uses a Gaussian atomic basis set for the construction of the molecular orbitals. In principle, it is the less empirical of the techniques used. In practice, its utilization implies very large computational possibilities frequently difficult to obtain. Nevertheless, calculations have been carried out by this procedure by B. Mély and A. Pullman [47] and by Clementi et al. [48] with a somewhat restricted basis set by the former authors, and the usual extended one by the latter.

It is thus obvious that we have available at present for the fundamental constituents of the nucleic acids, their purine and pyrimidine bases, a large number of calculations carried out with a wide variety of computational techniques, starting from the simple procedures limited to π electrons and culminating in refined all-electrons calculations. It is essential to realize that all these techniques are approximation methods as there is no possibility at present to solve rigorously the Schrödinger equation for large molecular systems. All of them involve at one stage or another, although to a different extent, some technical approximations, the validity of which can be best ascertained through the comparison of the theoretical results with experimental data. This situation leads us thus directly to the question of the general scope of the calculations and particularly of the impact of this development of the techniques of the calculations on the nature and significance of the results. There are numerous aspects of this problem related to the many types of results. We cannot of course treat all of them here, and shall therefore consider one or two representative examples.

III. ELECTRONIC CHARGES AND DIPOLE MOMENTS

Let us look first at the problem of the distribution of electronic charges and at the closely related measurements more accessible to a direct experimental check of the molecular dipole moments. Figures 1 and 2, which present the distribution of, respectively, the σ and the π charges along the molecular periphery of cytosine as obtained by a series of calculations carried out in the different previously enumerated methods, illustrate the general aspect of the phenomenon as observed in all the bases. Its principal features are:

1) Appreciable <u>differences in the absolute values</u> of the charges of the different atoms.
2) A striking <u>similarity in the overall pattern</u> of charge distribution obtained by these greatly different procedures.

Now in fact, the comparison of "charges" is really a complicated problem if only because their theoretical definitions are not equivalent in the different procedures. Also, they are not directly measurable quantities. A somewhat more significant and, in my opinion, more striking aspect of the results is therefore indicated by comparing the dipole moments (values and directions) obtained by the different methods. This comparison is illustrated in Figure 3.

The principal conclusion which may be drawn from this figure is again the overall similarity of the results obtained by the different procedures. The absolute values of the moments are again different in the different methods but their relative ordering is the same in all of them. Thus, all methods predict greater dipole moments for guanine and cytosine than for uracil, which in turn should have a slightly greater moment than adenine. In fact, what is really remarkable is the near identity even in the absolute values of the results obtained by the classical method of adding σ charges (calculated in the Hückel type Del Re-Berthod-Pullman procedure) to π charges (whether calculated in a Pariser-Parr-Pople SCF approximation or in the Hückel approximation) with those obtained in the all valence electrons CNDO procedure or in the *ab initio* all electrons procedure. Moreover, the comparison of the theoretical values with the experimental ones (available, it is true, only for simple derivatives of adenine and uracil) indicates

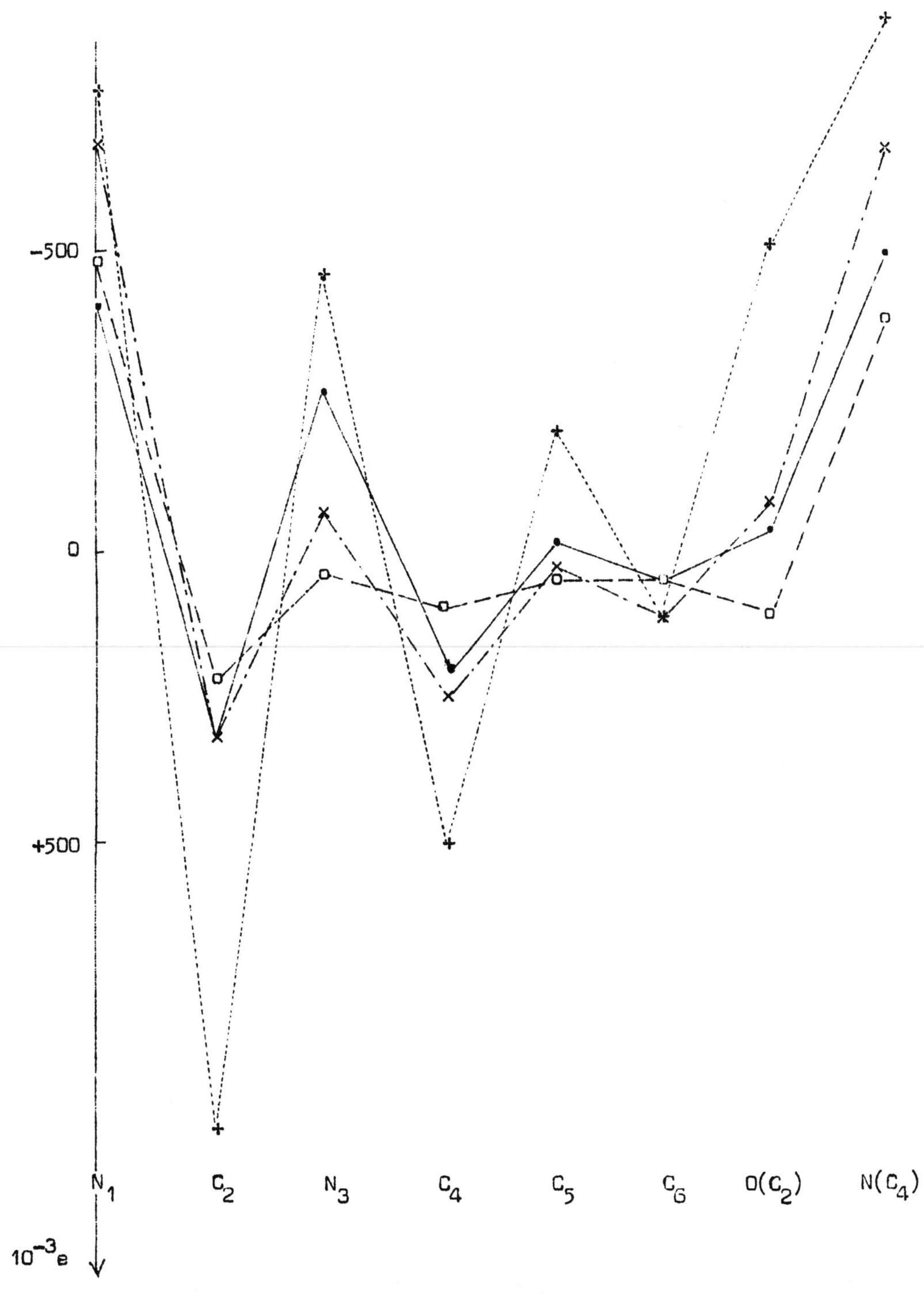

FIGURE 1. Plot of σ charges (10^{-3}e) along the molecular periphery in cytosine (•——— DRBP; +----- EHT; x—•—•—• IEHC; o— — — — CNDO)

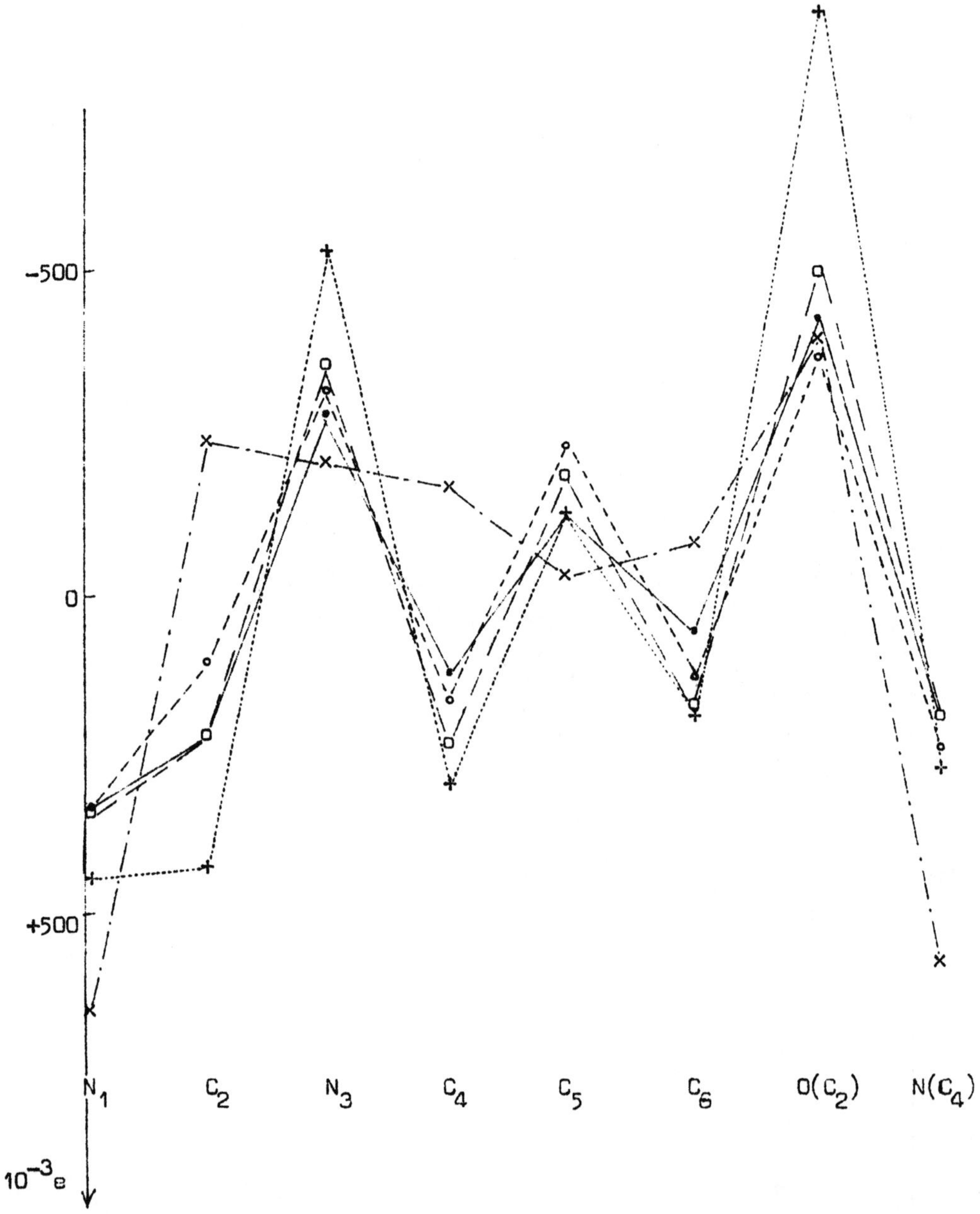

FIGURE 2. Plot of π charges (10^{-3}e) along the molecular periphery in cytosine (•——— PPP; +----- EHT; x—•—•— IEHC; o— — — — CNDO; o---- *ab initio*)

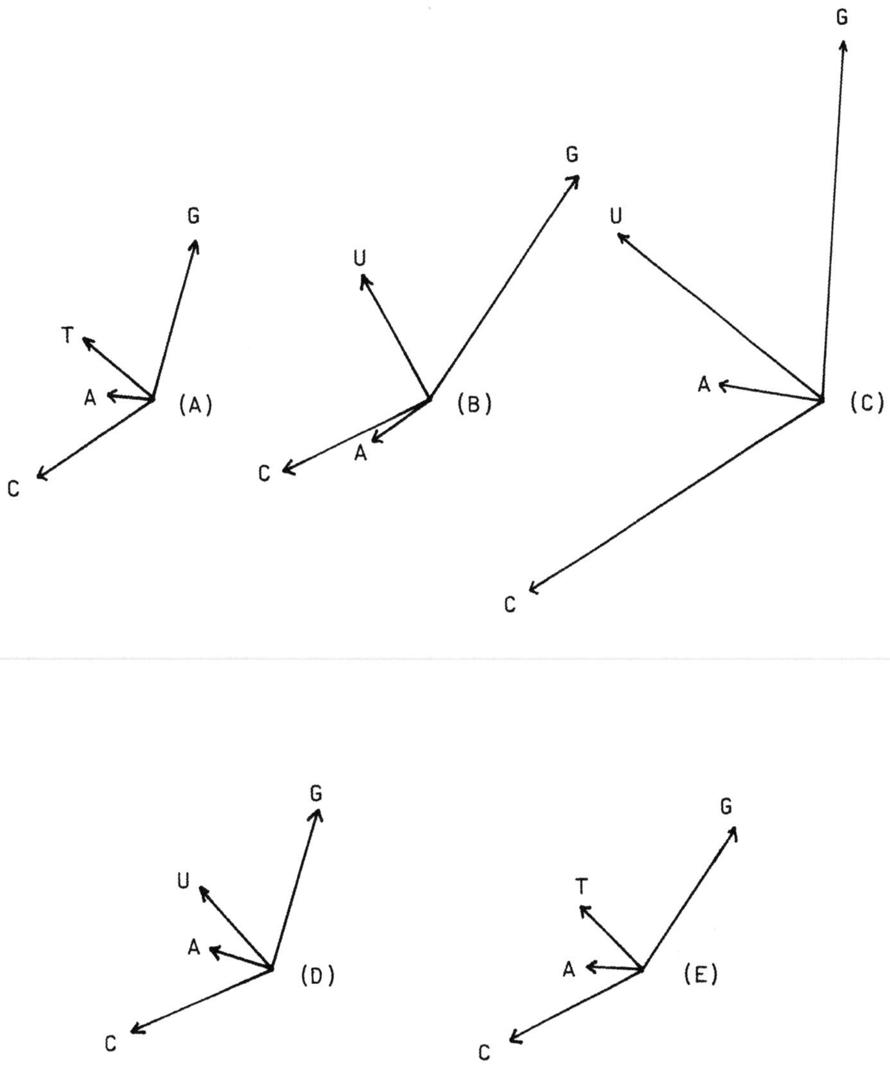

FIGURE 3. Values and directions of the dipole moments in cytosine. (A) $\sigma + \pi$; (B) IEHC; (C) EHT; (D) CNDO; and (E) *ab initio* methods

that these last types of calculations are in very satisfactory agreement with experiment too (Table 1). It may therefore reasonably be expected that the values predicted for G and C in these procedures are quite reliable.

TABLE 1. DIPOLE MOMENTS (DEBYE UNITS)

	σ/π_1 (a)	σ/π_2 (b)	EHT	IEHT	CNDO	*AB INITIO*	Expl. value (c)
A	3.2	2.0	6.1	4.4	2.9	2.8	3.0
U	3.6	3.3	12.2	7.6	4.6	4.2	3.9
G	6.8	7.2	17.2	13.6	7.5		-
C	7.2	7.1	17.3	12.9	7.6	6.7	-

(a) π-moment obtained from the best Hückel parameters and added to the σ-moments evaluated as in [34].

(b) π-moment obtained by the Pariser-Parr-Pople computations [30] and added to the same σ-moment.

(c) For 9-methyladenine and 1,3-dimethyluracile [10].

Another most striking feature of these results is the complete similarity in the directions of the dipoles, this similarity extending even to the EHT and IEHT methods which indicate too large absolute values of the moments. It seems most interesting to report that recent experimental studies of this problem by Mrs. Weiler-Feichenfeld in the laboratory of Professor Bergmann in Jerusalem [49], using a series of substituted purines, have confirmed quantitatively the theoretical predictions of the directions in two fundamental purine skeletons (purine and xanthine).

IV. MOLECULAR ORBITALS AND IONIZATION POTENTIALS

It must, of course, be acknowledged that for some electronic properties the contributions of the refined methods may be more fundamentally important. This is the case, for instance, for the problem of the energies of molecular orbitals. Table 2 gives, as an example, the energies of the occupied molecular orbitals in cytosine as calculated by different all-valence electron methods, and by the *ab initio* procedure.

TABLE 2. OCCUPIED ENERGY LEVELS IN CYTOSINE (eV). UNLABELED ORBITALS ARE σ-LEVELS.

PPP	EHT	IEHT	CNDO	*AB INITIO*
				565.42
				429.28
				428.79
				428.35
				315.09
				314.55
				313.73
				311.55
	37.03	31.35	52.36	39.46
	31.39	28.56	44.91	36.84
	29.51	26.76	41.69	35.48
	27.29	23.87	38.85	32.63
	25.42	22.89	36.61	31.24
	20.25	18.94	31.66	26.55
	19.87	18.28	27.75	25.71
	π 18.14	16.92	25.74	23.37
	17.90	16.23	π 25.53	22.58
	17.67	15.63	25.45	21.78
	16.78	π 15.25	20.96	20.31
	16.16	14.28	20.01	19.09
	15.44	13.72	π 19.91	π 18.73
	π 15.27	π 13.68	18.40	18.51
	14.86	13.11	17.91	π 16.27
	14.40	π 12.99	π 17.20	16.17
π 14.23	π 14.40	11.17	15.56	π 14.44
π 12.23	13.83	10.86	13.68	11.89
π 11.25	π 13.51	π 10.54	π 13.21	π 11.45
π 9.33	12.58	π 10.39	11.81	11.40
π 8.16	π 12.50	9.07	π 10.78	π 9.79

The most striking feature of the all valence and all electrons computations is undoubtedly the indication of a large intermingling of the σ and π levels with no appearançe of a supperficial "π-shell", as is implicitly assumed in π-electron calculations. This result is a definite new contribution of the refined techniques and an important one. But even here it may nevertheless be observed that the particularly significant, highest occupied molecular orbital (HOMO) is in all these calculations (with probably the artifact exception of IEHC) a π one. If we consider therefore, as seems highly plausible, that the highest occupied π molecular orbital is the one which gives, in fact, the measure of the first ionization potential of the molecule, the order of its increasing energy is, in absolute values

$$G < A \approx C < U.$$

Thus, in all cases, guanine appears as the best π-donor and uracil as the worst one among the four bases, the most refined calculations confirming the oldest, most primitive ones. It is very rewarding that the recently measured values of the ionization potentials of the base, carried out ten years after the first predictions, are in the order [50]

$$A \approx C < T < U$$

(values: Adenine 8.91 eV; Cytosine 8.90 eV; Thymine 9.43 eV; Uracil 9.82 eV). The measurements for guanine are unfortunately missing. However, a strong electron donor ability of this compound seems indicated by its easy charge-transfer complexation with chloranil [51].

As to the absolute values of the ionization potentials, they are overestimated in the all-valence and in the all-electrons calculations and somewhat underestimated in the SCF calculation.

In the presence of this situation, I cannot refrain from quoting a statement from Clementi [52] who, on the basis of his studies on a few very simple conjugated heterocycles (pyridine, pyrrole, etc.), issued the following judgment: "Much of the previous and present empirical work on large molecules, and, in particular, on the aromatic molecules of biological significance is at best open to question, not only on its quantitative validity but even on its qualitative validity!"

One has the impression that the author of this statement does not seem to have looked carefully at the previous results. The situation is much simpler and much more classical than he claims. The extension of the calculations to all electrons represents an important improvement of the available techniques, a step in the evolution of quantum chemistry, but apparently not a revolution.

V. INTERBASE INTERACTIONS

The difficulty with an introductory review lecture is that one would like to say a word about everything. One cannot, of course, but I would like to mention, at least, some other aspects of research dealing with the electronic properties of the nucleic acids and their constituents. Among these aspects one seems particularly important to me if only because of the amount of work which has been devoted to it in a number of laboratories including our own. I am thinking about the field of intermolecular interactions between the purines and pyrimidines, whether horizontal (hydrogen bonding) or vertical (stacking), whose fundamental importance to the understanding of the nature of the forces responsible for the ordered structure and stability of the nucleic acids needs hardly to be underlined.

In this problem, again, there is a succession of technical developments which have been introduced progressively in the course of time and particularly during the last few years. I have noticed from the program that Dr. Rein is devoting his whole talk to the problem of the purine-pyrimidine interactions and I suppose therefore that he will be talking about the technical refinements to which he has himself contributed greatly. I would like therefore rather to stress some outstanding aspects of the results concerning some particularly important problems, which have been dealt with in our laboratory. Outstanding among those seems to me to be the one concerned with the exclusivity of hydrogen-bonded pairing between the Watson-Crick complementary bases.

Thus, a large series of recent studies on the co-crystallization of derivatives of the nucleic acid bases, carrying a substituent at their glycosylic nitrogen [53,56] and on their interaction in nonaqueous solvents, e.g., deuterochloroform, CCl_4, or dimethylsulphoxide [57,63] point to the striking result that hydrogen-bonded pairs are being formed exclusively between bases showing complementarity in the Watson-Crick sense, namely between adenine and thymine (uracil) or guanine and cytosine. In the case of the A-T (or A-U) interactions, the pairing appears to be different from that occurring in the nucleic acids; in the case of the G-C interactions, it is similar to it. On the contrary, no interactions whatsoever seem to occur in these circumstances between guanine and thymine or adenine and cytosine, or between cytosine and thymine or guanine and adenine. This result seems surprising at first sight, because it is easily seen that hydrogen bonds can in principle be established in all these cases.

It was the merit of theoretical calculations on the intermolecular forces operating in such associations to have proposed a possible explanation for this situation, somewhat prior to its substantiation by experimental findings. The forces referred to and which we shall call broadly the Van der Waals-London interaction forces correspond to the summation of the electrostatic (monopole-monopole), polarization (monopole-induced dipole) dispersion and short range repulsion components. As I said, they may be evaluated in different degrees of technical refinements and Dr. Rein will certainly say more about it. Insofar as we know and insofar as our problem is concerned, they all lead, however, to the same general result. This result is summarized in Table 3, which indicates for each pair of considered bases the total interaction energy corresponding to the strongest conformation of the association.

It can then be observed that, in principle, all these associations, whether complementary or noncomplementary in the Watson-Crick sense, should involve considerable stabilization energies. A distinct difference appears, however, between the two classes of base pairs when the interaction energies of the cross-associations are compared with those of the self-associations of the constituent molecules. Thus, it may be observed that the stabilization of the A-T association, although relatively moderate, is nevertheless greater than that of the A-A or T-T self-associations. Similarly, although the stabilization of the G-G and C-C self-associations is relatively strong, that of the G-C association is still stronger. On the contrary, all the remaining cross-associations appear always weaker than the self-association of one of their constituents, G or C. It may be easily verified that the same result prevails when the values of the cross-associations are compared with the mean values of the corresponding two self-associations instead of being compared with the values of the strongest self-association.

This general situation points to the conclusion that it is the relatively great strength of the G-G and C-C self-interactions which may possibly be responsible for preventing the in-plane association of the noncomplementary bases.

TABLE 3. IN-PLANE INTERACTION ENERGIES FOR HYDROGEN-BONDED PAIRS (KCAL/MOLE)

A-A	-5.8	A-T	-7.0
T-T	-5.2		
G-G	-14.5	G-C	-19.2
C-C	-13		
A-A	-5.8	A-C	-7.8
C-C	-13		
G-G	-14.5	G-T	-7.4
T-T	-5.2		
C-C	-13	C-T	-6.5
T-T	-5.2		
A-A	-5.8	A-G	-7.5
G-G	-14.5		

A-T	>	A-A, T-T
G-C	>	G-G, C-C
A-C	<	C-C
G-T	<	G-G
C-T	<	C-C
A-G	<	G-G

These results need a few complementary remarks.

1) In the first place it may be useful to indicate that all the essential aforementioned theoretical indications on the relative energies of interaction have been confirmed recently by experimental studies on the interaction of bases in nonaqueous solvents. The available experimental results are summarized in Table 4 from which it may be observed that the only disagreement between theory and experiment concerns the relative order of the U-U *vs* A-A interaction energies, both of which are relatively small and close to each other, so that this reversal is not significant. It is important to realize that this situation indicates that although the calculations have been carried out for systems in vacuum, they seem nevertheless to be valid also insofar as the relative strength of the interactions are concerned for systems in solution.

2) Still more recently the values of the enthalpies of association, in chloroform solution, have been established for the principal self- and cross-associations of the nucleic acid bases [62,63,67,68]. The values are listed in Table 5. Compared with the theoretical values of Table 4 they appear generally appreciably smaller. This situation is in no way astonishing, because one cannot, of course, expect a numerical agreement between calculations carried out for systems in vacuum and measurements in solution. One immediately obvious possible reason for the disparity between the two sets of values could simply be the adoption of a dielectric constant of 1 in the calculation of the electrostatic component of the interaction energies, a component which represents the greatest part of this energy in hydrogen-bonded systems. Following the indication of Scheraga [69] a value close to 3 (close to 2 following Ramachandran [70]) for the dielectric constant would be more appropriate at the interatomic distances under consideration. The adoption of such a value would immediately bring the theoretical values in much closer agreement indeed with the experimental ones.

3) Finally, a mention must be made on some very recent crystallographic results indicating the possible formation in crystals of

TABLE 4. EXPERIMENTAL RESULTS ON HYDROGEN BONDING BETWEEN NUCLEIC ACID BASES

RESULT	REFERENCES	SOLVENT (AND METHOD)	
A-U > A-A or U-U	[57]	$CDCl_3$	(IR)
	[61]	CCl_4	(IR)
	[64]	$CDCl_3$	(IR)
	[62]	$CHCl_3$	(calorimeter)
G-C > G-G or C-C	[58]	$CDCl_3$	(IR)
	[65]		
	[63]	DMSO	(NMR)
G-C > A-T or A-U	[58]	DMSO + $CHCl_3$	(NMR)
	[60]	$CHCl_3$	(IR)
	[59]	DMSO	(NMR)
	[63]	DMSO	(NMR)
G-G > C-C	[65]	$CHCl_3$	(IR)
U-U > A-A	[64]	$CHCl_3$	(IR)
	[67]	$CHCl_3$	(calorimeter)
No interaction between noncomplementary nucleic acid bases	[56] [59] [65]	No co-crystallization	
No interaction between complementary bases unsubstituted at the glycosydic nitrogens.	[66]		

TABLE 5. ENTHALPIES OF HYDROGEN BONDING (KCAL/MOLE) [67]

G-G	8.5-10	G-C	10-11.5
C-C	6.3		
U-U	4.3	A-U	6.2
A-A	4.0		

noncomplementary base associations. Such associations have been established between 5-fluorouracil on one hand and cytosine or 1-methylcytosine or 9-ethylhypoxanthine on the other [71,72,73]. It must be understood that these results are not in contradiction to our previous proposals concerning complementary base pairings. One of the essential characteristics of the noncomplementary crystals resides in the fact that, probably due in a large extent to the absence of a methyl group on the glycosylic nitrogen of 5-fluorouracil, this molecule may form a more extended hydrogen bonded system than 1-methyluracil or 1-methyl-5-fluorouracil. The calculations leading to the complementarity theory are related to dimer formation and cannot be applied without reinvestigation to the formation of more extended networks. Thus, for instance, in the case of the 5-fluorouracil-9-ethylhypoxanthine complex the molecules form a sheet structure in which pairs of fluorouracil molecules are held together by two hydrogen bonds, with the 9-ethylhypoxanthine residues filling up the rest of the molecular sheet by forming single hydrogen bonds with each uracil pair. In the case of 5-fluorouracil and 1-methylcytosine, one observes cyclic hydrogen bonded dimers which are in turn connected by pairs of hydrogen bonds to form large arrays in the crystal. Clearly, these situations are much more complex than the dimer formation to which the previously quoted calculations apply. We are trying to investigate these more complex systems presently. (Very recently another noncomplementary association has been found between 9-ethyl-8-bromoadenine and 9-ethyl-8-bromohypoxanthine [74] which also deserves investigation.)

We are trying presently to investigate interaction energies in dimers involving base analogues, such interactions possibly being of importance for the understanding of the mechanism of action of some mutagens or drugs. Thus we have, for instance, compared the interaction energies of the guanine-cytosine pair with those of the hypoxanthine-cytosine and xanthine-cytosine pair (Table 6). The theoretical results predict a decrease of interaction energy in the two last pairs with respect to the G-C pair, the decrease being particularly strong in the case of xanthine (which may possibly be produced *in situ* from guanine by the action of the mutagen NO_2H). This decrease is substantiated by direct measurement of the enthalpy of base pairing in the case of the hypoxanthine-cytosine pair [67] and more indirectly for the xanthine-cytosine base pair by the absence of complexation between xanthylic acid and polycytidylic acid as opposed to complexations observed between polyguanylic acid or polyinosinic acid and polycytydylic acid [75]. On the other hand interactions stronger than those calculated for the A-U complexes are predicted for adenine-barbituric acid complexation (Table 7), a result of particular significance in connection with recent findings [76,77] of a specific and relatively strong hydrogen bonding of a series of barbiturates to adenine derivatives which may be of importance for the mechanism of action of these drugs.

On the other hand, it must also be recorded that calculations on base interactions have in no way been limited to in-plane interactions, through hydrogen bonding, but have been extended also to vertical interactions between stacked molecules. The most significant result of such calculations was probably to show that the two modes of interaction could be accounted for in a completely homogeneous way by the action of the same type of forces, the previously quoted Van de Waals-London forces, it being only the relative values of their components which change somewhat following the conformation of the association. Thus, the calculations indicate, e.g., that the two types of interaction, horizontal and vertical, contribute in a comparable way to the overall stability of DNA and thus offer an

TABLE 6. INTERACTION ENERGIES OF HYDROGEN BONDING (KCAL/MOLE)

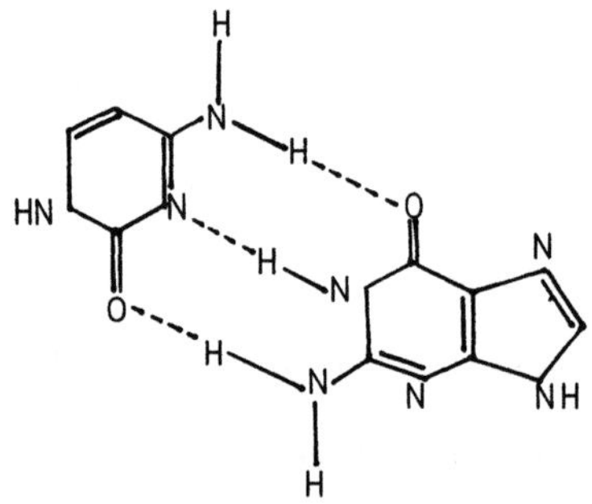 Guanine-cytosine	-19.18
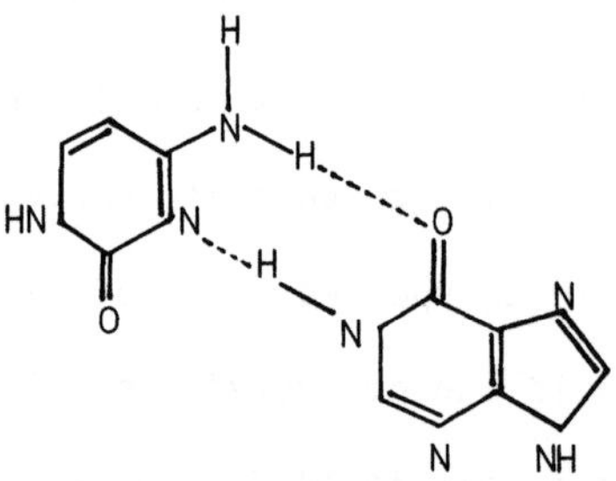 Hypoxanthine-cytosine	-14.24
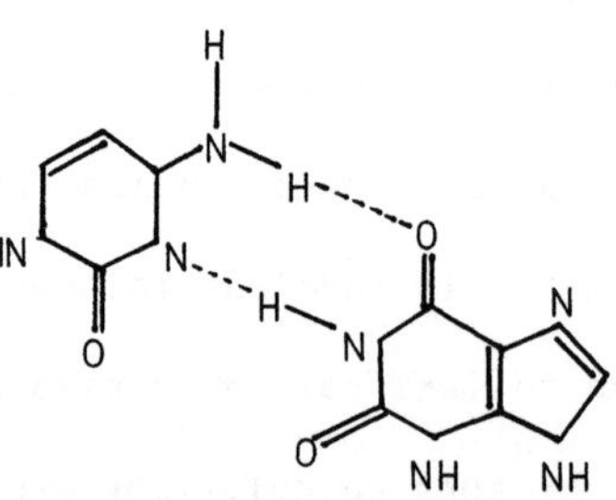 Xanthine-cytosine	-6.54

TABLE 7. INTERACTION ENERGIES FOR HYDROGEN-BONDED COMPLEXES OF ADENINE-URACIL AND ADENINE-BARBITURIC ACID (KCAL/MOLE)

	ENERGY
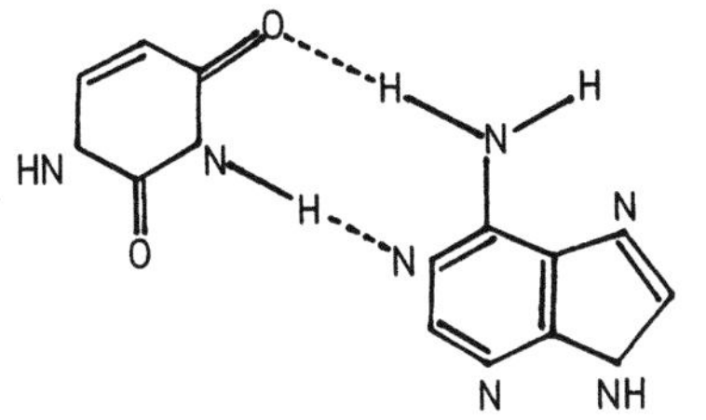	-5.1
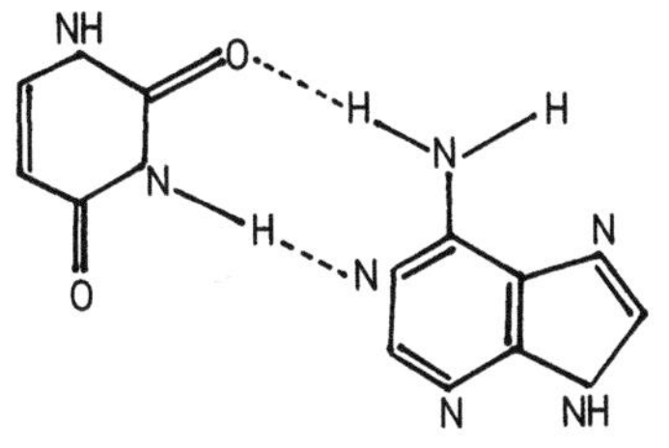	-4.7
Adenine-uracil	
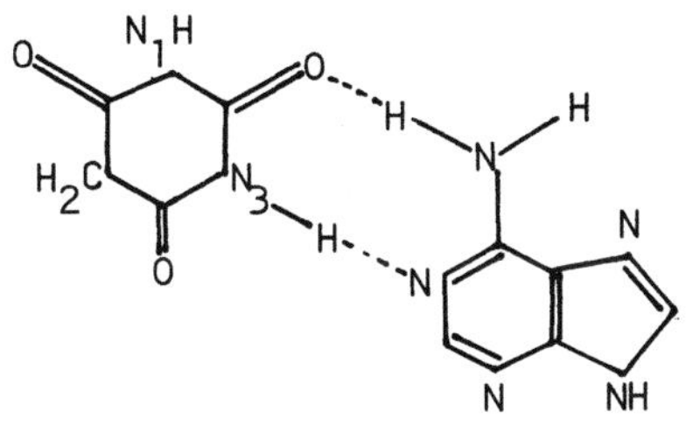	-5.4
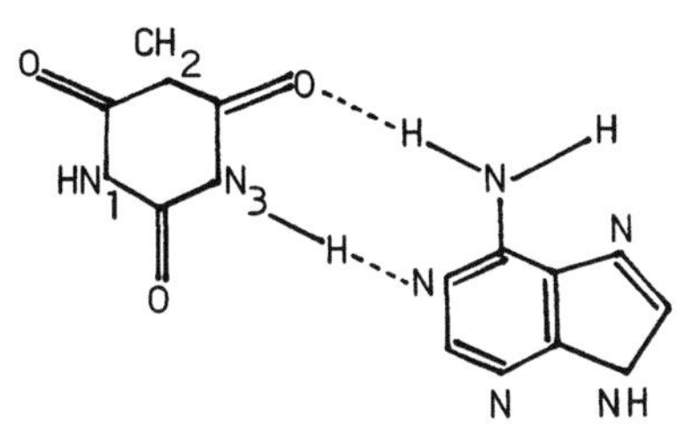	-5.3
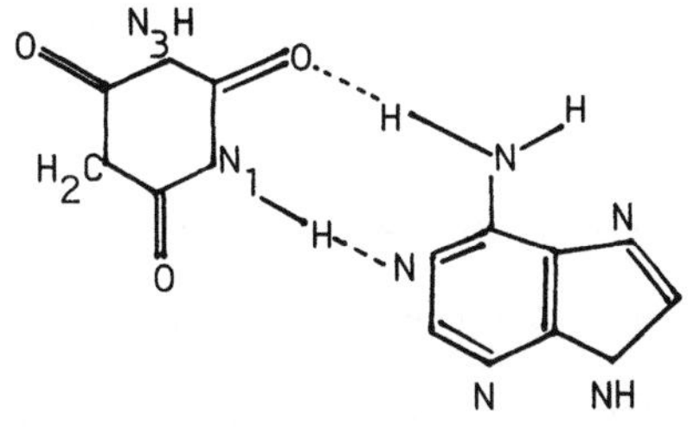	-5.6
Adenine-barbituric acid	

answer to the long debated question of the preeminence of one or the other of these interactions in the nucleic acids [27,78,79].

VI. TAUTOMERISM

Another problem upon which we have been working during the last months concerns the existence and the electronic properties of different tautomeric forms of the purines and the pyrimidines, in particular of the purines which offer a somewhat broader variety of possibilities. The problem itself of the tautomerism of these bases may be of fundamental biological importance, as it is highly possible, following a suggestion contained in the historical notes of Watson and Crick in *Nature*, that it represents one of the available mechanisms for mutations. Thus, it is easily seen that the existence of the bases in the rare tautomeric forms, imine and lactim, instead of the usual amine and lactam ones, may lead to miscouplings of the bases and thus through the perturbation of their sequence along the axis of DNA, to a perturbation of the genetic code. We have investigated already, some time ago, some of the essential energetic and electronic aspects of such miscouplings [80]. More recently we have gone deeper into the examination of the electronic properties of the different possible tautomeric forms of the purines of which there are many more possibilities than it is generally realized. To some extent our interest in this problem has been revived by the recent discovery that the crystal of purine [81] involves long chains of molecules, linked together by single hydrogen bonds, in the way illustrated in I (in Figure 4) for a dimer. The surprising feature of this configuration is that a proton is attached to $N_{(7)}$ rather than to $N_{(9)}$ of the purine skeleton, while in most biological derivatives of purines including the nucleosides and nucleotides the substituent is fixed at $N_{(9)}$.

Similarly, it must be realized that there are in fact two more possible prototropic tautomers III and IV (in Figure 4) corresponding to the fixation of the proton at N_1 and N_3 of the purine skeleton. This type of tautomerism seems to be constantly intermingled in more complex purine derivatives with the amine-imine and lactam-lactim ones. In some purine analogues, such as 8-azapurines, some of

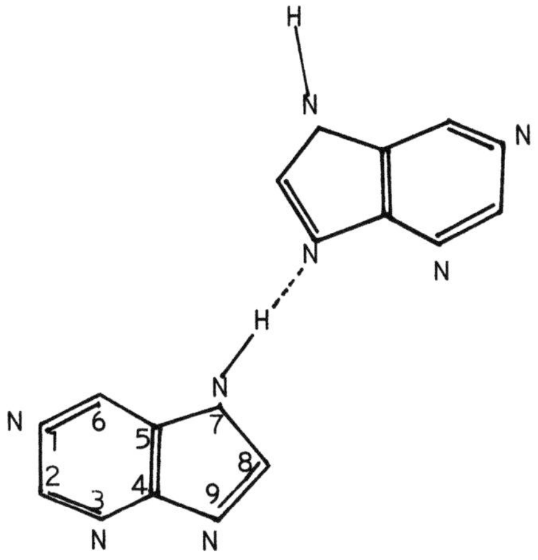

I

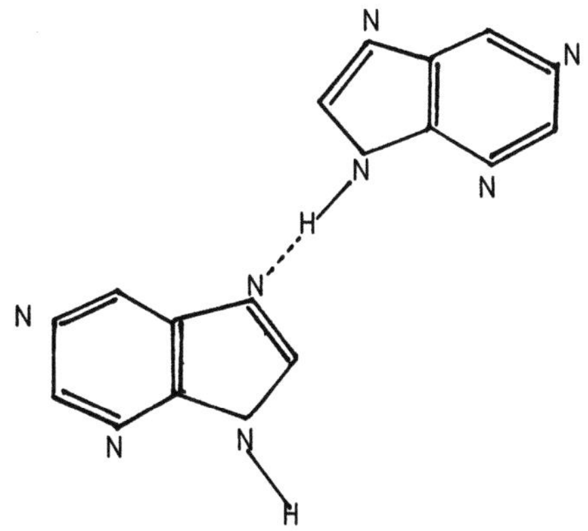

II

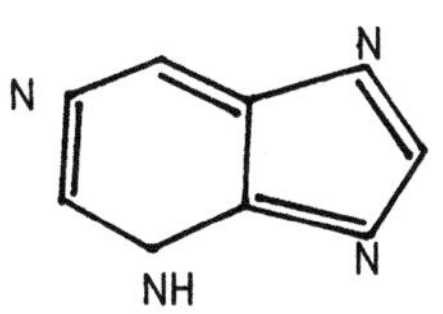

III

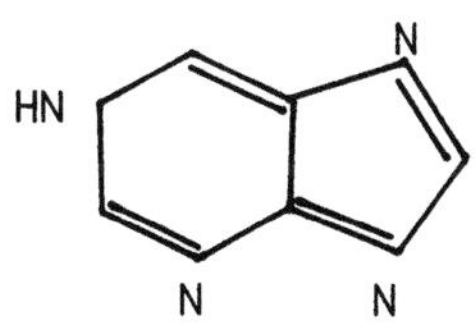

IV

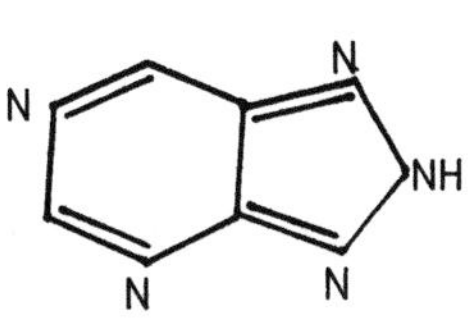

V

FIGURE 4. Tautomers of Purine Derivatives

which are important in mutagenesis or in cancer chemotherapy, there appears the supplementary possibility of the fixation of the proton at N_8, V (in Figure 4). There is a fascinating variety of problems linked with this situation [82] upon which unfortunately we cannot dwell here. The advent of the all-valence electrons method, and in particular of CNDO/2, rendered possible an essential progress in this field: by enabling the calculation of the total molecular energy $(\sigma + \pi)$, it enabled direct predictions on the relative stabilities of the tautomers. An elegant example of the achievement of the procedure is illustrated in Figure 5, which is concerned with the relative stabilities of the amine-imine tautomers of adenine [83]. It predicts that while the amine form should be the most stable one for the $N_{(3)}H$, $N_{(7)}H$, and $N_{(9)}H$ prototropic tautomers, the imine form should be the most stable for the $N_{(1)}H$ tautomer, a delicate prediction verified experimentally on the corresponding methylated derivatives.

Another interesting prediction of the calculations which has important practical consequences concerns the existence of large differences in the dipole moments of such prototropic tautomers, much more significant than the differences in other physico-chemical properties, with the result that the determination of such moments and their comparison with theory may represent one of the ways of identifying the tautomers.

VII. CONCLUSION

In this extremely vast subject of the electronic properties of the nucleic acids and their constituents, we have been able here to touch only upon some of its most striking aspects or at least those which seem among the most striking to us. We left many others untouched. Table 8 contains a list of some of these remaining problems related in one way or another to electrons in nucleic acids and which have been more or less, following the case, treated by quantum-mechanical methods.

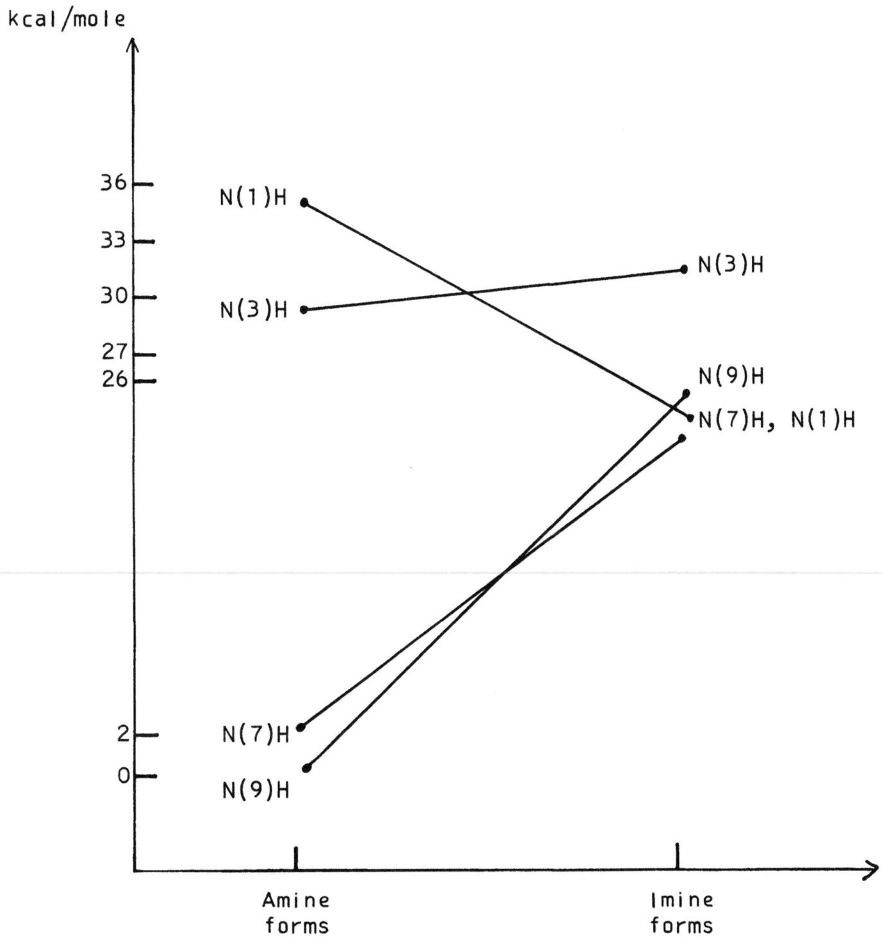

FIGURE 5. Energies of the associated amine and imine forms of adenine tautomers relative to the most stable form (for more details see [82,83])

TABLE 8. PROBLEMS DEALT WITH QUANTUM-MECHANICALLY IN THE FIELD OF THE ELECTRONIC PROPERTIES OF THE NUCLEIC ACIDS AND THEIR CONSTITUENTS

Electronic distribution and chemical reactivity
Basicity
Electron affinity
Polarography
Interactomic distances
Electronic transitions
Properties of the triplet states
Hypochromicity
Optical rotatory dispersion
Interactions with conjugated aromatics (aminoacridines and carcinogenic conjugated hydrocarbons)
Solvents effects
Involvement in charge transfer complexes
Proton tunnelling and the structure of the hydrogen bonds
Conformational problems
Radiosensitivity
Photobiology
Diamagnetic anisotropy, ring currents, proton shifts
Spin densities in free radicals
Semiconductivity
Coding
Mass spectroscopy
Degradation by xanthine oxidase
Structure of analogues

REFERENCES

[1] Pullman, B., and Pullman, A., *Quantum Biochemistry*, Wiley-Interscience, New York (1963).

[2] Pullman, A., Pullman, B., and Berthier, G., *Compt. Rend. Acad. Sci. Paris*, 243, 380 (1956).

[3] Pullman, B., and Pullman, A., *Biochim. Biophys. Acta*, 36, 343 (1959).

[4] Pullman, A., and Pullman, B., *Bull. Soc. Chim. France*, 766 (1958).

[5] Pullman, A., and Pullman, B., *Bull. Soc. Chim. France*, 594 (1959).

[6] Nakajima, T., and Pullman, A., *J. Chim. Phys.* 55, 793 (1958).

[7] Nakajima, T., and Pullman, B., *Bull. Soc. Chim. France*, 1502 (1958).

[8] Nakajima, T., and Pullman, B., *Bull. Soc. Chim. France*, 663 (1959).

[9] Pullman, B., and Pullman, A., *Nature*, 189, 725 (1961).

[10] De Voe, H., and Tinoco, I., Jr., *J. Mol. Biol.*, 4, 500 (1962).

[11] Pullman, A., *Compt. Rend. Acad. Sci. Paris*, 256, 5435 (1963).

[12] Fernandez-Alonso, J. I., p. 3 in *The Structure and Properties of Biomolecules and Biological systems*, edited by J. Dechesne, Wiley-Interscience, New York (1964).

[13] Ladik, J., p. 203 in *Electronic Aspects of Biochemistry* edited by B. Pullman, Academic Press, New York (1964).

[14] Veillard, A., and Pullman, B., *Compt. Rend. Acad. Sci. Paris*, 253, 2277 (1961).

[15] Veillard, A., and Pullman, B., *J. Theor. Biol.*, 4, 37 (1963).

[16] Nesbet, R. K., *Biopolymers Symp.*, 1, 129 (1964).

[17] Nagata, C., Imamura, A., Tagashira, Y., and Kodama, M., *Bull. Chem. Soc. Japan*, 38, 1638 (1965).

[18] Ladik, J., and Appel, K., *Theoret. Chim. Acta*, 4, 132 (1966).

[19] Tanaka, M., and Nagakura, S., *Theoret. Chim. Acta*, 6, 320 (1966).

[20] Kuprievich, V. A., *Intern. J. Quantum Chem.*, 1, 515 (1967).

[21] Imamura, A., Fujita, H., and Nagata, C., *Bull. Chem. Soc. Japan*, 40, 522 (1967).

[22] Pullman, A., p. 515 in *The Triplet State*, edited by A. B. Zahlan, Cambridge University Press, London (1967)

[23] Kwiatkowski, J. S., and Wasilewski, J., *Mol. Phys.*, 13, 229 (1967).

[24] Danilov, V. I., Kuprievich, V. A., and Shramko, O. V., *Biophysics*, 12 213 (1967).

[25] Danilov, V. I., Kuprievich, V. A., and Shramko, O. V., *Biophysics*, 12, 701 (1967).

[26] Kwiatkowski, J. S., *Theoret. Chim. Acta*, 10, 47 (1968).

[27] Pullman, A., and Pullman, B., *Adv. Quantum Chem.*, 4, 267 (1968).

[28] Fraga, S., and Valdemoro, C., *Struct. Bonding*, 4, 1 (1968).

[29] Fujita, H., Imamura, A., and Nagata, C., *Bull. Chem. Soc. Japan*, 41, 2017 (1968).

[30] Berthod, H., Giessner-Prettre, C., and Pullman, A., *Theoret. Chim. Acta*, 5, 53 (1966).

[31] Berthod, H., Giessner-Prettre, C., and Pullman, A., *Compt. Rend.*, 262, 2657 (1966).

[32] Berthod, H., Giessner-Prettre, C., and Pullman, A., *Intern. J. Quantum Chem.*, 1, 123 (1967).

[33] Denis, A., and Pullman, A., *Theoret. Chim. Acta*, 7, 110 (1967).

[34] Berthod, H., and Pullman, A., *J. Chim. Phys.*, 62, 942 (1965).

[35] Berthod, H., and Pullman, A., *Biopolymers*, 2, 483 (1965).

[36] Bradley, D. F., Lifson, S., and Honig, B., p. 7 in *Electronic Aspects of Biochemistry*, edited by B. Pullman, Academic Press, New York (1964).

[37] Del Re, G., *J. Chem. Soc.*, 4031 (1958).

[38] Del Re, G., p. 221 in *Electronic Aspects of Biochemistry*, edited by B. Pullman, Academic Press, New York (1964).

[39] Jordan, F., and Pullman, B., *Theoret. Chim. Acta*, 9, 242 (1968).

[40] Pullman, A., Kochanski, E., Gilbert, M., and Denis, A., *Theoret. Chim. Acta*, 10, 231 (1968).

[41] Giessner-Prettre, C., and Pullman, A., *Theoret. Chim. Acta*, 9, 279 (1968).

[42] Rein, R., Fukuda, N., Clarke, G. A., and Harris, F. E., *J. Theoret. Biol.*, 21, 88 (1968).

[43] Pullman, A., *Ann. N. Y. Acad. Sci.*, 158, 65 (1969).

[44] Pullman, A., *Intern. J. Quantum Chem.*, Suppl. 2, 187 (1968).

[45] Clementi, E., and Davis, D. R., *J. Comput. Phys.*, 1, 223 (1966).

[46] Clementi, E., Clementi, H., and Davis, D. R., *J. Chem. Phys.*, 46, 4725 (1967).

[47] Mély, D., and Pullman, A., *Theoret. Chim. Acta*, 13, 278 (1969).

[48] Clementi, E., André, J. M., André, M. C. L., Klint, D., and Hahn, D., (private communication).

[49] Weiler-Feichenfeld, H., and Neiman, S., *Proceedings of the Jerusalem Symposium on Quantum Aspects of Heterocyclic Compounds in Chemistry and Biochemistry, April 1969*, in press.

[50] Lifschitz, C., Bergmann, E. D., and Pullman, B., *Tetrahedron Letters*, 46, 4583 (1967).

[51] Machmer, P., and Duchesne, J., *Nature*, 206, 618 (1965).

[52] Clementi, E., *Chem. Rev.*, 341 (1968).

[53] Hoogsteen, K., *Acta Cryst.*, 16, 907 (1963).

[54] Mathews, F. S., and Rich, A., *J. Mol. Biol.*, 8, 89 (1964).

[55] Haschemeyer. A. E. V., and Sobell, H. M., *Proc. Nat. Acad. Sci. Wash.*, 50, 872 (1963).

[56] Haschemeyer, A. E. V., and Sobell, H. M., *Nature*, 202, 969 (1964).

[57] Hamlin, R. M., Jr., Lord, R. C., and Rich, A., *Science*, 148, 1734 (1965).

[58] Katz, K., and Penman, S., *J. Mol. Biol.*, 15, 220 (1966).

[59] Shoup, R. R., Miles, H. T., and Becker, E. D., *Biochem. Biophys. Res. Commun.*, 23, 194 (1966).

[60] Pitha, J., Jones, R. N., and Pithova, P., *Can. J. Chem.*, 4, 1045 (1966).

[61] Küchler, E., and Derkosch, J., *Z. Naturforsch.*, *b*, 21, 209 (1966).

[62] Binford, J. S., Jr., and Holloway, D. M., *J. Mol. Biol.*, 31, 91 (1968).

[63] Newmark, R. A., and Cantor, C. R., *J. Amer. Chem. Soc.*, 90, 5010 (1968).

[64] Kyogoku, Y., Lord, R. C., and Rich, A., *J. Amer. Chem. Soc.*, 89, 497 (1967).

[65] Kyogoku, Y., Lord, R. C., and Rich, A., *Science*, 154, 518 (1966).

[66] Miller, J. H., and Sobell, H. M., *Proc. Nat. Acad. Sci. U. S.*, 55, 1201 (1966).

[67] Kyogoku, Y., Lord, R. C., and Rich, A., *Biochim. Biophys. Acta*, 179, 10 (1969).

[68] Hammes, G. G., and Park, A. C., *J. Amer. Chem. Soc.*, 90, 4151 (1968).

[69] Poland, D., and Scheraga, H. A., *Biochemistry*, 6, 3791 (1967).

[70] Ramachandran, G. N., *Intern. J. Protein Res.*, 1, 5 (1969).

[71] Voet, D., and Rich, A., *J. Amer. Chem. Soc.*, 91, 3069 (1969).

[72] Kim, S. H., and Rich, A., *J. Mol. Biol.*, 42, 87 (1969).

[73] Kim, S. H., and Rich, A., *Science*, 158, 1046 (1967).

[74] Sakore, T. D., and Sobell, H. M., *J. Mol. Biol.*, 43, 77 (1969).

[75] Michelson, A. M., and Monny, C., *Biochim. Biophys. Acta*, 129, 460 (1966).

[76] Kyogoku, Y., Lord, R. C., and Rich, A., *Nature*, 218, 69 (1968).

[77] Hammes, G. G., and Park, A. C., *J. Amer. Chem. Soc.*, 91, 956 (1969).

[78] Pullman, B., and Pullman, A., *Progr. Nucleic Acid Res. Mol. Biol.*, 9, 327 (1969).

[79] Pullman, B., p. 1 in *Molecular Associations in Biology*, edited by B. Pullman, Academic Press, New York (1968).

[80] Pullman, A., p. 135 in *Electronic Aspects of Biochemistry*, edited by B. Pullman, Academic Press, New York (1964).

[81] Watson, D. G., Sweet, R. M., and Marsh, R., *Acta Cryst.*, 19, 573 (1965).

[82] Pullman, B., in *Quantum Aspects of Heterocyclic Compounds in Chemistry and Biochemistry, Proceedings of the 2d Jerusalem Symposium, April 1968*, in press.

[83] Pullman, B., Berthod, H., and Dreyfus, M., *Theoret. Chim. Acta*, 15, 265 (1969).

SEMIEMPIRICAL MO THEORIES: A CRITIQUE AND A REVIEW OF PROGRESS

by

James R. Hoyland*

I. INTRODUCTION

The basic principles and methods of quantum mechanics have gradually become familiar to an increasingly large number of scientists working in many diverse areas of research. At the present time, application of quantum mechanical methods to such problems as protein structure, drug design, hydrogen bonding, and many other phenomena important in biological studies is becoming common. Nearly all such applications to phenomena of biological interest are made by means of some type of semiempirical formulation. Therefore it seems of interest to review these semiempirical methods and to discuss in detail their advantages and shortcomings. This chapter is an attempt at such a review and will be restricted to a discussion of empirical and semiempirical molecular orbital (MO) approaches. Emphasis will be placed on recent all-valence electron approaches and no discussion of the older methods will be given since these latter formulations have already been exhaustively reviewed elsewhere.

II. THE SELF-CONSISTENT FIELD METHOD

The basic problem in considering a chemical system, such as a molecule, by means of quantum mechanics is the solution of the Schrödinger equation

$$H\psi = E\psi \qquad (1)$$

which, coupled with the Pauli exclusion principle, provides in theory all required information for a complete description of the system in the absence of external

*Battelle Memorial Institute, Columbus Laboratories, 505 King Avenue, Columbus, Ohio 43201.

fields and relativistic effects. Assuming that the Born-Oppenheimer separation has been carried out, the Hamiltonian operator, H, in atomic units for a chemical system is given by

$$H = \sum_i -1/2\nabla_i^2 - \sum_i \sum_N Z_N/r_{iN} + \sum_{i<j} \sum 1/r_{ij} + \sum_{M<N} \sum Z_M Z_N/r_{MN} \quad . \tag{2}$$

Subscripts i and j refer to electrons, M and N to nuclei, ∇^2 is the Laplacian operator, Z_N the charge on nucleus N, and $r_{k\ell}$ ($k,\ell = i,j,M$, or N) is the distance between particles k and ℓ. Because of the electron-electron repulsion terms, r_{ij}, Equation (1) can be solved exactly for a wavefunction, ψ, and corresponding energy, E, only if a single electron and not more than two nuclei are present. In all other cases an approximate wavefunction Φ must be constructed and its goodness tested by how closely the computed energy,

$$\overline{E} = \langle\Phi|H|\Phi\rangle = \int \Phi^* H \Phi d\tau, \tag{3}$$

approximates the true energy of the system. The variation theorem guarantees that $\overline{E} \geq E$ for the ground state. The problems encountered in the construction of very accurate wavefunctions are many and complex, and need not concern us here. It is sufficient to point out that terms must be included in Φ which take into account the fact that because of the r_{ij} terms in H, electrons will tend to move in such a way so as to avoid each other as much as possible. This latter effect is known as correlation.

If correlation were a significant factor in the calculation of properties of atoms and molecules, then little progress could be made except on systems containing only a very small number of electrons. Fortunately, however, correlation terms do not greatly influence computed molecular properties which depend only on the coordinates of one electron at a time. These are known as one-electron properties and comprise such physical observables as the dipole moment, diamagnetic susceptibility, polarizability, shielding constants, quadrupole coupling constants, and the like. Thus, for most calculations in which only one-electron ground-state properties are desired or qualitative trends are sought, a simpler procedure can be followed which is known as the self-consistent field (SCF) or Hartree-Fock formulation. This method was originated by Hartree [1] and improved by Fock [2]. The basic assumptions are that an electron in an atom or molecule can be considered to move in the potential field of the nuclei and the average potential of all of the other electrons in the molecule and that the wavefunction can be taken as a properly antisymmetrized product of one-electron spin orbitals.

Most molecules are closed-shell systems in that the wavefunction can be considered as an antisymmetrized product of doubly occupied orbitals. This means that each orbital of the system is occupied by two electrons, one with α-spin and the other with β-spin. In this case, the Hartree-Fock equations have an especially simple form: [3]

$$\psi = \mathcal{G}\phi_1^{\alpha}(1)\phi_1^{\beta}(2)\phi_2^{\alpha}(3) \; \ldots . \; \phi_n^{\beta}(2n) \tag{4}$$

$$F(1)\phi_i(1) = \epsilon_i\phi_i(1) \tag{5}$$

$$F(1) = H^{\circ}(1) + G(1) \tag{6}$$

$$H^{\circ}(1) = -1/2\nabla^2(1) - \sum_N Z_N/r_{1N} \tag{7}$$

$$G(1) = \sum_{k=1}^{n} \left\{ 2 \int dV_2 \frac{\phi_k^*(2)\phi_k(2)}{r_{12}} - \int dV_2 \frac{\phi_k^*(2)P_{12}\phi_k(2)}{r_{12}} \right\} \; . \tag{8}$$

In the above equations, $\mathcal{G}$ is an antisymmetrizer, F the Hartree-Fock operator, ϵ_i the Hartree-Fock energy levels, and P_{12} is the permutation operator which interchanges the coordinates of electrons 1 and 2. The energy levels, ϵ_i, are approximately equal to the negative of the ionization potential required to remove an electron found in the Φ_i from the molecule. [4] Finally the total energy of the system is given by:

$$E = \sum_{i=1}^{n} \left\{ \epsilon_i + \int \phi_i^*(1)H^{\circ}(1)\phi_i(1) \right\} + \sum_{M<N}\sum \frac{Z_M Z_N}{r_{MN}} \; . \tag{9}$$

The solution of the SCF or Hartree-Fock equation is an iterative one in that one must construct G in order to compute F. Since G requires a knowledge of the ϕ_i, one starts with a reasonable set of ϕ_i and computes F, giving a new set of ϕ_i, and proceeds in this way until convergence is attained. For atoms, the SCF equation can be solved numerically because of the spherical symmetry. This is not possible for molecules, however, and for these systems one makes the further assumption that the SCF-MO's, ϕ, can be written as a linear combination of a given, fixed basis set, χ: [3]

$$\phi_i = \sum_j C_{ji} \chi_j \quad . \tag{10}$$

Minimization of the energy with respect to the coefficients C_{ji} leads to the solution of the equation

$$\left(\underset{\sim}{F} - \epsilon \underset{\sim}{S}\right) \underset{\sim}{C} = 0 \quad . \tag{11}$$

The elements of the matrices $\underset{\sim}{F}$ and $\underset{\sim}{S}$ are given by

$$F_{pq} = \langle \chi_p(1) | H^{\circ}(1) | \chi_q(1) \rangle + \sum_r \sum_s D_{rs} \left\{ 2(pq|rs) - (ps|rq) \right\} \tag{12}$$

$$D_{rs} = \sum_{i=1}^{n} C_{ri} C_{si} \tag{13}$$

$$(km|\ell n) = \int dv_1 dv_2 \chi_k^*(1) \chi_\ell^*(2) \; 1/r_{12} \chi_m(1) \chi_n(2) \tag{14}$$

$$S_{pq} = \langle \chi_p | \chi_q \rangle = \int \chi_p^*(1) \chi_q(1) dv(1) \quad . \tag{15}$$

The quantities S_{pq} are known as the overlap integrals.

Much progress has been made in recent years in the construction of approximate molecular wavefunctions using this expansion technique. Since it is not the purpose of this article to review such calculations, it is sufficient to mention that it is now possible to perform *ab initio* calculations on molecules as large as naphthalene and azulene [5] with a relatively modest sized basis set of Gaussian orbitals.

III. ALL-VALENCE ELECTRON CALCULATIONS

A. The Need for Semiempirical Methods

The problems encountered in applying the Hartree-Fock method to molecular systems are purely mathematical or computational in nature, and arise from the necessity of evaluating electron repulsion integrals. Mathematical difficulties are inherent in the evaluation of these integrals if Slater orbitals are used as the basis set and the molecule contains more than two nuclei. This problem is being overcome at the present time but progress has been slow. The mathematical difficulty of integral evaluation can be avoided if a basis set of Gaussian orbitals (functions with an exponential dependence $\exp[-\alpha r^2]$) is utilized but this generates a new problem. The radial dependence of a Gaussian renders it unsuitable for use as a basis orbital and many Gaussians must be included to compute an accurate wavefunction. Since the number of electron repulsion integrals increases as the fourth power of the number of basis orbitals, the use of Gaussians requires sophisticated data handling techniques and a computer capable of rapid buffered input and output to or from peripheral storage devices. *Ab initio* calculations on relatively modest molecules, such as benzene, therefore require several hours of computer time on rapid large-scale computers and are hopeless on more modest machines. It is reasonable to expect that if progress is to be made on large molecules or routine calculations are desired on many smaller systems, approximations must be made in order to simplify the work required and drastically reduce the amount of computer time utilized.

Many methods have been proposed for carrying out empirical or semi-empirical calculations on molecules. Only a few of these have, or seem to have, the potential to withstand the tests of general utility, simplicity, and the capability of producing reasonable results. The remainder of this section will be directed toward a detailed examination of these latter methods.

B. Extended Hückel Theory

The extended Hückel theory (EHT) proposed by Hoffman [6] can be viewed as a logical extension of the ordinary Hückel method [7], allowing a treatment of both the σ- and π-electrons in the same manner. EHT can also be considered as a simple attempt to approximate the elements of a self-consistent field matrix, $\underset{\sim}{F}$, in which only the valence electrons are considered.

The EHT basis is a minimal Slater orbital set of valence-electron atomic orbitals. Thus for hydrogen only the 1s orbital is considered, for lithium through fluorine the 2s and 2p orbitals only are included, etc. The diagonal elements of the EHT matrix, $\underset{\sim}{\hat{H}}$, are given by the negative of the valence-state ionization potentials. A variety of expressions have been utilized for the off-diagonal elements, the most frequently utilized being:

$$\hat{H}_{ij} = KS_{ij}(\hat{H}_{ii} + \hat{H}_{jj})/2 \qquad (16)$$

$$\hat{H}_{ij} = K'S_{ij}(\hat{H}_{ii}\hat{H}_{jj})^{1/2} \qquad (17)$$

$$\hat{H}_{ij} = S_{ij}(2 - |S_{ij}|)(\hat{H}_{ii} + \hat{H}_{jj})/2 \quad , \tag{18}$$

where S_{ij} is the overlap integral between orbitals i and j. The equation $(\underset{\sim}{\hat{H}} - \underset{\sim}{S}\varepsilon)\underset{\sim}{C} = 0$ is then solved and the total energy of the system found by summing the energies of the occupied orbitals taking into account their occupancy numbers. The matrix $\underset{\sim}{C}$ contains the MO coefficients.

We wish to critically examine the procedures given above in relation to the effectiveness of the EHT method in approximating the SCF matrix. The first deficiency which should be pointed out is, perhaps, a subtle one which has not received the attention which its importance dictates. For simplicity, consider as an example a carbon atom in a molecular system. The EHT basis set for this atom is a 2s Slater orbital and the three 2p orbitals. The carbon 1s orbital is ignored and the effective nuclear charge of the carbon is lowered from 6 to 4. This procedure is not valid since the 2s Slater orbital is not orthogonal to the 1s. For a carbon atom the overlap integral $S_{1s,2s}$ is, furthermore, non-negligible, having a magnitude of 0.2205 if Slater orbital exponents are used. A proper choice for the form of the 2s orbital must be one which is orthogonal to the core 1s electrons. A reasonable choice for such a function is the orbital

$$2s^* = [(2s) - S_{1s,2s}(1s)][1 - S^2_{1s,2s}]^{-1/2} \tag{19}$$

which for carbon has the following numerical form:

$$2s^*(C) = 1.0252(2s) - 0.2261(1s) \quad . \tag{20}$$

Use of such an orbital will not greatly effect the overlap integrals for the calculation of the off-diagonal elements, but it is essential to use this form for the 2s function if one wishes to compare the EHT matrix elements with the *ab initio* results. This point has apparently been overlooked by Boer et al. [7] in their comparison of matrix elements for BH_3 and B_2H_6. For example, the EHT 2s - 2s diagonal element for carbon must be compared with the following combination of Hartree-Fock matrix elements:

$$\langle 2s^*|F|2s^*\rangle = 1.0511 \langle 2s|F|2s\rangle + 0.0511 \langle 1s|F|1s\rangle - 0.46354 \langle 1s|F|2s\rangle \quad . \tag{21}$$

The diagonal matrix elements in EHT are taken to be the negative of the valence state ionization potentials (VSIP). The most commonly employed values are -13.6 eV for hydrogen, -21.4 eV for carbon 2s, -11.4 eV for carbon 2p,

-26.0 eV for nitrogen 2s, -13.4 eV for nitrogen 2p, -32 to -35.3 for oxygen 2s, and -14.8 to -17.8 for oxygen 2p. Table 1 presents a tabulation of diagonal SCF matrix elements for carbon and hydrogen in several different molecules.

TABLE 1. DIAGONAL SCF MATRIX ELEMENTS FOR CARBON AND HYDROGEN[a]

Molecule	$<2s^*\|F\|2s^*>$	$<2p_\sigma\|F\|2p_\sigma>$	$<2p_\pi\|F\|2p_\pi>$	$<1s_H\|F\|1s_H>$
CH_4	-23.3	- 9.50		-13.8
C_2H_2	-24.1	-20.4	-4.60	-15.3
C_2H_4	-24.2	-14.9[b] -11.2[c]	-3.97	-14.6
C_2H_6	-23.8	-10.5[b] - 9.63[c]		-13.6
HCN	-25.9	-23.6	-5.77	-16.1

(a) All values are in eV.
(b) Matrix element for the $2p_\sigma$ orbital parallel to the C-C axis.
(c) Matrix element for the $2p_\sigma$ orbital perpendicular to the C-C axis.

These results are taken from the work of Palke and Lipscomb [8], who have used a minimal Slater orbital set with Slater exponents for carbon and nitrogen but with an exponent of 1.2 for hydrogen rather than 1.0. It is seen that the 2s* - 2s* diagonal element is relatively constant but somewhat larger in absolute magnitude than the VSIP of -21.4 usually utilized in EHT. Likewise the $1s_H$ - $1s_H$ values are in reasonable agreement with the EHT value of -13.6. The main source of disagreement between EHT and SCF diagonal matrix elements is found in the carbon 2p orbitals. The values for the saturated molecules (methane and ethane) are about the same and not too different from the EHT value of -11.4. Difficulties are encountered in the unsaturated systems in which an extremely pronounced anistropy is noted. In general, the $2p_\sigma$ - $2p_\sigma$ matrix elements are larger in absolute magnitude than the EHT value, while the $2p_\pi$ - $2p_\pi$ elements are much smaller. This effect is especially apparent in C_2H_2 and HCN in which the carbon atom has a classical hybridization of sp. It appears that the $2p_\sigma$ - $2p_\sigma$ diagonal elements increase in absolute magnitude at a rapid rate as the hybridization changes from

sp^3 to sp. The effect of binding the carbon to the more electronegative nitrogen in HCN further enhances the value of the $2p_\sigma - 2p_\sigma$ element. A similar trend appears in the $2s^* - 2s^*$ matrix element in HCN.

A similar situation exists in borane and diborane. The SCF $2s^* - 2s^*$ matrix elements are -16.7 eV and -19.8 eV in BH_3 and B_2H_6, respectively, compared to an EHT value of about -15.2. A large anisotropy occurs in the $2p - 2p$ elements in diborane, these being -11.9 eV for the $2p_\sigma - 2p_\sigma$ orbitals parallel to the B-B bond, -10.6 eV for the $2p_\sigma - 2p_\sigma$ orbitals perpendicular to this bond, and -4.98 eV for the "$2p_\pi - 2p_\pi$"-like orbitals. The $2p_\sigma - 2p_\sigma$ value for BH_3 is -9.39 eV, while the VSIP is about 8.5 eV. Large differences in $1s_H - 1s_H$ matrix elements between bridge and in-plane hydrogens also occur, these elements for B_2H_6 being -16.1 eV (bridge) and -12.6 eV (in-plane). The corresponding $1s_H - 1s_H$ matrix element in BH_3 is -12.7 eV.

Finally, we examine the nitrogen diagonal elements in NH_3 and HCN. The $2s^* - 2s^*$ values are -27.5 eV and -29.7 eV for NH_3 and HCN, respectively, in reasonable agreement with the usual Hückel values of -26.0 eV. The $2p_\sigma - 2p_\sigma$ elements for NH_3 are -8.92 eV for the two equivalent $2p$ orbitals and -9.69 eV for the other. The EHT value of -13.4 is therefore in extremely poor agreement with the SCF result in NH_3. For HCN, the nitrogen $2p_\sigma - 2p_\sigma$ element is -17.9 eV while the $2p_\pi - 2p_\pi$ value is -5.41 eV. Again there is a very large anisotropy but what is perhaps more disturbing is that the carbon $2p_\sigma - 2p_\sigma$ and $2p_\pi - 2p_\pi$ SCF matrix elements are <u>larger in absolute magnitude</u> than those for nitrogen! We must therefore conclude that the VSIP approximation is of limited utility and cannot be relied upon to give reasonable results. It is also evident that the anisotropy in $2p - 2p$ matrix elements for unsaturated molecules must be taken into account.

We next turn our attention to the off-diagonal elements, examining first the expression given by Equation (16). The basis for this equation is the Mulliken approximation for two-center charge distributions [9], originally formulated in terms of integrals and subsequently assumed to arise from the following [10]:

$$\chi_a\chi_b \approx S_{ab}\ (\chi_a^2 + \chi_b^2)/2 \quad . \tag{22}$$

In the above equation, χ_a and χ_b are atomic orbitals centered at nuclei a and b and S_{ab} is the overlap integral $\langle\chi_a|\chi_b\rangle$. It is then assumed that this approximation can be thought of as giving rise to the expression

$$\langle\chi_a|f|\chi_b\rangle \approx S_{ab}[\langle\chi_a|f|\chi_a\rangle + \langle\chi_b|f|\chi_b\rangle]/2 \quad , \tag{23}$$

where f is a one-electron operator. This procedure is approximately valid if f is not a differential operator. In the case that f is the kinetic energy operator, $-1/2\nabla^2$, the approximation cannot hold. Newton, Boer, and Lipscomb have studied the Mulliken approximation for the off-diagonal matrix elements in methane within the context of the following equation:

$$\langle\chi_a|f|\chi_b\rangle = K_{ab}S_{ab}[\langle\chi_a|f|\chi_a\rangle + \langle\chi_b|f|\chi_b\rangle]/2 \quad . \tag{24}$$

Deviations of K_{ab} from unity then measure the extent to which the Mulliken approximation is invalid. Their results are reproduced in Table 2. As expected, the Mulliken approximation is not valid for the kinetic energy terms, and hence for the total SCF Hamiltonian. It does hold reasonably well, however, for the potential energy terms. Equation (16) is usually used with a value of 1.75 for K in EHT calculations, which can be viewed as a compromise which may be accurate for some matrix elements but can be expected to be quite poor for others.

TABLE 2. K_{ab} FOR TWO-CENTER MATRIX ELEMENTS OF METHANE

	$F^{(a)}$	Kinetic Energy	Potential Energy	Nuclear Attraction Energy	Two-Electron Interaction Energy
K_{1sH}	2.04	−0.01	0.83	0.92	1.14
K_{2sH}	1.46	0.37	1.05	1.00	0.98
K_{2pH}	2.10	0.54	1.00	0.93	0.91
$K_{HH'}$	2.95	−0.04	1.19	1.09	1.05

(a) Total Hartree-Fock Hamiltonian.

The second expression for off-diagonal elements, Equation (17), can be thought of as arising from the use of a Mulliken-type approximation using a geometric rather than an arithmetic mean. This equation was introduced by Ballhausen and Gray [12] for calculations on inorganic complexes and has been utilized by Allen and Russell [13] in their EHT studies of several small molecules. There would seem to be no advantage to using this expression in favor of Equation (16). Again using the methane matrix elements for the total SCF Hamiltonian, a wide range of K values are needed, these being $K_{1sH} = -5.03$, $K_{2sH} = -1.66$, $K_{2pH} = -2.14$, and $K_{HH'} = -2.95$. Because of this fact, and since the geometric mean formulation is seldom used outside of the treatment of inorganic complexes, no more will be said concerning it at this time.

The final expression extensively used for off-diagonal elements in EHT, Equation (18), is due to Cusachs [14] and can be viewed as an attempt to take into account the dependence of the kinetic energy with overlap. Unfortunately, this method does not do very well in approximating the SCF matrix elements. Again we compare the CH_4 matrix elements by giving the values of $R_{ij} = F_{ij}$ (actual)/F_{ij} (Equation 18). These values are $R_{1sH} = 1.05$, $R_{2sH} = 0.98$, $R_{2pH} = 1.22$ and $R_{HH'} = 1.62$. At first glance the agreement seems much better than for Equation (16), but this is not true. Using a value of $K = 1.75$, the same R_{ij} values for matrix elements calculated from this expression are 1.17, 0.83, 1.20, and 1.69. The improvement brought about by the use of the Cusachs formulation is hardly remarkable. This has also been noted by Newton [15] who has pointed out another difficulty which arises from the use of Cusachs' formula. If the latter equation is used, the energy of the system is dependent upon the choice of the coordinate system. This violation of rotational invariance does not arise if either of the other two expressions are used, providing the p-orbital diagonal elements are all taken to be equal. Cusachs [16] has given a method for avoiding this difficulty and it is recommended that this latter formulation be used if the off-diagonal elements are to be computed by Equation (18).

A further point of criticism of the EHT method can be raised in that matrix elements between 2s and $2p_\sigma$ orbitals centered at the same nucleus are always set equal to zero, whereas nonzero matrix elements occur in the SCF formulation except in cases where symmetry considerations dictate them to be identically zero, as in methane. These matrix elements are not always small. For example, in HCN [8] the SCF matrix elements $F_{C2s,C2p_\sigma}$ and $F_{N2s,N2p_\sigma}$ have numerical values of -6.31 eV and 7.59 eV, respectively. These are considerably larger than many matrix elements which are included in EHT.

The calculation of the molecular energy in the EHT formalism simply involves the summing up of the energies of the various occupied MO's, taking into account the occupation of each MO. For a closed shell system, this reduces to

$$E_{EHT} = 2 \sum_{j}^{occ} \epsilon_j \quad . \tag{25}$$

It must be emphasized that this is not an approximation to the true energy of the system in which the 1s electrons are collapsed into the core. The correct expression for the total energy of the system is given by Equation (9). If the EHT energy levels can be regarded as an approximation to the SCF valence-electron eigenvalues, then one can write

$$E_{EHT} \approx 2 \sum_{j}^{val} \epsilon_j^{SCF} = E_{SCF} - 2 \sum_{j}^{core} \epsilon_j^{SCF} + V_{ee} - V_{nn} \quad , \tag{26}$$

where V_{ee} is the total electron-electron interaction energy and V_{nn} is the nuclear-nuclear repulsion. If E_{EHT} is to parallel E_{SCF}, then V_{ee} must effectively cancel V_{nn}. One would expect that $\sum_{j}^{core} \epsilon_j^{SCF}$ will be nearly constant for small changes in geometry. We shall return to these points later.

Another discussion given by Blyholder and Coulson [17] is of interest since it approaches the comparison of the SCF and EHT formalisms in another manner. These authors study the conditions under which the SCF matrix can be approximated by the methods of extended Hückel theory. The original paper should be consulted for details.

In view of the above discussions, one expects that, at best, MO's and charge distributions found by EHT will be of marginal value. This is not always true, saturated hydrocarbons being a counter-example, but will in general be correct if the molecule contains several different atoms with widely diverse electronegativities, such as acetamide. The use of VSIP's as diagonal matrix elements results in an unbalanced charge distribution in which too much electron density is shifted toward the more electronegative centers. Such an effect is not present in SCF theory since a large build-up of charge at a center gives rise to an increase in electron-electron repulsions, thereby decreasing the electronegativity of that atom. This can be thought of as a balancing effect between the electron-electron repulsion and bare nuclear portions of the SCF Hamiltonian, the proper charge distribution being that which minimizes the energy of the system. Since EHT does not explicitly consider the electron repulsion terms, this balancing does not occur. One can make allowance for the electron-electron repulsion terms in an empirical manner, however, by allowing the diagonal matrix elements to be functions of the charge distribution. This gives rise to the iterative extended Hückel theory (IEHT), examples of which have been proposed by several workers. These methods will be discussed below.

The first attempt to construct an iterative extended Hückel formulation was made by Rein, Fukuda, Win, Clarke, and Harris [18] who assign values of α_0 and $\Delta\alpha$ to each atomic orbital. The procedure is then an iterative one in which the diagonal elements, α, are given by

$$\alpha_{n+1} = (1 - \lambda)\alpha_n + \lambda(\alpha_0 + q_n\Delta\alpha) \tag{27}$$

where q_n is the total net charge on the atom at which the orbital in question is centered after the nth iteration. The value of λ was taken to be 0.1 in order to damp out violent oscillations. The parameters for H, C, N, and O originally used by Rein et al. [18] are given in Table 3, along with an alternate set given in a later paper [19]. The use of the iterative method has been found by Rein and coworkers to considerably smooth out the electron density, leading to better agreement with SCF charge distributions and good dipole moments. We will return to a discussion of these matters in the next section.

Pullman and coworkers [20] have used a slightly different parameterization for calculations on purine and pyrimidine bases. These investigators have not given the damping procedure used in the iteractions, although their final expression is

$$\alpha_n = \alpha_0 + q_n \Delta\alpha \tag{28}$$

for the diagonal matrix elements, along with the Cusachs formula for the off-diagonal elements. Their parameters are given in Table 4. Bloor, Gilson, and Billingsley [21] have also used the Pullman procedure for studies of several systems.

TABLE 3. REIN PARAMETERS FOR IEHT CALCULATIONS

Orbital	$\zeta(1)^{a,b}$	$\alpha_0(1)$,[b] eV	$\Delta\alpha(1)$,[b] eV	$\zeta(2)^{a,c}$	$\alpha_0(2)$,[c] eV	$\Delta\alpha(2)$,[c] eV
H, 1s	1.00	-13.60	-14.00	1.200	-11.60	-14.0
C, 2s	1.608	-21.20	-11.90	1.625	-25.00	-11.0
C, 2p	1.568	-11.40	-11.90	1.625	-10.00	-11.0
N, 2s	1.924	-27.40	-13.70	1.950	-30.00	-12.0
N, 2p	1.917	-14.40	-13.70	1.950	-11.50	-12.0
O, 2s	2.246	-30.70	-15.95	2.275	-33.00	-15.0
O, 2p	2.227	-15.84	-15.95	2.275	-14.00	-15.0

(a) Orbital exponent.
(b) Parameter set from [18].
(c) Parameter set from [19].

TABLE 4. PULLMAN PARAMETERS FOR IEHT CALCULATIONS

Orbital	α_0	$\Delta\alpha$
H, 1s	-13.8	-14.3
C, 2s	-21.2	-11.9
C, 2p	-11.4	-11.9
N, 2s	-25.5	-13.7
N, 2p	-14.4	-13.7
NH, 2s	-27.4	-13.7
NH, 2p	-14.4 (-12.5 for $2p_\pi$)	-13.7
O, 2s	-32.0	-15.2
O, 2p	-16.45	-15.2

Duke [22] has used a quadratic dependence of the diagonal elements with charge, and also advocates adjustment of the orbital exponents, ζ, with q. These refinements are probably not justified in so crude a method as EHT, especially since the overlap integrals must be recalculated at each cycle.

In review, then, it is felt that EHT matrix elements cannot be regarded as an approximation to the valence-state SCF matrix. The gross exaggeration of charges in the EHT method is also disturbing. We can only quote Duke [22] in saying that "the main justification for the method is that it works". The iterative methods are a considerable improvement in that the charge distribution is more reasonably predicted. The diagonal elements in IEHT will undoubtedly be somewhat more similar to the SCF minimal basis set values except for unsaturated molecules. We expect little or no improvement in off-diagonal elements since they are generated by the same procedures as in EHT.

C. "Nonempirical" Molecular Orbital Theories

The methods which are to be discussed in this section have been developed by Lipscomb and coworkers and are designated by the acronym NEMO meaning non-empirical molecular orbital methods. They are designated nonempirical because no experimental data is introduced, parameter evaluation being made by using SCF calculations on model molecules with a minimal Slater orbital basis set to establish matrix elements. These methods have not received the attention which they deserve, possibly due to the erroneous assumption that they are much more difficult to utilize than other semiempirical schemes or that they are more costly in terms of computer time. It should be most strongly emphasized that neither of these assumptions is true. The computer time required for a NEMO calculation is only slightly more than for an EHT calculation and considerably less than for an IEHT study. The use of NEMO methods does require somewhat higher routine effort on the part of the user but only for parameter choice. The better results generally justify this greater effort in setting up the calculation.

The original NEMO method, designated as NEMO 1, was developed by Newton, Boer, and Lipscomb [11] in an effort to correct some of the poorer features of EHT, these being the use of VSIP's for diagonal elements, use of the Mulliken approximation for matrix elements involving the kinetic energy operator, and neglect of nonzero one-center s-p_σ matrix elements. Inner shells, such as the carbon 1s, are also included in NEMO so that one need not be concerned about orthogonality problems.

We discuss first the choice of diagonal elements. Choosing these for atomic orbitals in a large molecule involves finding *ab initio* calculations for small molecules in which the atom in question is surrounded by a similar environment. For example, parameters for the carbon and nitrogen atoms of a nitrile are taken from a calculation on HCN, those for a carbonyl group in a ketone or aldehyde from a formaldehyde calculation, etc. For planar molecules, sacrifice of complete rotational invariance is made by allowing an anisotropy to occur between $2p_\pi$ and $2p_\sigma$ diagonal elements. This is a small price to pay for improved eigenvalues and wavefunctions. The $2p_\sigma$ diagonal elements for unsaturated systems are given the average value of the two components, while for three-dimensional molecules the average of the three $2p_\sigma$-values is taken. An exception to the latter evaluation is in substituted π-electron systems in which the parameters for the π-electron moiety are evaluated as for planar systems. Diagonal matrix elements for many types of molecules are discussed by Newton, Boer, and Lipscomb [11,23].

The evaluation of the off-diagonal elements represents another great improvement over EHT calculations. These elements are evaluated by first computing the exact kinetic energy contribution and then using a modified Mulliken-type approximation for the potential energy terms. This is summarized by the following equation:

$$F_{ij} = T_{ij} + K_{ij}S_{ij}(U_{ii} + U_{jj})/2 \quad , \qquad (29)$$

where T_{ij} is the kinetic energy contribution, K_{ij} is a constant for a particular type of interaction, S_{ij} is the overlap integral, and U_{kk} is the potential energy part of the diagonal matrix element F_{kk}. We note that U_{kk} is found by simply subtracting T_{kk} from F_{kk}. For matrix elements of the type 2p − 2p, this expression is modified slightly to read

$$F_{ij}(2p - 2p) = T_{ij} + (K^\sigma_{ij}S^\sigma_{ij} + K^\pi_{ij}S^\pi_{ij})(U_{ii} + U_{jj})/2 \quad . \qquad (30)$$

Use of this expression does not violate rotational invariance [11] and provides a more accurate evaluation by separating the 2p - 2p interactions into σ- and π-components. A list of various K_{ij} values for model molecules is given in Table 5. Inspection of this table indicates a remarkable constancy of K-values for the various types of interactions considered. The anomalous $K_{2p_\pi 2p_\pi}$ for B_2H_6 need not concern us since biologically important molecules do not contain boron, and the value of K_{HH} in acetylene can be ignored since the matrix element U_{HH} is negligibly small.

TABLE 5. K_{ij} VALUES FOR MODEL MOLECULES[(a)]

	CH_4	C_2H_2	C_2H_4	C_2H_6	HCN	H_2CO	NH_3	BH_3	B_2H_6
K_{1s2s}(one-center)	0.66	0.66	0.66	0.66	0.66	0.66	0.66	0.66	0.66
K_{1s2s}	--	0.82	0.81	0.80	0.81	0.81	--	--	0.81
K_{1s2p}	--	0.82	0.82	0.81	0.82	0.82	--	--	0.82
K_{2s2s}	--	1.08	1.02	0.94	1.07	1.00	--	--	1.05
K_{2s2p}	--	1.09	1.06	1.00	1.11	1.05	--	--	1.11
$K_{2p_\sigma 2p_\sigma}$	--	1.12	1.05	0.99	1.17	1.07	--	--	1.13
$K_{2p_\pi 2p_\pi}$(b)	--	1.07	1.10	--	1.05	1.05	--	--	--
$K_{2p_\pi 2p_\pi}$(c)	--	--	0.73	0.69	--	0.74	--	--	1.14
K_{1sH}	0.83	0.83	0.83	0.83	0.83	0.83	0.84	0.81	0.81
K_{2sH}	1.05	1.07	1.05	1.04	1.07	1.04	1.06	1.05	1.04
K_{2pH}	1.00	0.95	0.98	0.99	0.92	0.94	1.02	1.02	1.05
K_{HH}	1.19	1.48	1.18	1.15	--	1.20	1.19	1.16	1.13

(a) Values are from Newton et al., Reference 11, and are weighted averages for each type of interaction in the same molecule found from the equation $K_{ab} = (\sum_{(ij)} K_{ij} |U_{ij}|)/(\sum_{(ij)} |U_{ij}|)$. All K's are for two-center interactions unless otherwise noted.

(b) K's are for π-electrons in planar or linear molecules.

(c) K's for in-plane π-π interaction except for B_2H_6 where it is the average of the two π-π interactions.

The above formulation does not give nonzero values to matrix elements between s and p orbitals on the same center so that a separate procedure is required for their calculation. The procedure recommended by Newton et al.[11] is to use the following equation:

$$F_{ij}^{ZO} = K_{ij}^{ZO} \sum_k S_{ik} S_{jk} F_{kk} \quad , \tag{31}$$

where the sum is over all basis orbitals, k. The only important nonzero sp-matrix elements for many molecules are those of the type $F_{2s,2p}$, and it is only these which are considered in NEMOI. Unfortunately the value of K_{ij}^{ZO} varies considerably from molecule to molecule, ranging from 0.22 in C_2H_6 to 0.86 in NH_3. An average value of 0.5 for K_{ij}^{ZO} is recommended. The rather large variation of this quantity is one of the more unsatisfactory aspects of the theory.

After evaluation of the matrix elements by the methods given above, the equation $\left(\underset{\sim}{F} - \epsilon \underset{\sim}{S}\right)\underset{\sim}{C} = 0$ is solved. Because of the way in which the matrix elements of $\underset{\sim}{F}$ are evaluated, it is expected that the energy levels and MO's will bear a closer relation to those resulting from an SCF calculation. Calculations have been carried out on a large number of systems by Newton, Boer, and Lipscomb [23], and this paper should be referred to for results and a summary of the values for diagonal elements.

As in EHT, the total energy of the system cannot be computed rigorously in NEMOI. In order to compute an approximate energy, use is made of the fact that the nuclear-nuclear repulsion for many molecules can be approximated by the relation

$$V_{nn} = 1/2 \sum_i^{electrons} [E_i^a - E_i^m] \quad , \tag{32}$$

where E_i^a and E_i^m are expectation values of kinetic energy plus nuclear attraction terms in the free atoms and in the molecule, respectively. This approximation implies that the energy of atomization, A, can be written as

$$A = 1/2 \sum_i^{electrons} (\epsilon_i^m - \epsilon_i^a)/2 \tag{33}$$

where the ϵ's are the SCF energy levels. The validity of this approximation can be tested by computing

$$\Delta = V_{nn} - 1/2 \sum_i^{electrons} [E_i^a - E_i^m] \tag{34}$$

for molecules for which the SCF results are available. As seen from Table 6 taken from Newton et al.[23], the approximation is fairly good. The value of Δ is generally about 2 percent or less of the value of V_{nn}. Assuming Δ to be zero, one can approximate the molecular energy by the expression

$$E = 1/2 \sum_i^{electrons} (\epsilon_i^a + \epsilon_i^m) \quad . \tag{35}$$

TABLE 6. VALUES FOR Δ FOR SEVERAL MOLECULES

Molecule	Δ, Atomic Units
CH_4	-0.044
C_2H_2	0.183
C_2H_4	0.102
C_2H_6	-0.058
H_2CO	0.313
HCN	0.388
BH_3	0.011
B_2H_6	0.326
NH_3	-0.074

Values for $\sum_i E_i^a$ in a.u. are -0.5 (H), -50.483 (C), -74.055 (N), and -103.541 (O). The necessity of approximating the total energy by Equation (35) is perhaps the weakest point of NEMO 1. It is therefore no better, fundamentally, for determination of molecular geometries than EHT.

Boyd and Lipscomb [24] have developed a variation of NEMO 1 in which a more unified approach for the evaluation of the matrix elements is used. This model is designated as NEMO 2. The initial procedure is the same as for NEMO 1 in that model molecules are used to determine parameters and the kinetic and potential energies are treated separately. In particular, we begin by selecting a set of diagonal matrix elements $\overline{F}_{kk}$ from model molecules and constructing a set of $\overline{F}_{kk}^{AV}$ by averaging over all the components of p- and d-orbitals. All overlap (S_{ij}) and kinetic energy (T_{ij}) integrals are then evaluated exactly for the basis set utilized (usually a minimal Slater orbital set) and diagonal T_{kk} values are subtracted from the corresponding $\overline{F}_{kk}^{AV}$ to give a set of $\overline{U}_{kk}^{AV}$. The molecular SCF energy matrix $\underset{\sim}{F}$ is then set equal to

$$\underset{\sim}{F} = \underset{\sim}{T} + \underset{\sim}{U} \quad , \tag{36}$$

where all elements of $\underset{\sim}{U}$ are constructed from the equation

$$U_{ij} = C_{ij} \sum_k S_{ik} \overline{U}_{kk}^{AV} S_{kj} \quad . \tag{37}$$

The usual secular equation is then solved for the NEMO 2 eigenvalues and eigenvectors.

The major problem in using NEMO 2 is to have a set of C_{ij} coefficients which span a large range of model molecules. Boyd and Lipscomb [24] have tabulated a large number of C-values and give an excellent, detailed discussion concerning anisotropies, rotational invariance problems, and the like. The amount of data is too voluminous to reproduce here and the reader is referred to the original paper [24] for details. The total energy of the molecule is computed in the same manner utilized for NEMO 1.

The choice of which variant of NEMO to use is not clear from examination of results already published. NEMO 1 has been more extensively utilized and more data as to its accuracy and general utility is available. Comparison of results for the same molecule obtained by the two methods indicates that perhaps NEMO 2 is slightly superior in overall performance.

The logical extension of the NEMO method is to compute all one-electron integrals exactly (kinetic and nuclear attraction) and approximate only the two-electron part of the F-matrix. Lipscomb and coworkers are attempting to do this [24] but no results have as yet been published. Such an approach has a number of advantages. The obvious one is that the less we approximate, the better our results should be. Such an approach also allows a calculation of the total energy of the system in the normal manner without resort to dubious approximations. If successfully parameterized, this method should prove very useful for conformational and other geometrical problems. A disadvantage is that more integrals must be computed exactly, among them the rather nasty three-center nuclear attraction terms. Evaluation of these latter quantities is not particularly difficult [25] but requires a good deal of programming effort and considerably more computation time than for the two-center integrals.

D. Methods Neglecting Differential Overlap

In NEMO and EHT attempts are made to compute molecular wavefunctions by using methods which allow the complete neglect of the electron repulsion integrals. As pointed out previously, these integrals are the main bottleneck in *ab initio* work, and it turns out that, in general, those integrals which are smallest in magnitude are the most difficult to compute if Slater orbitals are used as the basis set. This observation led Pariser and Parr [26] and Pople [27] to propose that in computing electron repulsion integrals, one could neglect differential overlap. The consequences of this assumption are given in the following equations:

$$\chi_p(1)\chi_q(1) = \delta_{pq}\chi_p\chi_p \tag{38}$$

$$\int \chi_p^*(1)\chi_r^*(2)\ {}^1/_{r_{12}}\chi_q(1)\chi_s(2)d\tau_1 d\tau_2 = (pq|rs) = \delta_{pq}\delta_{rs}(pp|rr) \tag{39}$$

$$\delta_{ij} = \begin{Bmatrix} 1 \text{ if } i = j \\ 0 \text{ if } i \neq j \end{Bmatrix} \tag{40}$$

The differential overlap formulation therefore eliminates all three- and four-center and most of the one- and two-center integrals, leaving only the so-called coulomb type, which are extremely simple to compute. This formulation was originally applied only to π-electron systems but has recently been extended to include all out-valence electrons. It is this latter extension which will be discussed in some detail below.

The basic formulation of the general theory for molecules, known as CNDO (complete neglect of differential overlap) was given by Pople and coworkers in a series of three papers [28,29,30]. We will discuss here only the revised version of the theory [30] known as CNDO/2.

The most important feature of the CNDO method, as implied by the name, is the complete neglect of differential overlap. The electron repulsion integrals are first subjected to neglect of differential overlap, resulting in Equation (39), and the further assumption is then made that, if only the valence electrons are considered, we can approximate all coulomb integrals between orbitals centered at the same two nuclei A and B by the common value, γ_{AB}:

$$(p^A p^A | q^B q^B) = \gamma_{AB} \quad . \tag{41}$$

Pople et al. suggest that the following expression be used for γ_{AB}:

$$\gamma_{AB} = (s^A s^A | s^B s^B) \quad , \tag{42}$$

where s^A and s^B are the appropriate Slater-type s-orbitals for the valence shell in question. The formulas given by Roothaan [31] are used for the evaluation of the γ_{AB}.

The integrals necessary for the evaluation of the one-electron part of the Hartree-Fock Hamiltonian are evaluated empirically or semiempirically. We first consider the quantity U_{rr} given by

$$U_{rr} = \langle \chi_r^A | - 1/2\nabla^2 - Z_A'/r_A | \chi_r^A \rangle \quad , \tag{43}$$

where Z_A' is the core charge on atom A, i.e., the nuclear charge minus the number of inner shell electrons. The quantity U_{rr} can be evaluated from atomic data by noting that in the CNDO approximation the energy of an atom or ion having m s-electrons and n p-electrons in its valence shall be written as

$$E(X, s^m p^n) = mU_{s,s} + nU_{p,p} + 1/2(m + n)(m + n - 1)\gamma_{XX} \quad . \tag{44}$$

We note that CNDO theory does not predict the splitting of atomic states so that the energy given by Equation (44) must be regarded as a weighted average of the energy of all states arising from the configuration $s^m p^n$. For the nitrogen atom, for example,

$$E(N, 2s^2 2p^3) = 1/5\, E(N, {}^4S) + 1/2\, E(N, {}^2D) + 3/10\, E(N, {}^2p) \quad , \tag{45}$$

the weighting factors being taken as proportional to the multiplicity of the state in question. The quantity U_{rr} is then related to either the ionization potential or the electron affinity of the orbital in question by the equations

$$-I_r = U_{rr} + (Z_A' - 1)\gamma_{AA} \tag{46}$$

$$-A_r = U_{rr} + Z_A'\gamma_{AA} \tag{47}$$

The value of U_{rr} is taken as the average of those given by the above equations:

$$U_{rr} = -1/2(I_r + A_r) - (Z_A' - 1/2)\gamma_{AA} \quad . \tag{48}$$

It is now noted that the one-electron part of a diagonal matrix element can be written as

$$H_{rr}^0 = \langle\chi_r^A|-1/2\nabla^2 - Z_A'/r_A - \sum_{B\neq A} Z_B'/r_B|\chi_r^A\rangle = U_{rr} - \sum_{B\neq A}\langle\chi_r^A|Z_B'/r_B|\chi_r^A\rangle \quad . \tag{49}$$

The term $\langle\chi_r^A|Z_B'/r_B|\chi_r^A\rangle$ is approximated by the relationship

$$\langle\chi_r^A|Z_B'/r_B|\chi_r^A\rangle = Z_B'\gamma_{AB} \quad . \tag{50}$$

This quantity was originally evaluated exactly but it was subsequently found that Equation (50) seems to provide a better balancing. From Equation (12) we can write that

$$F_{rr} = H_{rr}^0 + \sum_p \sum_q D_{pq}\{2(rr|pq) - (rq|pr)\} \quad , \tag{51}$$

which, after neglecting differential overlap can be written as

$$F_{rr} = H_{rr}^0 + \sum_p 2D_{pp}(rr|pp) - D_{rr}(rr|rr) \quad . \tag{52}$$

This equation can be further simplified by use of the γ_{AB} approximation, resulting in

$$F_{rr} = H_{rr}^0 + \sum_B 2D_{BB}\gamma_{AB} - D_{rr}\gamma_{AA} \quad , \tag{53}$$

where

$$D_{BB} = \sum_{p\ni B} D_{pp} \quad . \tag{54}$$

The symbol $p \ni B$ denoting that orbital p is centered at nucleus B. Pople's notation is somewhat different from that used here in that he defines his equations in terms of the quantities P_{pq}, analogous to the bond orders of Hückel theory. Since $P_{pq} = 2D_{pq}$, Equation (53) can be rewritten as

$$F_{rr} = H_{rr}^0 + \sum_B P_{BB}\gamma_{AB} - 1/2\, P_{rr}\gamma_{AA} \quad . \tag{55}$$

The off-diagonal matrix elements are evaluated by using an empirical expression for the one-electron part, namely

$$H_{rs}^0 = \langle\chi_r^A|-1/2\,\nabla^2 - \sum_C Z_C'/r_C|\chi_s^B\rangle = 1/2(\beta_A^0 + \beta_B^0)S_{rs} \quad , \tag{56}$$

where β_A^0 and β_B^0 are known as bonding parameters and are constant for each atomic species. This is a modified type of Mulliken approximation, the β's being chosen in such a way so as to reproduce as accurately as possible the SCF wave-functions for diatomic molecules. We note that H^0_{rs} for r and s centered at the same nucleus is set equal to zero. Finally, the total off-diagonal element of the F-matrix is written as

$$F_{rs} = H^0_{rs} + \sum_p \sum_q D_{pq} [2(rs|pq) - (rq|ps)] \quad , \tag{57}$$

which reduces to

$$F_{rs} = H^0_{rs} - D_{rs}(rr|ss) = H^0_{rs} - 1/2 \, P_{rs}(rr|ss) \tag{58}$$

if differential overlap is neglected.

Since the CNDO/2 procedure is an iterative one, an initial estimate of the molecular orbitals is made by setting $F^{(0)}_{rr} = -1/2(I_r + A_r)$ and $F^{(0)}_{rs} = 1/2(\beta^0_A + \beta^0_B)S_{rs}$. Cycling then proceeds as in SCF theory until input and output MO's agree to a predetermined accuracy. The total energy is then computed via the relationship

$$E_T = \sum \epsilon_j + 1/2 \sum \sum P_{rs}H^0_{rs} + \sum_{A<B} \sum \frac{Z'_A Z'_B}{r_{AB}} \quad . \tag{59}$$

Note that in solving the secular equation, the matrix $\underset{\sim}{S}$ is set equal to the unit matrix of appropriate dimension. Parameter values for CNDO/2 calculations [30] are given in Table 7.

TABLE 7. PARAMETERS FOR CNDO/2 CALCULATIONS IN eV

Atom	$1/2\ (I_s + A_s)$	$1/2\ (I_p + A_p)$	$-\beta^0$
H	7.18	--	9
Li	3.11	1.26	9
Be	5.95	2.56	13
B	9.59	4.00	17
C	14.05	5.57	21
N	19.32	7.27	25
O	25.39	9.11	31
F	32.27	11.08	39

Because of the neglect of differential overlap, it is difficult to compare the matrix elements of the CNDO/2 method with those taken from an SCF calculation. The usual interpretation [29] is to assume that the CNDO calculation can be compared with an *ab initio* one using a set of Löwdin-orthogonalized orbitals [32]. Letting $\underset{\sim}{\phi}'$ denote a column matrix of unorthogonalized basis functions, the Löwdin orbitals are given by

$$\underset{\sim}{\phi} = \underset{\sim}{\phi}'\underset{\sim}{S}^{-1/2} \tag{60}$$

where $\underset{\sim}{S}$ is the overlap matrix. Thus it is easier to compare the CNDO/2 MO's with those found from an SCF calculation by transforming the CNDO basis set, $\underset{\sim}{\phi}_{CNDO}$, using the transformation

$$\underset{\sim}{\phi} = \underset{\sim}{\phi}_{CNDO}\underset{\sim}{S}^{1/2} \tag{61}$$

and rewriting the CNDO MO's in terms of the $\underset{\sim}{\phi}$ basis set.

The CNDO/2 procedure has many strong points in its favor. It avoids the complete neglect of electron repulsion terms, and although most of the electron repulsion integrals are ignored, the important ones are included. The method is simple enough to be generally useful and avoids the great multiplicity of parameters inherent in the NEMO techniques. Furthermore, nuclear-nuclear repulsions are included in a reasonable way and the zero overlap matrix elements neglected in EHT appear in CNDO/2 because of the two-electron terms. The prediction of bond angles with CNDO/2 is another strong point, as is the reasonable electron distribution. This is not to imply that the method has no inherent faults. We expect that the use of an isotropic p-orbital value for the H^0_{rr} component of F_{rr} will lead to difficulties in π-electron systems, and this point will be discussed shortly in more detail. Bond lengths are generally not predicted as well as the angles [33] and stretching force constants and binding energies are grossly exaggerated. Finally, the detailed balancing of the various terms entering the calculated total energy is not quite correct in that eclipsed and *gauche* conformations are generally predicted to be too stable relative to staggered conformations.

Attempts to re-parameterize CNDO theory have been made by several investigators. Unfortunately, as with other semiempirical theories, a given parameterization which is suitable for the calculation of one property is generally found to be poor for the calculation of others. Sichel and Whitehead [34-36] have made the most extensive changes in CNDO parameters in order to compute more reasonable ionization potentials and binding energies. These authors make more extensive use of atomic data for parameter evaluation and have made studies in which correlation effects have been empirically included by use of electron repulsion terms which are somewhat smaller than those computed theoretically. In computing dissociation energies, it is further assumed that the nuclear-nuclear repulsion term should be approximated by

$$V_{nn} = \sum_{A<B}\sum Z_A' Z_B' \gamma_{AB} \quad . \tag{62}$$

Bonding parameters are chosen so as to reproduce the observed dissociation energies of H_2 and the hydrides AH_n. Computed binding energies and ionization potentials are in good agreement with experiment. However, no mention is made of attempts to compute molecular geometries.

Del Bene and Jaffe' [37] have modified the CNDO/2 method in order to compute reasonable spectroscopic transition energies and oscillator strengths. These investigators assign a value to γ_{AA} of $(I_A - A_A)p$ for elements other than hydrogen and $(I_A - A_A)_{1s}$ for the latter. A distinction is made between π- and σ-electrons by writing

$$H^0_{ij} = 1/2\, K(\beta^0_M + \beta^0_N) S_{ij} \quad , \tag{63}$$

where $K = 1$ if S_{ij} is an overlap integral between σ-orbitals, and $K = 0.585$ if S_{ij} involves the overlap between π-orbitals. The extrapolation technique of Pariser and Parr [38] is used to evaluate the two-center integrals γ_{AB}. Slightly different values of the bonding parameters are also used. This method, coupled with limited configuration interaction, has been successful for spectroscopic considerations [37,39,40], but is not as good as the Pople-Segal form of CNDO/2 for bond angles and dipole moments.

Wiberg [41] has used modified parameters for hydrogen and carbon and has scaled the binding energies computed for hydrocarbons by an empirical factor to obtain reasonable agreement with experiment.

Application of the CNDO technique to molecules containing second row atoms has not met with a great deal of success since the 3d orbitals centered on these latter atoms must be included [42] if dipole moments are to be computed. The orbital independent parameterization was found to be poor for 3d orbitals necessitating a change in the basic CNDO philosophy.

Dixon [43] and Pople, Beveridge, and Dobosh [44] have proposed a modification of CNDO known as INDO (intermediate neglect of differential overlap) which transcends the basic assumptions of CNDO in that electron repulsion integrals of the form $(ij|ij)$ are not neglected if orbitals χ_i and χ_j are centered on the same atom. The inclusion of these terms complicates the calculations to a slight extent since we now have more integrals to consider and also since the one-center coulomb integrals are not given an isotropic value. The basic relations are given below:

$$(ss|ss) = (ss|p_\mu p_\mu) = F^0 = \gamma_{AA}, \ (\mu = x,y,z) \tag{64}$$

$$(sp_\mu|sp_\mu) = 1/3\ G^1, \ (\mu = x,y,z) \tag{65}$$

$$(p_\mu p_\nu|p_\mu p_\nu) = 3/25\ F^2, \ (\mu \neq \nu, \ \mu,\nu = x,y,z) \tag{66}$$

$$(p_\mu p_\mu|p_\mu p_\mu) = F^0 + 4/25\ F^2 \ (\mu = x,y,z) \tag{67}$$

$$(p_\mu p_\mu|p_\nu p_\nu) = F^0 - 2/25\ F^2 \ (\mu \neq \nu, \ \mu,\nu = x,y,z) \quad . \tag{68}$$

The parameters G^1 and F^2 are taken from spectral data although they may be evaluated from Slater orbitals. The values of G^1 and F^2 used by Pople et al. [44] are given in Table 8. The core integrals U_{ss} and U_{pp} are somewhat different in the INDO formulation since the one-center exchange terms are included. The following equations apply to the evaluation of these quantities:

$$\text{Hydrogen:} \quad U_{1s,1s} = -1/2(I + A)_{1s} - 1/2\gamma_{HH} \tag{69}$$

$$\text{Lithium:} \quad \begin{aligned} U_{2s,2s} &= -1/2(I + A)_{2s} - 1/2\ F^0 \\ U_{2p,2p} &= -1/2(I + A)_{2p} - 1/2\ F^0 + 1/12\ G^1 \end{aligned} \tag{70}$$

$$\text{Beryllium:} \quad \begin{aligned} U_{2s,2s} &= -1/2(I + A)_{2s} - 3/2\ F^0 + 1/2\ G^1 \\ U_{2p,2p} &= -1/2(I + A)_{2p} - 3/2\ F^0 + 1/4\ G^1 \end{aligned} \tag{71}$$

Boron to $U_{2s,2s} = -1/2(I + A)_{2s} - (Z' - 1/2)F^0 + 1/6(Z' - 3/2)G^1$

Fluorine $U_{2p,2p} = -1/2(I + A)_{2p} - (Z' - 1/2)F^0 + 1/3\ G^1 + 2/25(Z' - 5/2)F^2$. (72)

TABLE 8. VALUES FOR G^1 AND F^2 FOR FIRST-ROW ATOMS[(a)]

Element	G^1, eV	F^2, eV
Li	2.5037	1.3569
Be	3.8286	2.4252
B	5.4222	3.5486
C	7.2845	4.7271
N	9.4157	5.9607
O	11.8157	7.2494
F	14.4844	8.5932

(a) Data taken from J. C. Slater, *Quantum Theory of Atomic Structure*, Vol 1, McGraw-Hill Book Company, New York (1960).

Finally, the matrix elements F_{rs} are given by

$$F_{rr}(r \ni A) = H^0_{rr} + \sum_{p \ni A} P_{pp} \{(rr|pp) - 1/2(rp|rp)\} + \sum_{B \neq A} P_{BB}\gamma_{AB} \tag{73}$$

$$H^0_{rr} = U_{rr} - \sum_{B \neq A} Z'_B \gamma_{AB} \tag{74}$$

$$F_{rs}(r \neq s,\ r \ni A,\ s \ni A) = P_{rs} \{(rs|rs) - 1/2(rr|ss)\} \tag{75}$$

$$F_{rs}(r \ni A,\ s \ni B) = 1/2(\beta^0_A + \beta^0_B)S_{rs} - 1/2P_{rs}\gamma_{AB} \quad . \tag{76}$$

The INDO method predicts molecular geometries as well as, if not better than, CNDO/2 and computed dipole moments are also improved. It is also capable of accurate prediction of esr hyperfine coupling constants.

A method similar to INDO has been developed by Dewar and coworkers [45, 46] for computing heats of formation. This method has been designated MINDO (modified INDO) and differs from INDO in that electron repulsion integrals are evaluated empirically, valence state ionization potentials are used to compute the terms U_{ss} and U_{pp}, a modified equation for the off-diagonal H^0_{rs} terms is used, and the nuclear-nuclear repulsions are evaluated in the same manner as suggested by Sichel and Whitehead [34]. Excellent agreement with experiment is obtained for heats of formation of many hydrocarbons, although the method fails to predict the relative stabilities of rotational isomers. For example the *cis* isomers of 2-butene and 1,3-butadiene are predicted to be more stable than the trans forms. It is also probable that the *gauche* conformations of butane and pentane will be predicted to be much too stable by MINDO. Dipole moments tend to be poor and electron distribution in molecules containing hetero-atoms is exaggerated. This is to be expected since the parameters were calibrated to reproduce heats of formation which require the use of low values of electron repulsion parameters to compensate for correlation effects.

IV. COMPUTED PROPERTIES FROM ALL-VALENCE ELECTRON SEMIEMPIRICAL METHODS

A. Molecular Geometry and Relative Conformational Energies

The nature of EHT and NEMO calculations renders these methods worthless for the prediction of bond lengths since these latter quantities are sensitive to the detailed balancing of one- and two-electron contributions, along with the nuclear-nuclear repulsion. Therefore, a discussion of predicted bond lengths must necessarily be limited to those calculations carried out by CNDO or INDO methods.

Segal [33] has examined bond lengths for several diatomic molecules using the CNDO/2 formulation. His results are shown in Table 9, along with the predicted and experimental value of the force constant, k. This latter quantity is proportional to $\partial^2E/\partial R^2|R = R_{eq}$ for a diatomic molecule, and therefore to the curvature of the total energy at the equilibrium distance. The computed force constants are all much too large, indicating that the curvature at the minimum is too great (i.e., the potential curve is not flat enough near the minimum). The computed equilibrium distances, on the other hand, are in fairly good agreement with experiment.

Gordon and Pople [47] have published a massive study on the computed geometry of a large number of molecules using the INDO method. The results for bond lengths are too numerous to present a complete tabulation, but some

TABLE 9. PREDICTED BOND LENGTHS AND FORCE CONSTANTS BY CNDO/2

Molecule	R_{eq}, A Observed	R_{eq}, A Calculated	% Error	k, mdyn/A Observed	k, mdyn/A Calculated
H_2	0.742	0.746	0.5	5.7	10.6
HF	0.917	1.004	9.5	9.7	19.7
OH	0.971	1.026	5.7	7.8	16.6
NH	1.038	1.062	2.3	6.0	14.9
N_2	1.094	1.140	4.2	23.0	53.8
N_2^+	1.116	1.113	0.3	20.1	52.2
CH	1.120	1.109	1.0	4.5	12.5
O_2^+	1.123	1.095	2.5	16.6	63.1
CO	1.128	1.190	5.5	19.0	43.6
NO	1.151	1.152	0.1	15.9	51.1
O_2	1.207	1.132	6.2	11.8	58.5
BH	1.233	1.193	3.2	3.0	9.3
BeH	1.343	1.324	1.4	2.26	5.07
LiH	1.595	1.568	1.7	1.03	1.92

representative results are given in Table 10. These values are not very encouraging. Particularly poor results are obtained for O-F and N-F bond lengths, and the O-H distances are consistently in error by 8-10 percent. Another discouraging feature of the INDO calculations is the insensitivity of predicted bond lengths for some types of bonds, irrespective of the molecule in which that bond is found. For example, the computed C-F bond distances in CH_3F, CF_4, FCN, C_2F_4, and C_2F_6 range from 1.32 to 1.35, whereas the experimental values vary from 1.26 in FCN to 1.385 in CH_3F. It is therefore probably not possible to use either CNDO or INDO for anything other than a rough prediction of bond lengths.

The calculation of equilibrium bond angles can be carried out very accurately, for the most part, by CNDO or INDO techniques and under certain conditions by extended Hückel-type procedures. We will discuss the latter

TABLE 10. PREDICTED BOND LENGTHS BY INDO

Molecule	Bond	R_{eq}, A Calc.	R_{eq}, A Exptl.	Molecule	Bond	R_{eq}, A Calc.	R_{eq}, A Exptl.
H_2O	O–H	1.03	0.96	H_2NOH	N–H	1.08	1.02
OF_2	O–F	1.18	1.41	H_2NOH	N–O	1.28	1.41
NH_3	N–H	1.07	1.019	H_2NOH	O–H	1.04	0.96
NHF_2	N–H	1.09	1.026	H_2CCH_2	C–H	1.11	1.086
NHF_2	N–F	1.25	1.400	H_2CCH_2	C–C	1.31	1.337
NF_3	N–F	1.25	1.371	H_2NNH_2	N–H	1.08	1.02
CH_4	C–H	1.116	1.093	H_2NNH_2	N–N	1.33	1.45
CH_3F	C–H	1.120	1.105	F_2CCF_2	C–F	1.34	1.30
CH_3F	C–F	1.348	1.385	F_2CCF_2	C–C	1.33	1.33
CF_4	C–F	1.338	1.317	F_2NNF_2	N–F	1.26	1.37
HCN	C–H	1.09	1.063	F_2NNF_2	N–N	1.36	1.47
HCN	C–N	1.18	1.155	H_3COH	C–O	1.37	1.434
FCN	F–C	1.32	1.262	H_3COH	O–H	1.04	0.937
HCCH	C–H	1.10	1.057	H_3CNH_2	C–N	1.40	1.474
HCCH	C–C	1.20	1.209	H_3CNH_2	N–H	1.07	1.011
HOOH	O–H	1.04	0.95	H_3CCH_3	C–H	1.12	1.108
HOOH	O–O	1.22	1.475	H_3CCH_3	C–C	1.46	1.536
H_2CO	C–H	1.12	1.116	F_3CCF_3	C–F	1.35	1.33
H_2CO	C–O	1.25	1.208	F_3CCF_3	C–C	1.49	1.51

computations first. If we can regard the EHT energy as an approximation to the sum of valence-state Hartree-Fock energies, we can set down reasonable guide lines as to the conditions which must be met in order for EHT to give a reasonable prediction of bond angles. Allen and Russell [13] have shown that $\sum_i^{val} \epsilon_i$ should give a reasonable prediction of bond angles if either of the following two inequalities hold:

$$\partial/\partial\theta(2 \sum_i^{val} \epsilon_i) \Big/ \partial/\partial\theta(V_{nn} - V_{ee} + 2 \sum_i^{core} \epsilon_i) > 0 \tag{77}$$

$$|\partial/\partial\theta(2 \sum_i^{val} \epsilon_i)| > |\partial/\partial\theta(V_{nn} - V_{ee} + 2 \sum_i^{core} \epsilon_i| \quad (78)$$

These inequalities do not hold for highly ionic species so that a poor prediction of bond angle is forthcoming from EHT calculations in such cases. A tabulation of Allen and Russell's results [13] are given in Table 11.

TABLE 11. PREDICTED BOND ANGLES BY EHT[(a)]

Molecule	*Ab Initio* Equilibrium Angle	EHT Equilibrium Angle
BeH_2	180	180
BH_2^+	180	180
BH_2^-	100	110
NH_2^+	120	120
H_2O	110	150
BeH_3^-	120	120
BH_3	120	120
CH_3^+	120	120
Li_2O	180	100
F_2O	102	100
LiOH	180	<60
FOH	100	<60

(a) Results taken from Allen and Russell [13].

The accurate prediction of bond angles is a strong point of either the CNDO or INDO methods. Pople and Segal [30] and Gordon and Pople [47] have extensively studied many molecules, and some of their results are given in Tables 12 and 13. The results speak for themselves. The only case in which CNDO or INDO is grossly in error is the triplet state of CH_2.

TABLE 12. PREDICTED BOND ANGLES BY CNDO[a]

Molecule	Bond Angle Calc.	Bond Angle, Exptl.
$CH_2(^1A_1)$	108.6	103.2
$CH_2(^3\Sigma g^- - {}^3B_1)$	141.4	180.0
H_2O	107.1	104.5
NO_2	137.7	132
NO_2^+	180.0	180.0
CO_2	180.0	180.0
CO_2^-	142.3	134
O_3	114.0	116.8
OF_2	99.2	103.8
NH_3	106.7	106.6
OH_3^+	113.9	117
CF_3	113.5	111.1

(a) Results taken from Pople and Segal[30].

TABLE 13. PREDICTED BOND ANGLES BY INDO[(a)]

Molecule	Angle	Bond Angle, Calc.	Bond Angle, Exptl.
$CH_2(^1A_1)$	HCH	106.0	103.2
$CH_2(^3\Sigma_g^- - ^3B_1)$	HCH	131.8	180.0
OF_2	FOF	106.6	103.3
NH_3	HNH	106.4	106.6
NHF_2	FNF	104.6	102.9
NHF_2	HNF	105.2	99.8
NF_3	FNF	104.2	102.2
FNO	FNO	111.6	110.0
HNO	HNO	111.2	108.6
HOOH	OOH	108.8	94.8
FNNF	NNF	116.0	114.5
FOOF	OOF	108.4	109.5
H_2NOH	HNO	110.2	106.0
H_2NOH	NOH	111.8	103.0
H_2CCH_2	HCC	124.3	121.3
H_2NNH_2	HNN	110.6	112.0
F_2NNF_2	FNN	106.7	104.0
H_3COH	HCH	108.2	109.5
H_3COH	HCO	110.7	109.5
H_3COH	COH	107.3	105.9
H_3CCH_3	HCH	106.6	108.8
H_3CCH_3	HCC	112.2	110.1

(a) Results taken from Gordon and Pople [47].

The problem of computing energetically preferred conformations is extremely important in biological systems. Most biologically important molecules are too large to be treated by even a rough *ab initio* calculation so that it is necessary to utilize a semiempirical scheme. If the prediction of the preferred conformation is to be made, it is imperative that the chosen method of calculation be tested on many systems of known conformation so that the proper degree of confidence in the computed result can be established.

The early studies of Hoffman [6] indicated that EHT can deal successfully with the prediction of preferred conformations in most hydrocarbon molecules but that the barriers to internal rotation are generally exaggerated, especially for larger systems. Also, *trans* conformations are disproportionately favored over *gauche*. The situation with CNDO calculations is somewhat different. Very little work has been reported on computations concerning internal rotation but it appears that there is an underestimation of steric factors, so that the barrier to internal rotation in ethane is too small and *gauche* conformations are predicted to be too low in energy relative to the *trans*. Thus for ethane EHT predicts a barrier to internal rotation of 4.02 kcal/mole [6], CNDO gives 2.3 kcal/mole [48], and the experimental value is 2.93 kcal/mole [49]. In propane, one has two methyl rotors which are coupled in their internal rotation. Hoyland [50] has shown from *ab initio* calculations and examination of the microwave spectra that the internal rotation in this molecule can be approximately described by the equation

$$E_{rel} = 1/2\ V_0(2 - \cos 3\alpha_1 - \cos 3\alpha_2) - 1/2\ V_1[1 - \cos 3(\alpha_1 + \alpha_2)] \quad , \qquad (79)$$

The experimental values of V_0 and V_1 being 3575 ± 100 cal/mole and 310 ± 40 cal/mole, respectively. The results reported by Hoffmann [6] lead to values for V_0 and V_1 of 6205 and 575 cal/mole, considerably larger than experiment, whereas CNDO calculations [51] predict these values to be 2449 and 344 cal/mole. It is interesting that V_1 is essentially correct, indicating that CNDO is more accurate in predicting long-range interactions than for the interaction of neighboring groups.

The trends noted above become even more striking in butane for internal rotation about the central C–C bond. If we denote the angle of rotation by α and set $\alpha = 0$ for the *trans* conformation, the *gauche* conformation occurs experimentally at $\alpha = \pm 112.5 \pm 1.1^{\circ}$ [52], with an energy difference between the *trans* and *gauche* conformations of 770 ± 90 cal/mole [53] and a barrier for transformation from *trans* to *gauche* of about 3.6-3.8 kcal/mole [54-56]. The barrier for direct interconversion of the two *gauche* conformations has been estimated to be 5.3-6.7 kcal/mole [55,56]. Table 14 summarizes the predicted energy changes for rotation about the central bond in butane as computed by EHT [6,51], CNDO/2 [51], and two *ab initio* calculations [57]. The *ab initio* calculations differ in the size of the Gaussian basis set utilized, the smaller set containing 64 orbitals and the larger 94 orbitals. Neither EHT or CNDO/2 is capable of providing even a qualitative picture of the energetics involved. The energy difference between *trans* and *gauche* is much too large in the EHT calculation, whereas CNDO/2 predicts that the *gauche* conformation is more stable than the *trans*. Likewise, the barrier hindering in the conversion of the *trans* and *gauche* conformations is greatly exaggerated by EHT and much too small by CNDO/2. We must therefore conclude that neither method is satisfactory for hydrocarbons.

TABLE 14. INTERNAL ROTATION ABOUT THE CENTRAL BOND IN BUTANE[(a)]

α, °	Relative E EHT	Relative E CNDO/2	Relative E[(b)] *Ab Initio* (1)	Relative E[(c)] *Ab Initio* (2)
0	0	0	0	0
30	3.56	1.06	1.751	---
60	7.29	1.89	3.536	3.619
90	4.34	0.51	1.851	---
100	3.48	0.03	1.140	---
105	3.48	-0.09	0.918	0.876
110	3.86	-0.11	0.824	0.766
115	4.66	-0.01	0.871	0.801
120	5.88	0.18	1.062	---
150	18.22	1.81	4.311	---
180	26.50	4.18	7.643	7.595

(a) Energies in kcal/mole relative to the *trans* conformation.

(b) Smaller Gaussian basis set.

(c) Larger Gaussian basis set.

Herndon, Feuer, and Hall [58] have studied the conformations of propene, 1-butene, acetaldehyde, propionaldehyde, formic acid, and acetic acid by CNDO/2 and have compared these results wherever possible with those found by EHT and also with experiment. Both CNDO/2 and EHT give reasonable results for propene and acetaldehyde, correctly predicting that a methyl C-H bond eclipses the double bond. For propionaldehyde, however, CNDO/2 fails completely, predicting a minimum near the experimental maximum in the potential curve. EHT correctly predicts the most stable conformation and also predicts a secondary minimum but at a position 20° away from the experimental value. The computed EHT barrier is (probably fortuitously) in almost exact agreement with experiment. In formic acid, CNDO correctly predicts the hydroxyl group conformation (a planar molecule with the hydroxyl *cis* to the carbonyl), whereas EHT predicts a *trans* orientation. However, the CNDO result for the barrier to internal rotation for the -OH group is 34.9 kcal/mole, more than twice the observed value of 13.4-17 kcal/mole [59,60]. For acetic acid, both CNDO and EHT predict the correct conformation of the methyl group for -OH *cis* to the carbonyl, but again EHT predicts a *trans* orientation.

The above discussion serves as an illustration of the diverse results which can be expected from CNDO/2- and EHT-computed conformations and emphasizes our warning that many model molecules should be studied in order to determine the probable correctness of any predicted preferred conformation. This should not be taken to imply that potentially useful conformation results cannot be obtained from either EHT or CNDO studies. Kier and coworkers [61-70] have studied a large number of molecules by EHT, including many of biological and pharmacological importance. Computed preferred conformations were found to agree with experimental data in most cases and low-lying secondary minima can be invoked to explain the dual pharmacological activity of histamine. These studies have led to a working hypothesis of drug-receptor interaction in which drug molecules having the same type of activity present a similar pattern of charged moieties to the receptor.

Several other conformational studies have been carried out with EHT or CNDO/2. Jordan and Pullman [71] have calculated the preferred conformations of uracil and thymine photodimers. It was later shown [72] that these studies led to several incorrect predictions. For example, Jordan and Pullman have computed that the most stable conformations are obtained with planar bases, the half-chair conformation being less stable by 80-100 kcal/mole. It has now been established by X-ray diffraction that the bases in the *trans-anti* thymine photodimer do assume a half-chair conformation [73]. For a further discussion of incorrect EHT predictions in these photodimers, see Reference 72.

Jordan and Pullman [74] have carried out EHT calculations of the preferred conformation of the nucleosides uridine, cytidine, adenosine, and guanosine. The computed stable conformations appear to be in agreement with experimental data. Other EHT studies include those of Giordano, Hamann, Harkins, and Kaufman [75] on 2-formyl N-methyl pyridinium (cation) oxime and that of Neely on α-D-glucopyranose [76]. Experimental data on these systems is vague so that nothing can be said concerning their correctness. Finally, Tinland has examined internal rotation in biphenyl by EHT and CNDO [77]. The CNDO/2 calculation predicts an angle of rotation of 90°, EHT gives 66° for this quantity, whereas the vapor phase angle is 42°.

In summary, it would appear that EHT is probably a better overall procedure than CNDO/2 for the calculation of preferred conformations, but still leaves much to be desired. No work has as yet been reported on IEHT conformational calculations and no data on the magnitude of computed barriers is available from INDO calculations. Finally, the entire area of conformational prediction by semi-empirical methods is not very satisfying and investigators in this field are urged to use more restraint in proclaiming the accuracy of computed conformations in the absence of experimental data.

B. Charge Distribution and Dipole Moments

The charge distribution in a molecule is usually defined in terms of gross charges on the various nuclei as defined in terms of a Mulliken population analysis [78]. For a closed-shell system in which the wavefunction is written as an antisymmetrized product of doubly occupied MO's $\phi_1 - \phi_m$ expanded in terms of a basis set $\chi_1 - \chi_n$, the net atomic population of a given orbital χ_j is defined as

$$p_j = 2 \sum_{i=1}^{m} c_{ji}^2 \qquad (80)$$

where we have written the MO's as

$$\phi_i = \sum_{k=1} c_{ki}\chi_k \quad . \qquad (81)$$

We further define the overlap population of the basis orbitals by the equation

$$o_{ij} = o_{ji} = 2 \sum_k c_{ik}c_{jk}S_{ij} = 2D_{ij}S_{ij} \quad , \qquad (82)$$

and write the gross population of orbital χ_j as

$$P_j = \sum_{i=1}^{n} o_{ij} \quad , \qquad (83)$$

noting that $p_j \equiv o_{jj}$. Finally, the total gross population at any nucleus n is given by

$$\overline{P}_n = \sum_{j \ni n} P_j \quad , \qquad (84)$$

the symbol $j \ni n$ meaning that orbital j is centered at nucleus n. The gross charge at nucleus n is then the nuclear charge minus $\overline{P}_n$.

The Mulliken scheme has the advantage of simplicity but is not above criticism. The main item of concern is partitioning of the overlap density equally between the two basis orbitals in question, whereas in reality some weighted average should be used. This fact makes the comparison of charge distributions for the same molecule calculated with different basis sets difficult, especially if one set is made up of Slater orbitals and the other of Gaussians.

Perhaps the most advantageous way to compare the overall accuracy of a molecular charge distribution is to compute the dipole moment for molecules in which it does not vanish by symmetry. For a neutral molecule the magnitude of the dipole moment is independent of the origin of coordinates, and is a vector quantity with components given (in atomic units) by

$$\mu_w = \sum_{\substack{j,\text{all} \\ \text{nuclei}}} Z_j w_j - \langle\Psi| \sum_{\substack{i,\text{all} \\ \text{electrons}}} w_i |\Psi\rangle, \quad w = x,y,z \qquad (85)$$

x, y, and z being measured from some arbitrary origin. The magnitude of the dipole moment is $(\overline{\mu} \cdot \overline{\mu})^{1/2}$. Again assuming that the total wavefunction Ψ for a closed shell molecule is an antisymmetrized product of MO's, ϕ, expanded in terms of $\chi_1 - \chi_n$, the expression for μ_w becomes

$$\mu_w = \sum_{\substack{j,\text{all}\\ \text{nuclei}}} Z_j w_j - 2 \sum_{i,j}\sum D_{ij} \langle\chi_i|w|\chi_j\rangle, \quad w = x,y,z \quad . \tag{86}$$

The charge distribution given by EHT is very exaggerated so that it is hopeless to compute dipole moments using wavefunctions generated by this method. IEHT wavefunctions, on the other hand, should lead to a much better description of the electron density which should be reflected in the computed dipole moments. Table 15 is a tabulation of dipole moments computed by EHT and IEHT [21], and a comparison with experiment. These results were computed using the rigorous definition of the dipole moment given above, with no approximations, other than the use of Z-value for the nuclei appropriately reduced by the number of inner-shell electrons. As expected the EHT values are completely unrealistic. The IEHT

TABLE 15. DIPOLE MOMENTS FROM EHT AND IEHT WAVEFUNCTIONS[a,b]

Molecule	μ, EHT	μ, IEHT	μ, Exp.
NH_3	2.987	1.583	1.47
H_2O	4.264	1.772	1.84
HCN	6.640	2.449	2.95
CO	3.469[c]	1.164	0.13
HF	3.743	1.657	1.82
H_2CO	7.154	1.848	2.17
HCOOH	4.422	1.905	1.53
$HCONH_2$	10.229	5.046	3.71
HCOF	6.325	1.776	2.02
Pyridine	4.324	2.157	2.20
Sydnone	14.353	6.781	7.31

(a) Data taken from Bloor, Gilson, and Billingsley, [21].

(b) All values are in debye units.

(c) Dipole moment vector incorrectly oriented by 180°.

results, however, are all in fairly good agreement with experiment except for carbon monoxide and formamide. Dipole moments have also been computed by Rein et al. [18] but an approximation was used in that the dipole moment was calculated by the equation

$$\mu_w = \sum_{\substack{i, \text{all} \\ \text{nuclei}}} (Z_i - \overline{P}_i) w_i \quad , \tag{87}$$

where $\overline{P}_i$ is the total gross electron population of nucleus i. Neglect of other contributions to the dipole moment renders their results of little value in many cases.

Some dipole moments have been computed from NEMO wavefunctions by Lipscomb and coworkers [23,24]. The results are not very good in most cases since dipole moments from minimal basis SCF calculations are unreliable and extremely sensitive to the basis set. NEMO calculations are not carried out with optimized sets and the dipole moments fluctuate randomly around experimental values to an alarming degree. This is a very negative aspect of NEMO.

Considerable success has been found in the calculation of dipole moments from CNDO/2 wavefunctions. These are computed using the relation

$$\mu_w(\text{CNDO}) = \sum_{\substack{A, \text{all} \\ \text{nuclei}}} \left[4.803 (Z'_A - P_{AA}) w_A - 7.337 \frac{P_A(2s, 2p)}{\zeta_A} \right], \quad w = x, y, z \quad , \tag{88}$$

where Z'_A and P_{AA} have been defined previously, $P_A(2s,2p_w)$ is the bond order between 2s and $2p_w$ orbitals centered at nucleus A, and ζ_A is the orbital exponent [i.e., $2s_A = N\, r_A \exp(-\zeta_A r_A)$]. The distances are measured in angstroms and the dipole moment is in debyes. Pople and Gordon [79] have compiled a large list of computed dipole moments, and we present some of these in Table 16. The agreement with experiment is excellent in most cases, ammonia and the methylamines being exceptions. Experimentally, the dipole moments of NH_3, CH_3NH_2, $(CH_3)_2NH$, and $(CH_3)_3N$ are 1.47, 1.33, 1.03, and 0.61 debyes, whereas the computed results are 1.97, 1.86, 1.76, and 1.68 debyes. The decreasing trend of the dipole moment with the number of methyl groups is correctly predicted but the magnitude of the change is not.

TABLE 16. DIPOLE MOMENTS FROM CNDO/2 WAVEFUNCTIONS[(a,b)]

Molecule	μ Calc.	μ Exptl.	Molecule	μ Calc.	μ Exptl.
Propene	0.36	0.364	Acetone	2.90	2.90
Isobutane	0	0.132	Acrolein(s-*trans*)	2.63	3.11
Isoprene	0.25	0.292	Ketene	1.30	1.414
Hydrogen fluoride	1.85	1.819	Formic acid	0.87	1.415
Fluoroform	1.66	1.645	Phenol	1.73	1.55
Ethyl fluoride	1.83	1.96	Ammonia	1.97	1.468
Vinyl fluoride	1.51	1.427	Methylamine	1.86	1.326
cis-1,2-Difluoroethylene	2.83	2.42	Hydrogen cyanide	2.48	2.986
2-Fluoro-1,3-butadiene	1.65	1.417	Nitrogen trifluoride	0.43	0.235
Fluorobenzene	1.66	1.66	Nitrous acid	2.27	1.85
Water	2.10	1.846	Nitric acid	2.24	2.16
Methanol	1.94	1.69	Formyl fluoride	2.16	2.02
Dimethyl ether	1.83	1.30	Formamide	3.79	3.71
Formaldehyde	1.98	2.339	Nitrobenzene	5.33	4.28

(a) Data taken from Pople and Gordon [79].

(b) All values are in debye units.

Sichel and Whitehead [80] have also computed dipole moments of several molecules using their parameterization of CNDO. The results are generally about as good as those for CNDO/2.

Finally, it is interesting to note that if we consider the CNDO MO's as being linear combinations of Löwdin orthogonalized AO's, an alternate approach to calculation of the dipole moments is to transform the MO's back to the nonorthogonal basis and compute the dipole moment by the rigorous formula. This has not been done and the results may prove quite interesting.

C. Miscellaneous Properties

The ionization potential (IP) of a closed-shell molecule is given approximately by the negative of the Hartree-Fock energy of the highest occupied MO [4]. This relation holds fairly well due to a fortuitous cancellation of the errors made in neglecting reminimization of the energy of the ion and the difference in correlation energies of molecule and ion. Similarly, higher ionization potentials should be related to the corresponding Hartree-Fock levels in the same way. It is interesting to compare the calculated IP's with experiment using the semiempirical methods discussed above to obtain the energy levels. The CNDO/2 method appears to be worthless for this purpose, especially for π-electron systems. The calculated ionization potentials are too large, and in many cases inversion of the correct ordering of the levels occurs. For example, the highest occupied σ-level in ethylene is predicted to be above the π-level. IP's computed from EHT are also usually poor, being consistently too large. Use of IEHT, however, appears to have some merit for the calculation of occupied energy levels, although π-electron MO's will probably not be given well since *ab initio* calculations, as mentioned previously, indicate that diagonal matrix elements for $2p_\pi$ - AO's are much smaller in absolute magnitude than for the $2p_\sigma$'s, and the off-diagonal elements between nearest neighbor $2p_\pi$ orbitals are much larger than predicted by IEHT or EHT. This factor, incidentally, is responsible for the very low-lying virtual orbital energies given by either EHT or IEHT. SCF calculations have indicated that the energy of the lowest lying virtual orbital is always positive while EHT or IEHT calculations on conjugated π-electron systems always give a significant negative value. Rein et al. [19] have given a compilation of IP's computed by IEHT, as have Bloor and coworkers [21].

Newton, Boer, and Lipscomb [23] have also tabulated a lengthy list of IP's computed by NEMO 1. These results are hardly spectacular in their agreement with experiment for conjugated systems larger than ethylene. It would appear that parameterization of the π-electron AO's using ethylene as a standard is a poor approximation. Computed IP's for molecules such as butadiene, benzene, azulene, etc., are much too small. This suggests that the diagonal elements for the

$2p_\pi$-orbitals should be somewhat larger (in absolute magnitude) than predicted by the ethylene calculation and the off-diagonal elements smaller.

Sichel and Whitehead [26] have computed IP's for a very large number of molecules using their parameterization of CNDO. The results are usually in good agreement with experiment and it would seem that their procedure is to be recommended if IP's are of concern.

Some success has been achieved in the area of hydrogen bonding using CNDO/2. Murthy and Rao [81] have studied the hydrogen bond in water using both EHT and CNDO/2 and have concluded that the latter method gives reasonable results. It was found that the computed hydrogen bond strength for the water dimer is 6.3 kcal/mole, in fair agreement with experiment [82]. This result has been confirmed by Hoyland and Kier [83], who have carried out extensive studies on various water polymers. It is interesting that the CNDO results on water are better than those found from an *ab initio* calculation of Morokuma and Pedersen [84] using a small Gaussian basis set.

Hoyland and Kier [83] have studied hydrogen bonding in a variety of molecules and ions. The hydrogen bond strength in ammonia is predicted to be 4.06 kcal/mole, the experimental value being 3.7-4.4 [82]. Studies on various polymers of HF seem to be qualitatively correct, although the hydrogen bond strengths are too large and the F–F distances somewhat too small. The CNDO calculations also predict an extremely enthalpically stable ring hexamer, as conjectured by Simons and Hildebrand [85] from PVT data but not confirmed by the electron diffraction studies of Bauer, Beach, and Simons [86]. Entropy effects are of great importance in this case so that little more can be said. Very reasonable results were also obtained for the interaction of NH_4^+ and $CH_3NH_3^+$ with water and for hydrogen bonding in methanol. The latter system has also been studied by Murthy, Davis, and Rao [87]. Neither of these calculations find any evidence that the methanol dimer is cyclic.

Studies on formic acid by Hoyland and Kier [83] and Murthy et al. are not in agreement for the calculated heat of formation of the cyclic dimer. The former authors find a stabilization energy of 22.96 kcal/mole whereas the latter workers predict this value to be 16.8 kcal/mole. Hoyland and Kier have repeated their calculations [88] using the geometry of Murthy and coworkers, but have failed to reproduce their results, the recalculated binding energy being 20.44 kcal/mole. These results for formic acid are not in good agreement with the experimental value of the heat of formation of the cyclic dimer of about -14.2 kcal/mole [82]. Also, the computed O-O separation of 2.42 Å is much shorter than the experimental value of 2.70 Å [88]. It is apparent that the large deviations from experiment in formic acid are due to hydrogen bonds involving carbonyl oxygens, indicating that some changes in parameterization may be necessary if a good account of hydrogen bond strengths is to be forthcoming. This effect was not noted by Pullman and Berthod [89] in their study of the dimerization of formamide since the energy of the dimer was computed with the experimental geometry in which the O----H bond distance is most probably longer than would be predicted by minimization of the dimer energy.

A small amount of work has been started on applying semiempirical all-valence electron methods to chemical reactions. Adam and Grimison [90] have considered nucleophilic substitution in pyridine, quinoline, and isoquinoline using EHT. The position of substitution is correctly predicted by the total charge densities and also by consideration of the energy of an intermediate in which the three molecules considered are attacked by a hydride ion to form a σ-complex. These authors have also considered electrophilic substitution in imidizole with some success using EHT [91].

Hermann [92] has considered electrophilic substitution in pyrrole, indole, furon, and benzofuran utilizing both EHT and CNDO/2, and considering a proton as the electrophile. Both methods correctly predict the preferred position of attack, but only CNDO/2 accounts reasonably well for the relative basicity of various positions of indole.

V. SUMMARY AND CONCLUDING REMARKS

The methods outlined in this chapter are, and will probably continue to be, utilized more generally than other specialized schemes and will be applied to more diverse problems in organic, inorganic, and biological chemistry. In view of this, it is unfortunate that none of the formulations is free from major defects and a thorough knowledge of points of breakdown is vital if efficient use is to be made of them. With this in mind, we present here a summary of the strong and weak points of the methods discussed.

Extended Hückel theory is the simplest of the methods considered and, as such, is the least satisfactory for anything other than very qualitative prediction. It is best suited to molecules in which the charge distribution is quite uniform (such as hydrocarbons), as shown by Blyholder and Coulson [17]. Since EHT neglects both electron-electron and nuclear-nuclear repulsions, it cannot be used to predict bond lengths, but is capable under certain conditions of yielding satisfactory angles [13]. The charge distribution as given by EHT is very unsatisfactory for molecules containing atoms with large differences of electronegativity, leading to grossly exaggerated dipole moments. EHT has been relatively successful in the prediction of preferred conformations and it may be that it is within this area that it has its greatest utility, in spite of the fact that predicted barriers to internal rotation are often quite bad. Finally, it is felt that application of EHT to unsaturated molecules must be undertaken with caution since the virtual orbital levels indicate that the π-system is not treated correctly.

The iterative Hückel schemes (IEHT) have been developed in an effort to overcome some of the shortcomings of EHT with regard to charge distribution. These methods appear capable of predicting adequate dipole moments, provided these are computed with the exact quantum mechanical prescription. Ionization potentials are usually predicted somewhat better by IEHT than by EHT, but application to unsaturated molecules is not warranted in its present form. Although no work has appeared on conformational calculations or on prediction of bond angles, it is felt that IEHT should be as good as EHT for conformation and somewhat superior for angles.

The NEMO methods have the definite advantage of a much better parameterization and attempt to include in a reasonable way all nonzero matrix elements. This leads to a rather large number of parameters which renders these methods more difficult and awkward to use compared to EHT. The separation of the kinetic energy is of great utility in providing a more accurate approximation to the matrix elements. Unfortunately, the NEMO scheme is based on SCF matrix elements of model compounds generated with a minimal Slater orbital set. Therefore one must have many SCF calculations available for the fixing of parameters. Furthermore, the unoptimized Slater sets utilized are far from ideal and do not in general lead to a good approximation of the SCF function. A better procedure would probably be to base the parameterization on a set of fully contracted Gaussian calculations. Such a procedure should prove advantageous if the scheme to estimate only the two-electron terms is implemented. SCF calculations with Gaussians are more easily carried out and are generally more accurate than minimal Slater calcalations if a modest set is utilized.

The NEMO methods have not received a wide following and little work has been done outside of the original papers. The wavefunctions computed by this procedure, however, will probably be a better overall description than with any other method. As pointed out previously, however, more attention needs to be paid to conjugated systems in which the π-orbital parameterization appears faulty on the basis of the energy levels.

Methods based on neglect of differential overlap, most notably CNDO and INDO, appear to be generally useful for computing dipole moments and geometry. The CNDO/2 procedure as outlined originally by Pople and Segal [30] generally overemphasizes bond strengths and does not lead to good potential functions for bond stretching or contraction. Furthermore, CNDO/2 does not give good energy levels, especially for unsaturated molecules, and conformational information is liable to be very poor. The Sichel-Whitehead parameterization [34-36] leads to better energy levels and has proved adequate for binding energies but cannot be used for the prediction of bond lengths since the nuclear-nuclear repulsion is not evaluated in the proper manner for such a calculation.

These faults and advantages also apply to INDO which has a further advantage in being able to adequately predict esr hyperfine coupling constants in radicals. It would appear that CNDO and INDO have many fine features and a more careful parameterization and a better system of integral evaluation may be able to cope with many of the difficulties of the original theories.

In view of the above discussion, it is difficult to recommend the use of one method for all types of calculation. It appears best to decide which formulation seems to be most adequate for the calculation of the properties of interest. Further work on all of these methods is needed to overcome some of the most glaring faults, especially with regard to unsaturated molecules. This necessarily means that complete rotational invariance must be sacrificed, as has been done in the NEMO formulations. This is a small price to pay for better accuracy in the energy levels.

More work should be done with IEHT directed toward building a set of rules for choosing appropriate diagonal elements for atoms in various molecular environments. This could lead to a method requiring no iteration and producing results of comparable value to a full IEHT calculation.

It is expected that within the next few years significant improvement in existing semiempirical methods will be made and new and better schemes devised which will be more generally applicable to the calculation of a wider variety of properties. Hopefully a greater amount of this effort will go into the prediction of chemical reactivities and a more fundamental understanding of such topics as linear free energy relationships, aromatic substitution, acidity and basicity, and other areas of greater interest to biochemists.

In closing, it should be pointed out that the author does not intend this chapter to be construed as an exhaustive review article, and many excellent papers have therefore not been cited. Rather, it is hoped that this exposition should serve as a guide to workers not familiar with the newer all-valence electron approaches and to point out the advantages and pitfalls of the most widely used or potentially useful methods.

VI. ACKNOWLEDGMENT

The author wishes to thank Dr. Lemont B. Kier for the use of his excellent collection of reprints on semiempirical calculations.

VII. REFERENCES

[1] D. R. Hartree, *Proc. Cambridge Phil. Soc.*, 24, 89, 111 (1928).

[2] V. Fock, *Z. Physik*, 61, 126 (1930); 62, 795 (1930).

[3] C. C. J. Roothaan, *Rev. Modern Phys.*, 23, 69 (1951).

[4] T. A. Koopmans, *Physica*, 1, 104 (1933).

[5] R. J. Buenker and S. D. Peyerimhoff, *Chem. Phys. Letters*, 3, 37 (1969).

[6] R. Hoffman, *J. Chem. Phys.*, 39, 1397 (1963).

[7] F. P. Boer, M. D. Newton, and W. N. Lipscomb, *Proc. Natl. Acad. Sci. U.S.*, 52, 890 (1964)

[8] W. E. Palke and W. N. Lipscomb, *J. Am. Chem. Soc.*, 88, 2384 (1966).

[9] R. S. Mulliken, *J. Chim. Phys.*, 46, 497, 675 (1949).

[10] For example, see R. G. Parr, *The Quantum Theory of Molecular Electronic Structure*, W. A. Benjamin, Inc., New York, New York, 1963.

[11] M. D. Newton, F. P. Boer, and W. N. Lipscomb, *J. Am. Chem. Soc.*, 88, 2353 (1966).

[12] C. J. Ballhansen and H. B. Gray, *Inorg. Chem.*, 1, 111 (1962).

[13] L. C. Allen and J. D. Russell, *J. Chem. Phys.*, 46, 1029 (1967).

[14] L. C. Cusachs, *J. Chem. Phys.*, 43, S157 (1965).

[15] M. D. Newton, *J. Chem. Phys.*, 45, 2716 (1966).

[16] L. C. Cusachs, *J. Chem. Phys.*, 45, 2717 (1966).

[17] G. Blyholder and C. A. Coulson, *Theoret. Chim. Acta. (Berl.)*, 10, 316 (1968).

[18] R. Rein, N. Fukuda, H. Win, G. A. Clarke and F. E. Harris, *J. Chem. Phys.*, 45, 4743 (1966).

[19] R. Rein, N. Fukuda, G. A. Clarke, and F. E. Harris, *J. Theoret. Biol.*, 21, 88 (1968).

[20] A. Pullman, E. Kuchanski, M. Gilbert, and A. Denis, *Theoret. Chim. Acta. (Berl.)*, 10, 231 (1968).

[21] J. E. Bloor, B. R. Gilson, and F. P. Billingsley, II, *Theoret. Chim. Acta. (Berl.)*, 12, 360 (1968).

[22] B. J. Duke, *Theoret. Chim. Acta. (Berl.)*, 9, 260 (1968).

[23] M. D. Newton, F. P. Boer, and W. N. Lipscomb, *J. Am. Chem. Soc.*, 88, 2367 (1966).

[24] D. B. Boyd and W. N. Lipscomb, *J. Chem. Phys.*, 48, 4955 (1968).

[25] For example, see J. R. Hoyland, *J. Chem. Phys.*, 40, 3540 (1964).

[26] R. Pariser and R. G. Parr, *J. Chem. Phys.*, 21, 466 (1953).

[27] J. A. Pople, *Trans. Faraday Soc.*, 49, 1375 (1953).

[28] J. A. Pople, D. P. Santry, and G. A. Segal, *J. Chem. Phys.*, 43, S129 (1965).

[29] J. A. Pople and G. A. Segal, *J. Chem. Phys.*, 43, S136 (1965).

[30] J. A. Pople and G. A. Segal, *J. Chem. Phys.*, 44, 3289 (1966).

[31] C. C. J. Roothaan, *J. Chem. Phys.*, 19, 1445 (1951).

[32] P. O. Löwdin, *J. Chem. Phys.*, 18, 365 (1950).

[33] G. A. Segal, *J. Chem, Phys.*, 47, 1876 (1967).

[34] J. M. Sichel and M. A. Whitehead, *Theoret. Chim. Acta. (Berl.)*, 7, 32 (1967).

[35] J. M. Sichel and M. A. Whitehead, *Theoret. Chim. Acta. (Berl.)*, 11, 220 (1968).

[36] J. M. Sichel and M. A. Whitehead, *Theoret. Chim. Acta. (Berl.)*, 11, 239 (1968).

[37] J. Del Bene and H. H. Jaffé, *J. Chem. Phys.*, 44, 759 (1966).

[38] R. Pariser and R. G. Parr, *J. Chem. Phys.*, 21, 767 (1953).

[39] J. Del Bene and H. H. Jaffé, *J. Chem. Phys.*, 48, 4050 (1968).

[40] J. Del Bene and H. H. Jaffé, *J. Chem. Phys.*, 50, 563 (1969).

[41] K. B. Wiberg, *J. Am. Chem. Soc.*, 90, 59 (1968).

[42] D. P. Santry and G. A. Segal, *J. Chem. Phys.*, 47, 158 (1967).

[43] R. N. Dixon, *Mol. Phys.*, 12, 83 (1967).

[44] J. A. Pople, D. L. Beveridge, and P. A. Dobosh, *J. Chem. Phys.*, 47, 2026 (1967).

[45] N. C. Baird and M. J. S. Dewar, *J. Chem. Phys.*, 50, 1262 (1969).

[46] N. C. Baird, M. J. S. Dewar, and R. Sustmann, *J. Chem. Phys.*, 50, 1275 (1969).

[47] M. S. Gordon and J. A. Pople, *J. Chem. Phys.*, 49, 4643 (1968).

[48] H. Fischer and H. Kollmar, *Theoret. Chim. Acta. (Berl.)*, 13, 213 (1969).

[49] S. Weiss and G. E. Leroi, *J. Chem. Phys.*, 48, 962 (1968).

[50] J. R. Hoyland, *J. Chem. Phys.*, 49, 1908 (1968).

[51] J. R. Hoyland, unpublished results.

[52] K. Kuchitsu, *Bull. Chem. Soc. Japan*, 32, 748 (1959).

[53] G. J. Szasz, N. Sheppard, and D. H. Rank, *J. Chem. Phys.*, 16, 704 (1948).

[54] K. S. Pitzer, *J. Chem. Phys.*, 8, 711 (1940).

[55] K. Ito, *J. Am. Chem. Soc.*, 75, 2430 (1953).

[56] J. E. Piercy and M. G. S. Rao, *J. Chem. Phys.*, 46, 3951 (1967).

[57] J. R. Hoyland, *J. Chem. Phys.*, 49, 2563 (1968).

[58] W. C. Herndon, J. Feuer, and L. H. Hall, *Tetrahedron Letters*, 2625 (1968).

[59] D. L. Bernitt, K. O. Hartman, and I. C. Hisatsune, *J. Chem. Phys.*, 42, 3553 (1965).

[60] R. G. Lerner, B. P. Dailey, and J. P. Friend, *J. Chem. Phys.*, 26, 680 (1957).

[61] L. B. Kier, *Tetrahedron Letters*, 1233 (1967).

[62] L. B. Kier, *Molec. Pharmacol.*, 3, 487 (1967).

[63] L. B. Kier, *Molec. Pharmacol.*, 4, 70 (1968).

[64] L. B. Kier, *J. Med. Chem.*, 11, 441 (1968).

[65] L. B. Kier, *J. Pharm. Sci.*, 57, 1188 (1968).

[66] L. B. Kier, *J. Med. Chem.*, 11, 915 (1968).

[67] L. B. Kier, *J. Pharmacol. Exp. Ther.*, 164, 75 (1968).

[68] L. B. Kier and M. W. Whitehouse, *J. Pharm. Pharmac.*, 20, 793 (1968).

[69] L. B. Kier, *J. Pharm. Pharmac.*, 21, 93 (1969).

[70] L. B. Kier and J. M. George, *Theoret. Chim. Acta. (Berl.)*, In Press.

[71] F. Jordan and B. Pullman, *Theoret. Chim. Acta. (Berl.)*, 10, 423 (1968).

[72] N. Cameron and S. C. Nyburg, *Theoret. Chim. Acta. (Berl.)*, 13, 162 (1969).

[73] E. Adam, M. P. Gordon, and L. H. Jensen, *Chem. Comm.*, 1019 (1968).

[74] F. Jordan and B. Pullman, *Theoret. Chim. Acta. (Berl.)*, 9, 242 (1968).

[75] W. Giordano, J. R. Hamann, J. L. Harkins, and J. J. Kaufman, *Mol. Pharmacol.*, 3, 307 (1967).

[76] H. B. Neely, *J. Med. Chem.*, 12, 16 (1969).

[77] B. Tinland, *Theoret. Chim. Acta. (Berl.)*, 11, 452 (1968).

[78] R. S. Mulliken, *J. Chem. Phys.*, 23, 1833, 1841 (1955).

[79] J. A. Pople and M. Gordon, *J. Am. Chem. Soc.*, 89, 4253 (1967).

[80] J. M. Sichel and M. A. Whitehead, *Theoret. Chim. Acta. (Berl.)*, 11, 254 (1968).

[81] A. S. N. Murthy and C. N. R. Rao, *Chem. Phys. Letters*, 2, 123 (1968).

[82] G. C. Pimentel and A. L. McClellan, *The Hydrogen Bond*, W. H. Freeman and Company, San Francisco, (1960).

[83] J. R. Hoyland and L. B. Kier, *Theoret. Chim. Acta. (Berl.)*, In Press.

[84] K. Morokuma and L. Pedersen, *J. Chem. Phys.*, 48, 2275 (1968).

[85] J. H. Simons and J. H. Hildebrand, *J. Am. Chem. Soc.*, 46, 2183 (1924).

[86] S. H. Bauer, J. Y. Beach, and J. H. Simons, *J. Am. Chem. Soc.*, 61, 19 (1939).

[87] A. S. N. Murthy, R. E. Davis, and C. N. R. Rao, *Theoret. Chim. Acta. (Berl.)*, 13, 81 (1969).

[88] L. Pauling and L. O. Brockway, *Proc. Natl. Acad. Sci. U.S.*, 20, 336 (1934).

[89] A. Pullman and H. Berthod, *Theoret. Chim. Acta. (Berl.)*, 10, 461 (1968).

[90] W. Adam and A. Grimison, *Tetrahedron*, 21, 3417 (1965).

[91] W. Adam and A. Grimison, *Tetrahedron*, 22, 835 (1966).

[92] R. B. Hermann, *Int. J. Quantum Chem.*, 2, 165 (1968).

MOLECULAR ORBITAL CONSIDERATION OF AMINO ACID CONFORMATION

by

Lemont B. Kier*

and

Jack M. George**

I. INTRODUCTION

The shape of a polypeptide molecule in aqueous solution is generally recognized as being governed by the conformational preference of the individual amino acid residues, the interaction of side chains, inter-residue hydrogen bonds, and solvent-polypeptide interactions. It has been suggested that the short-range interactions, i.e., the individual residue conformations may dominate polypeptide conformational preference as a result of the balancing of the other effects [1].

The influence of short-range interactions on polypeptide conformations has recently been examined in some detail by Scheraga [2]. The study was made using peptide geometries calculated by a summation of energy components such as nonbonded interactions, barriers to internal rotation, dipole-dipole interactions, and hydrogen bonding [3]. These calculated geometries were compared with geometries of the same peptide as found in a polypeptide of known structure. It was found that the predicted geometries correlated with the ability of the peptide to influence the helicity of the experimentally determined structure.

Further, it was reported that the conformation of the backbone of a particular peptide was essentially the same regardless of the nature of the side chain on adjacent residues in the calculated model [2]. Thus the conformation of a peptide may be significantly independent of interactions with neighboring side chains.

---

* Columbus Laboratories, Battelle Memorial Institute, Columbus, Ohio.

** College of Medicine, Ohio State University, Columbus, Ohio.

The study supports the view that the short-range interaction of the side chain with the backbone in the same peptide is the dominant factor in determining the conformation of that peptide.

If this were the case, then it could conceivably be possible to determine the conformation of segments of the polypeptide, say the individual amino acid residues, and to assemble these into the correct order to obtain a rough approximation of the polypeptide geometry. The crudeness of this approximation must be stressed, particularly for large polypeptides, where nonbonded interactions across chain segments and large entropy effects could be quite influential on the final geometry. The value in such an operational hypothesis would be in the use of such an approximation of the conformation of a small polypeptide as a starting point for further refinement.

This intriguing possibility has prompted us to pursue a course of study in which we seek to predict conformations of amino acid residues with the hope that the proper assemblage of these residues may result in a structure which has some significance as far as the peptide conformation.

II. METHODS

Theoretical predictions of amino acid conformational preference have centered around the minimization of a total energy obtained as a summation of the weighted contributions of several components [3-6]. The energy components considered have been barriers to internal rotation, nonbonded interactions, dipole-dipole interactions, and hydrogen bonding. These calculations have frequently been successful in correlating with experimental peptide structures.

Quantum mechanics effects a unification of these classical energy components into a single molecular energy which varies as a function of geometry. A simple varient of this has been introduced by Hoffmann and is known as extended Hückel theory [7]. The method is based on a one-electron Hamiltonian but apparently the matrix elements are a good approximation of more sophisticated calculations, since the conformations predicted frequently mirror physical experience. Hoyland has shown that extended Hückel theory leads generally to good approximations of equilibrium conformations, and that the method is superior, in this respect, to CNDO-type methods [8]. It is not possible to dissect the calculated total energy into recognizable components but the behavior of this energy indicates that these components must be present. This is evident from the appearance of calculated rotational barriers, the energy increase from the proximity of nonbonded groups, the presence of electronic effects as evidenced by the planarity calculated for amide groups and the good approximation of the hydrogen bond potential.

Extended Hückel theory develops from the L.C.A.O. approximation

$$\Psi_i = \Sigma_j C_{ij} \Phi_j$$

where Ψ_i is the molecular orbital and Φ_j the atomic orbitals. The C's are the appropriate coefficients. Upon minimization, a set of equations is generated

$$\Sigma_j (H_{ij} - ES_{ij}) C_j = 0$$

treating all of the valence electrons of each atom, i.e., the 2s and 2p electrons of carbon. H_{ii} is the diagonal matrix element and is taken to be the value of the valence state ionization potential. All off-diagonal Hamiltonian matrix elements H_{ij} are considered and are calculated

$$H_{ij} = K \frac{H_{ii} + H_{jj}}{2} S_{ij}$$

with $K = 1.75$. All overlap integrals, S_{ij} are computed, using the appropriate Slater exponents and coordinates of each atom. The parameters used for the valence state ionization potentials are H (1s) = -13.6 eV; C (2s) = -21.4 eV; C (2p) = -11.4 eV; N (2s) = -26.0 eV; N (2p) = -13.4 eV; O (2s) = -35.3 eV; O (2p) = -17.76 eV.

The application of this method to the prediction of the preferred conformation of relatively small drug molecules has occupied our attention for several years [9]. Over the past two years we have been studying the conformations predicted by extended Hückel theory for amino acids in peptide form. A preliminary report of some of these findings has recently been published [10]. Hoffmann and Imamura have also recently published some results of extended Hückel theory calculations on two amino acid residues [11].

Our calculations have been made on model compounds simulating the immediate environment of the amino acid in a nonterminal position. The model calculated in each case has been the N-acetyl amide.

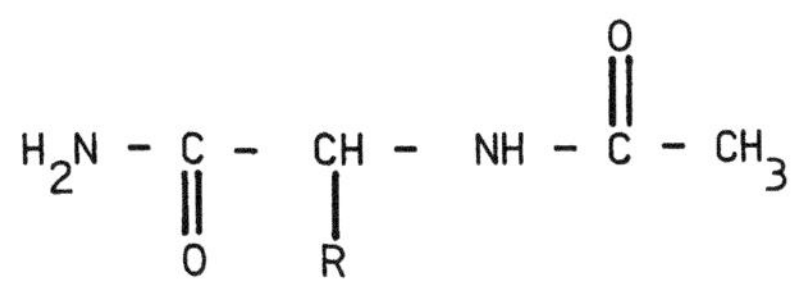

The neglect of more remote atoms in our model is, of course, the hypothesis we described earlier, but this can also be supported on quantum mechanical grounds [12] and has served as a basis for our treatment of some large molecules.

A number of assumptions were necessary to bring the calculations into manageable proportions. It was assumed that the amide groups were planar and trans substituted. The acetyl methyl group was held constant with one hydrogen atom eclipsing the carbonyl group. In the case of the glycine model then there are only two rotors which need be considered and a complete two-dimensional energy contour map can be calculated. The same is true for alanine if it is assumed that the side chain methyl group staggers nearest neighbor groups.

In the case of the other amino acids, however, there is at least one more single bond rotation possible in the side chain and frequently more than one. The number of computations necessary to generate a complete 3- or 4-dimensional contour map would make such an effort impracticable if it were not for some simplifying features which can be employed.

It is possible to eliminate regions in a contour map from consideration as containing a minimum energy conformation, by the judicious application of intuition. Those regions where there is pronounced nonbonded interaction of atoms and groups will be regions of high energy. As these groups approach each other, the repulsion energies will increase as a function of distance. Therefore, ranges of rotational angles can be excluded from the possibility of containing an energy minima. This intuition can be assisted by employing a scale model of the molecule under study.

The situation is well illustrated by correlating this intuition with the energy levels calculated and displayed in a two-dimensional map, see Figure 1.

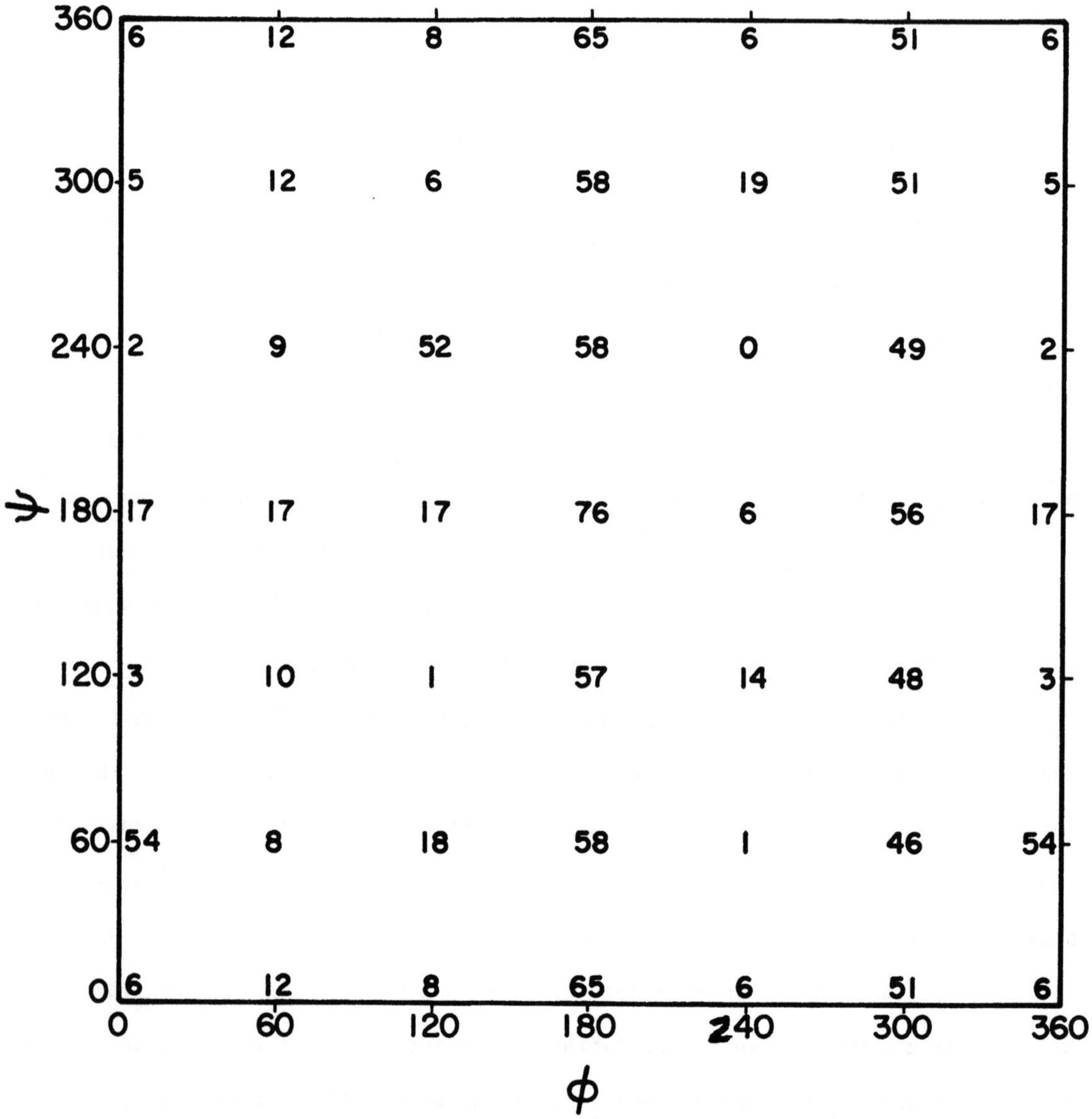

FIGURE 1. Two dimensional plot of Φ, Ψ angles for alanine showing relative calculated energies (kcal) above the minimum.

In this case, we have performed a series of calculations on N-acetyl alanine amide. The convention for designating the angles is that proposed by Edsall [13], Figure 2.

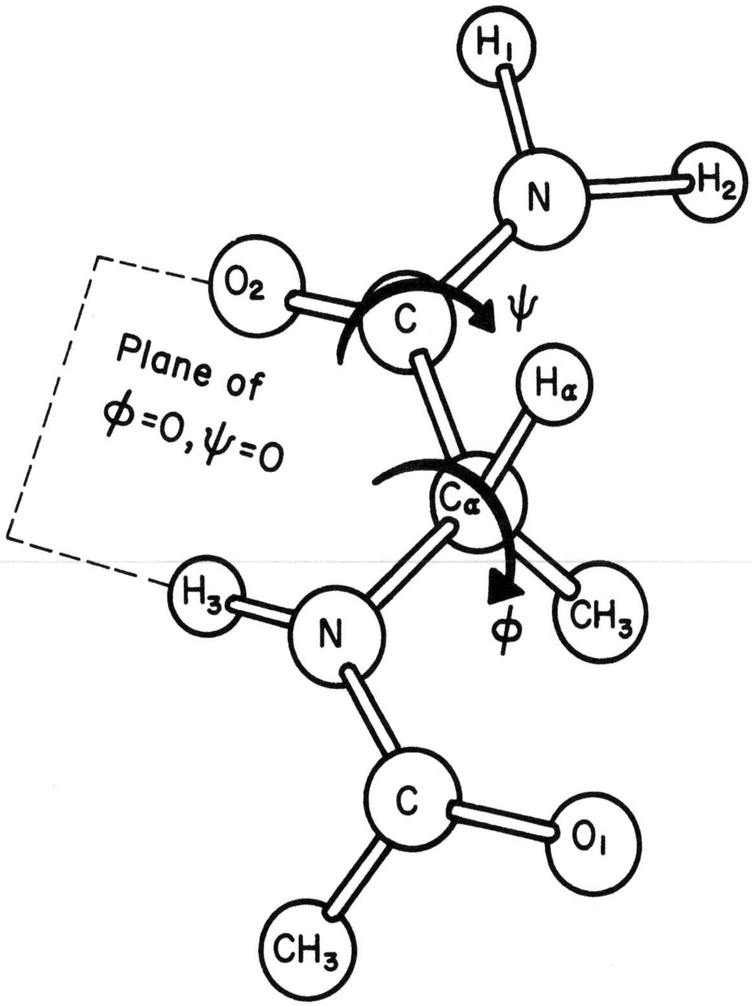

FIGURE 2. N-acetyl alanine amide at $\Phi = 0^\circ$, $\Psi = 0^\circ$. Ψ is the clockwise angle of rotation of the CO group and Φ is the clockwise angle of rotation of the CHR group [13].

From an inspection of the scale model of this compound, it is apparent that as we hold $\Phi = 0^\circ$ and increase Ψ, the amide hydrogen H_2 approaches the side chain methyl and is closest at $\Psi = 60^\circ$. On the contour map our prediction of high energy at $\Phi = 0^\circ$, $\Psi = 60^\circ$ is borne out. The interaction of amide hydrogens H_2 and H_3 is predicted at $\Phi = 0^\circ$, $\Psi = 180^\circ$, which is substantiated by the high energy calculated at this point of the map. With $\Phi = 180^\circ$, $\Psi = 0^\circ$ to 360°, a substantial amount of interaction would be predicted due to oxygen O_1 interacting with the methyl group, O_2, and the α hydrogen. On the map this is reflected as a high-energy ridge at $\Phi = 180^\circ$ and $\Psi = 0^\circ - 360^\circ$. Similarly for $\Phi = 300^\circ$, $\Psi = 0^\circ$ to 360°, the O_1 oxygen would be quite close to the side chain, hence, all values of Ψ would give a high energy. In support of this, the map reveals another high-energy ridge at $\Phi = 300^\circ$ and $\Psi = 0^\circ - 360^\circ$.

It is thus possible to accumulate a volume of experience on these high-energy relationships based upon inspection of models and checking by calculation. This experience leads to an intuition which permits the exclusion of significant portions of an angle vs. energy profile map from consideration. This is true for molecules with added flexibility in the side chain as well.

We have employed this technique in greatly reducing the number of calculations performed on our model residue molecules. It must be emphasized that we have exercised considerable caution in this approach and have always calculated conformations in which there was any doubt.

In the angular regions near low calculated energies, the angular increments were refined to 30° to locate more accurately the energy minimum. Energy minima within 1 kcal or less of each other were considered as being significant contributions to an equilibrium and are reported as a range of angles for the predicted conformations. Bond lengths and angles were adopted from Pauling and Cory [14].

Using a statistical mechanical approach to calculate the allowed regions of a conformational map, Ramachandran has predicted that only 7.5 percent of the total area would be fully allowed [15]. This is consistent with our approach to the allowed regions.

III. RESULTS AND DISCUSSION

Glycine

The model compound used in the calculation of the glycine (peptide form) conformation was N-acetyl glycine amide, see Figure 3. The rotation of the

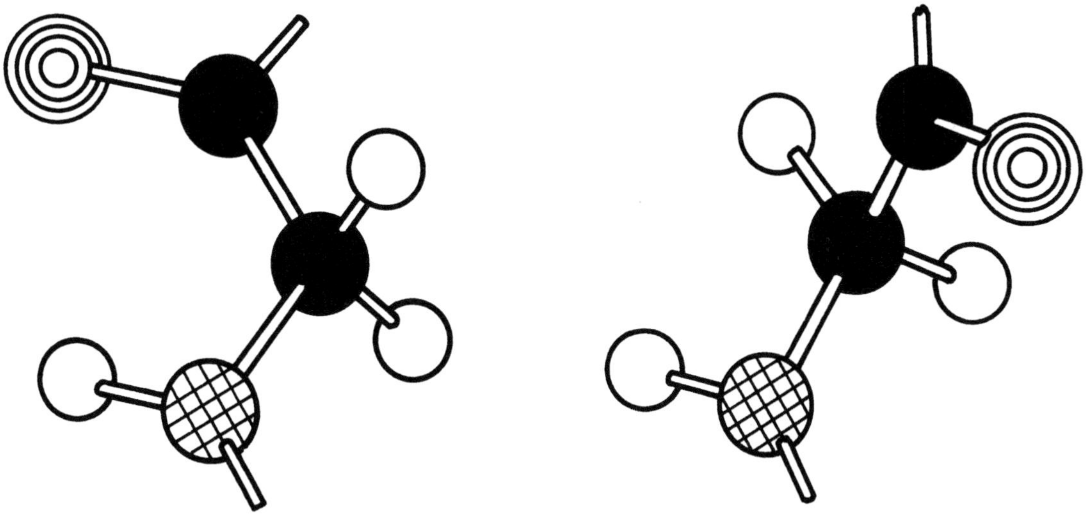

(a) (b)

FIGURE 3. (a) Calculated conformation of glycine residue at $\Phi = 0^\circ$, $\Psi = 0^\circ$; (b) calculated conformation for the same residue at $\Phi = 0^\circ$, $\Psi = 120^\circ$. ● = carbon, ◎ = oxygen, ◍ = nitrogen, ○ = hydrogen.

N-C bond, Φ, was calculated to be quite free for angles of $\Phi = 0^\circ$ to 120°, which from the symmetry of the molecule would also include $\Phi = 0^\circ$ to 240°. Throughout this two-thirds of a cycle for Φ, the value of Ψ at the minima was approximately 0°. Thus in the range $\Phi = 120^\circ$ to 240°, $\Psi = 0^\circ$, a barrier exists in excess of 1 kcal over the minimum energy. The source of this barrier, as suggested from the model, is very probably the interaction of the two carbonyl oxygen atoms.

A reasonable comparison with experimental conformations can be made with the poly-L-amino acids. Polyglycine is known to occur in two forms. Polyglycine I exists in the β form [16], which is a non-helical pleated sheet structure. This β form has been found to be an anti-parallel arrangement in which the individual residues would have a standard set of angles, $\Phi = 38^\circ$, $\Psi = 325^\circ$ [17], see Table I. The conformation designated by these angles is in good agreement with our calculated values, adopting the criterion suggested by Phillips [18] that residues within 40° of the standard Φ, Ψ values be considered as describing the particular structural category.

TABLE 1. STANDARD Φ, Ψ VALUES FOR RESIDUE STRUCTURAL TYPES [17]

Structural Type	Φ	Ψ
Fully extended chain	0°	0°
Rα helix	132°	123°
Lα helix	228°	237°
Parallel pleated sheet	61°	293°
Antiparallel pleated sheet	38°	325°
Polyglycine II	100°	330°
Collagen	120°	340°

Polyglycine II has a conformation resembling the triple helical fold in collagen [19], namely $\Phi = 100^\circ$, $\Psi = 330^\circ$. This again is in satisfactory agreement with the calculated predictions.

A third comparison can be made with an infrared study of the conformation of the two crystalline forms of N-acetylglycine-N-methylamide [20]. Of the conformations found, $\Phi = 120^\circ$, $\Psi = 0^\circ$ and $\Phi = 120^\circ$, $\Psi = 180^\circ$, the former is in agreement with the theoretical calculations.

Alanine

The two dimensional map for the alanine model, N-acetyl alanine amide, is shown in Figure 1. The high energy areas have been discussed in the previous section. The energy minimum at $\Phi = 240^\circ$, $\Psi = 240^\circ$ appears to be unique, being at least 1 kcal below low energy points at $\Phi = 120^\circ$, $\Psi = 120^\circ$ and $\Phi = 240^\circ$, $\Psi = 60^\circ$. The conformation at the minimum is shown in Figure 4. The two carbonyl bonds in this conformation are virtually parallel. The side chain conformation is designated $\chi_1 = 60^\circ$ using the convention of Edsall [13].

Currently, the available experimental studies on alanine indicate that the residue can assume either an antiparallel pleated sheet [21] or an α-helix [22].

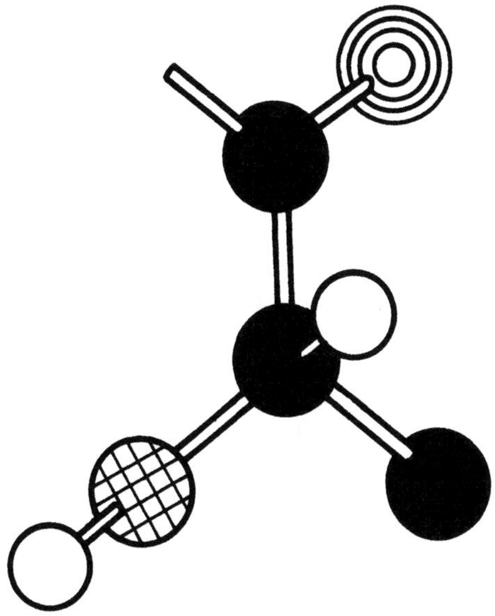

FIGURE 4. Conformation of alanine residue at calculated energy minimum $\Phi = 240^\circ$, $\Psi = 240^\circ$.

The chirality of the α-helix is right handed. Our minimum energy calculation indicates a preference for a left-handed α-helix with the right-handed α-helix, $\Phi = 120^\circ$, $\Psi = 120^\circ$, lying 1 kcal above the minimum.

Phenylalanine

This first peptide of a more complex nature in our studies was handled according to the tenents laid down in the discussion under methods. The backbone conformation was found to have a minimum energy at $\Phi = 30^\circ$, $\Psi = 330^\circ$, see Figure 5. It is evident from a consideration of scale models that most values of Ψ would be denied, except those near 0°, due to the interaction of the ring and the benzyl hydrogens with the carbonyl and N-hydrogens of the Ψ rotor. The same restrictions are evident on the Φ angle, due to interactions of the carbonyl group and the N-hydrogen. In the minimum energy conformation, the carbonyl and N-H bonds of the peptide residue are about parallel. The phenyl ring lies over and equidistant between these two bonds. The side chain designation is thus $X_1 = 60^\circ$, $X_2 = 90^\circ$.

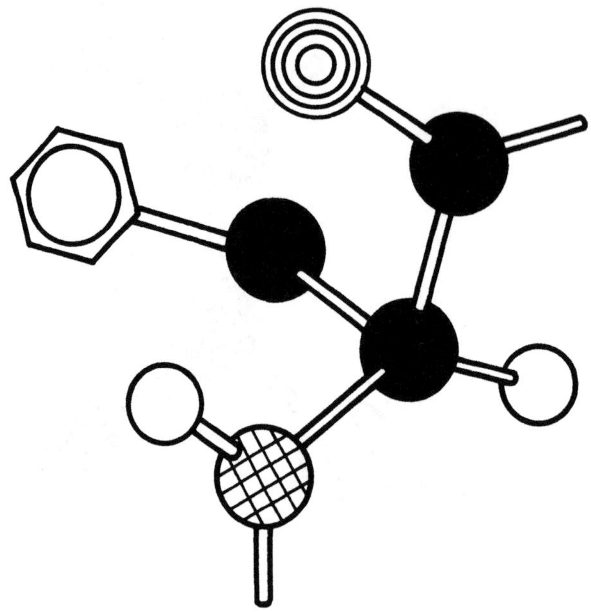

FIGURE 5. Conformation of phenylalanine residue at calculated energy minimum $\Phi = 30^\circ$, $\Psi = 330^\circ$.

Experimental studies on poly-L-phenylalanine indicate that the molecule can assume a right-handed α-helix [23]. A parallel chain pleated sheet conformation has been reported for the crystal of the tripeptide glycyl-L-phenylanalylglycine [24]. The calculated conformation of the phenylalanine model is within the range of this latter finding, which would have values near $\Phi = 61^\circ$, $\Psi = 293^\circ$ (see Table 1), although the calculations are certainly closer to antiparallel pleated sheet standard angles of $\Phi = 38^\circ$, $\Psi = 325^\circ$.

Proline

The model compound, N-acetyl proline amide was found to have a lower energy when the N-acetyl group was positioned trans; that is, the carbonyl group is directed toward the carboxamide group on the α carbon atom, see Figure 6. The carboxamide group was found to prefer an angle of $\Psi = 330^\circ$ at the energy minimum. The calculated energy minimum coordinates are thus $\Phi = 120^\circ$, $\Psi = 330^\circ$.

Poly-L-proline is known to exist in two forms designated I and II. Form I has the amide group in the cis position, while form II is in the trans position, the latter arrangement agreeing with our calculations. Conformation studies on the crystals of two different tripeptides with proline as the central residue indicate a conformation for proline in good agreement with our calculations [25,26]. The conformation of proline in poly-L-proline leads to an ordered chain which rotates about its axis once every three residues [27].

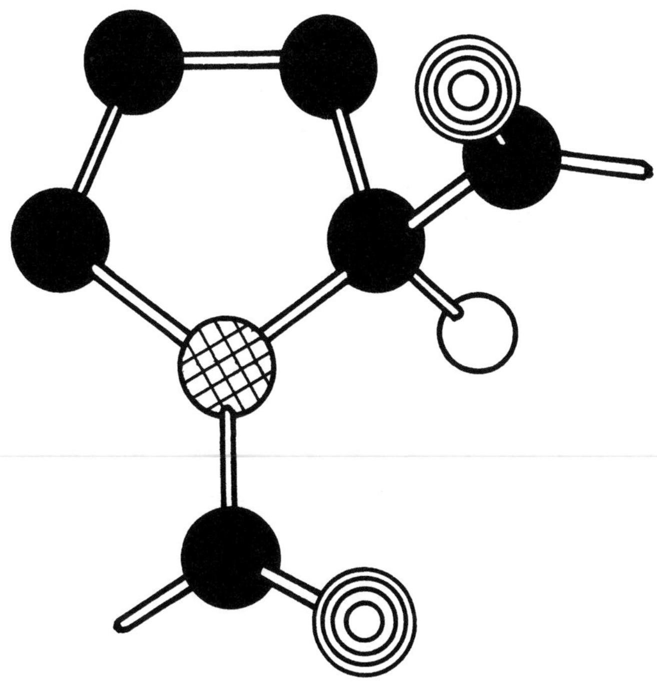

FIGURE 6. Conformation of N-acetyl proline residue at calculated energy minimum $\Phi = 120°$, $\Psi = 330°$ with N-acetyl group trans.

Serine

The serine model compound, N-acetyl serine amide was calculated to have an energy minimum at $\Phi = 60°$ to $120°$, and $\Psi = 330°$. The side chain C-O bond is trans to the C-H bond, see Figure 7. The side chain is thus designated $\chi_1 = 60°$, $\chi_2 = 0°$.

A study of poly-L-serine using optical rotatory dispersion and infrared measurements indicated that it is in the β form [28]. The calculated energy minimum would fit well with either the parallel chain pleated sheet ($\Phi = 61°$, $\Psi = 293°$), or the antiparallel pleated sheet ($\Phi = 38°$, $\Psi = 325°$).

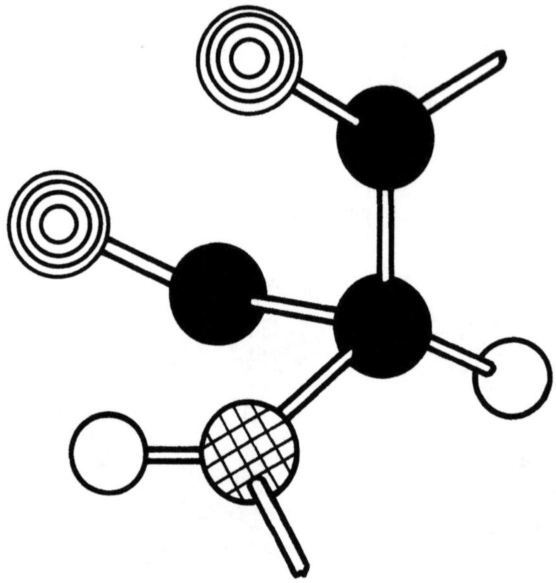

FIGURE 7. Conformation of serine residue at calculated energy minimum $\Phi = 90^\circ$, $\Psi = 330^\circ$.

Leucine

The leucine model compound N-acetyl leucine amide was calculated to have a minimum energy conformation at $\Phi = 60^\circ$, $\Psi = 0^\circ$, Figure 8. In the side chain, the C_β-C_γ bond was found to be trans to the C-C_α bond of the backbone. The methyl groups on the C_γ atom are symmetrically disposed around the C, C_α, C_β, C_γ plane. The side chain designation is $\chi_1 = 60^\circ$, $\chi_{3,1} = 240^\circ$, $\chi_{3,2} = 120^\circ$.

Some experimental data on leucine ir peptide form is available from a study of Gramicidin-S using nuclear magnetic resonance [29]. The conformation of leucine in Gramicidin-S was found to be $\Phi = 30^\circ$, $\Psi = 0^\circ$, and while there may be constraints on leucine due to the cyclic nature of Gramicidin-S, it is noteworthy that the observed conformation agrees with the calculated energy minimum at Ψ and is within 30° at Φ. Poly-L-leucine has also been reported to be in an α-helix in 100 percent dichloroacetic acid [30].

Isoleucine

The model compound N-acetyl isoleucine amide was calculated to have an energy minimum at $\Phi = 60^\circ$ to 90°, $\Psi = 300^\circ$, see Figure 9. The three-carbon

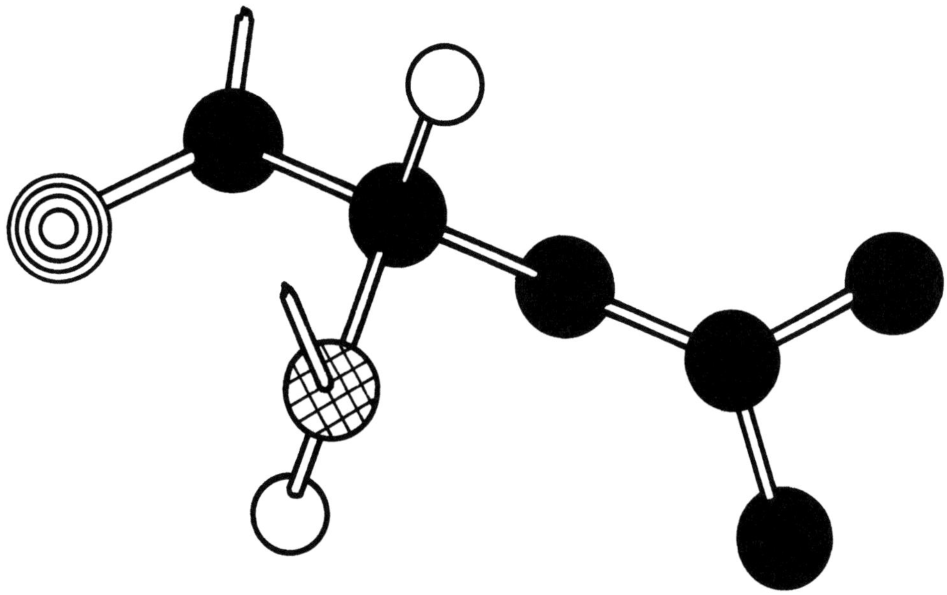

FIGURE 8. Conformation of leucine residue at calculated energy minimum $\Phi = 60^{\circ}$, $\Psi = 0^{\circ}$.

fragment of the side chain is in a staggered conformation relative to the C-C_{α} bond. The side chain is designated $X_1 = 300^{\circ}$, $X_{2,1} = 180^{\circ}$. The two carbonyl groups and the two N-H bonds are all parallel.

Studies on poly-L-isoleucine using optical rotatary dispersion (ORD) have shown that this polymer exists in the β-conformation [31]. This finding is in agreement with our calculations.

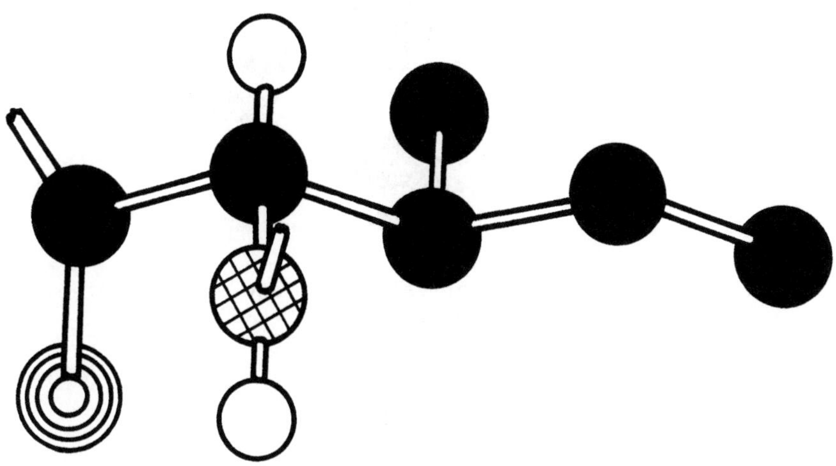

FIGURE 9. Conformation of isoleucine residue at calculated energy minimum $\Phi = 60^{\circ}$, $\Psi = 300^{\circ}$.

Valine

The model compound, N-acetyl valine amide was calculated to exist in a conformation of $\Phi = 60^\circ$ to 90°, $\Psi = 300^\circ$, see Figure 10. A side chain methyl group is calculated to be trans relative to $N\text{-}C_\alpha$ bond, and the other methyl group is calculated to be trans to the $C\text{-}C_\alpha$ bond. The side chain designation is $\chi_1 = 300^\circ$. The two carbonyl groups and the two N-H bonds are all parallel.

Poly-L-valine has been studied in solution using optical rotatory dispersion and circular dichroism. The evidence suggests that this polypeptide can exist as either a right-handed α-helix or in the β conformation [32]. The conformation in the β structure, particularly the parallel chain pleated sheet ($\Phi = 61^\circ$, $\Psi = 293^\circ$) fits well with the calculated energy minimum.

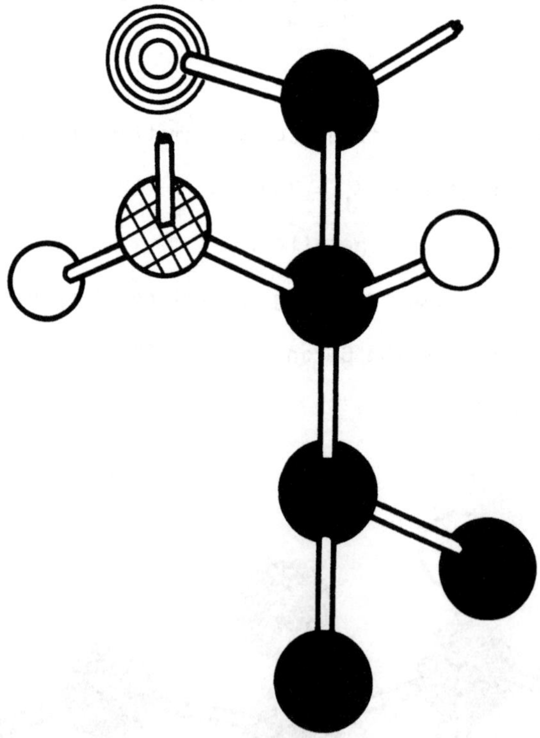

FIGURE 10. Conformation of valine residue at calculated energy minimum $\Phi = 90^\circ$, $\Psi = 300^\circ$.

Arginine

For the purposes of assembling the calculated model peptides into the sequence found in the polypeptide bradykinin, it is necessary to calculate the conformation of arginine as an N-terminal and as a C-terminal residue, as is found in bradykinin.

The arginine calculations were simplified by adopting results calculated for a model of the side chain, namely the propyl guanidinium ion, Figure 11. This fragment was found to prefer an all-trans conformation with the charged guanidinium group planer. This is in agreement with four studies of different arginine derivatives [33]. Assuming that the guanidinium group is sufficiently far removed from the arginine backbone in this all-trans side chain conformation (>6Å separates the guanidine central carbon atom from the C_α of the backbone), it was assumed that its effect on the backbone conformation would be negligible. The main influence of the side chain atoms on the backbone conformation were assumed to come from the C_β and C_γ of the side chain in subsequent calculations.

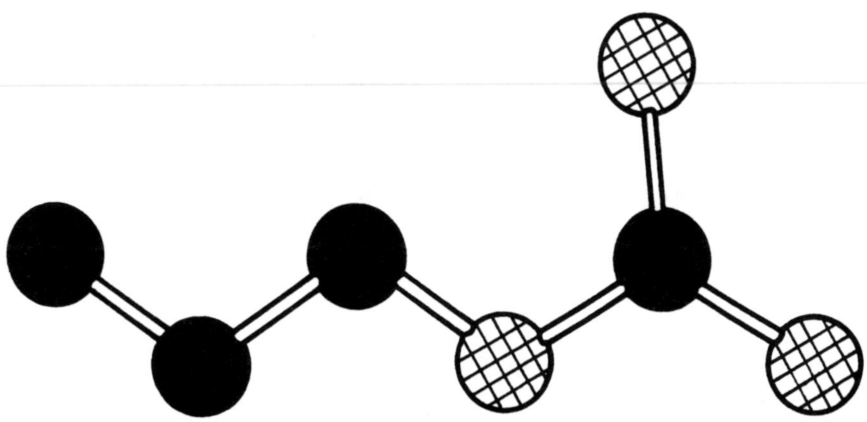

FIGURE 11. Conformation calculated for propylguanidinium model for the arginine side chain.

Arginine N-terminal

The model compound used for the N-terminal arginine residue was 2-carboxamido-propylammonium. The side chain was treated using the same assumptions just described.

In the minimum energy calculation, the Ψ angle is in the range of 330° to 0°, see Figure 12. The side chain is all trans to the $C-C_\alpha$ bond of the backbone. The side chain designation is thus $\chi_1 = 300°$, $\chi_2 = 180°$, $\chi_3 = 180°$, $\chi_4 = 180°$, $\chi_5 = 180°$, $\chi_{61} = 0°$.

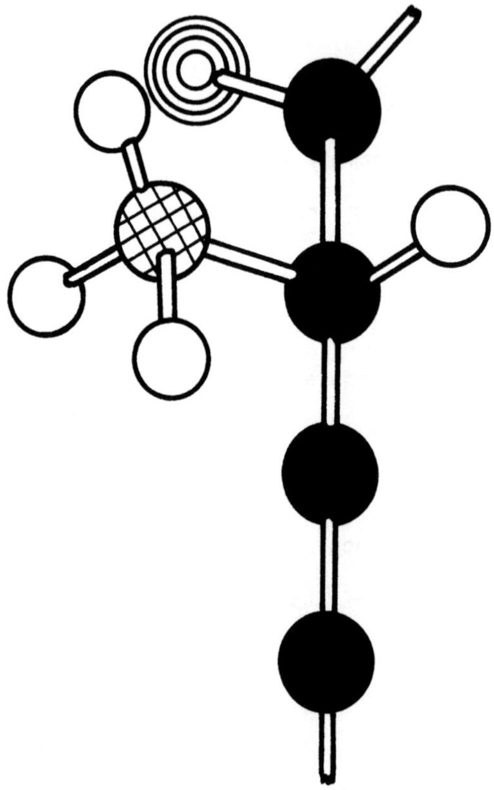

FIGURE 12. Conformation of the N-terminal arginine residue model at calculated energy minimum $\Psi = 330^\circ$.

Arginine C-terminal

The model used for this calculation was N-acetyl homo alanine carboxylate. The energy minimum was found for the angles $\Phi = 60^\circ$, $\Psi = 0^\circ$ with the side chain trans to the C-C_α bond, see Figure 13. The side chain designation is $\chi_1 = 60^\circ$, $\chi_2 = 180^\circ$, $\chi_3 = 180^\circ$, $\chi_4 = 180^\circ$, $\chi_5 = 180^\circ$, $\chi_{61} = 0^\circ$.

An examination of Table 2 reveals agreement between the calculation of the conformation of a model compound and some experimental data in all cases but alanine. The calculations do not predict all experimental conformations nor is it possible to decide whether the calculations are more relevant to crystal or solution experimental conditions. This relevance is probably an imponderable at this time, although it has been suggested that quantum mechanical calculated conformations are more closely related to dilute solution phenomena [34].

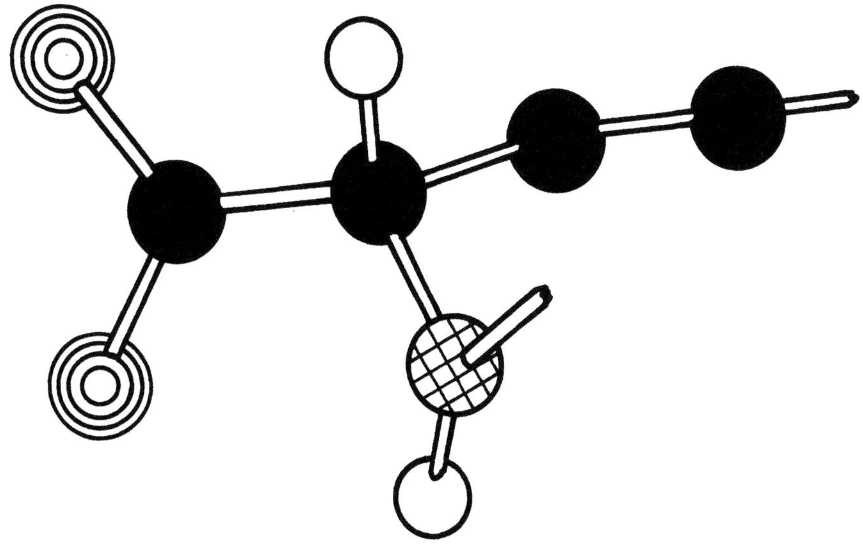

FIGURE 13. Conformation of the C-terminal arginine residue model at calculated energy minimum $\Phi = 60^\circ$, $\Psi = 0^\circ$.

It is interesting to note that practically all of the calculations predict a minimum energy for a β structure for the amino acid residues as if they were part of a homogeneous polymer. The prevalence of this structure among the residues calculated suggests that, in the cases where the residues are known experimentally to form an α-helix, additional stabilizing factors are present which are not accounted for in the calculations. These factors would include hydrogen bonding, side chain interactions, or solvent effects. All of the residues shown in Table 2 are known experimentally to form a β structure (except proline). The question as to whether the β structure is energetically preferred over the α-helix when both are known to exist experimentally, cannot be answered at this time.

It should certainly be noted that the calculations could be further refined using smaller angular increments. Further, the assumption of planarity of the amide bond is not strictly valid. Deviations of a few degrees have been noted experimentally. Nevertheless, we feel that the general agreement of the calculations with conformations obtainable experimentally indicates that the calculations give an approximation of a conformation which is achieveable in reality.

TABLE 2. SUMMARY OF CALCULATED AND EXPERIMENTAL Φ, Ψ ANGLES OF RESIDUES

Residue	Calculated (°) Φ	Ψ	Experimental Conformations (°) Structural Type	Φ, Ψ[(a)]
Glycine	0-120,	0	I β-antiparallel pleated sheet	38, 325
			II Collagen-like	100, 330
Alanine	240,	240	Right-handed α-helix	132, 123
			β-antiparallel pleated sheet	41, 315
Phenylalanine	30,	330	Right-handed α-helix	132, 123
			β parallel pleated sheet	61, 293
Proline	120,	330	I	300, 300
			II	120, 330
Serine	60-120,	330	β parallel pleated sheet	61, 293
Leucine	60,	0	In Gramicidin	30, 0
			Right-handed α-helix	132, 123
Isoleucine	60-90,	300	β-form	38-61, 293-325
Valine	60-90,	300	β-form	38-61, 293-325
			Right-handed α-helix	132, 123

(a) Angles quoted are from standard values, Table 1, when specific values are not reported.

Bradykinin

If the calculated conformations of the residues have any relationship to reality, and if our operational hypothesis of the relative independence of the residue conformations from neighboring residue influence, is, in any measure valid, it should be possible to assemble the calculated residues into a polypeptide order and obtain thereby an approximation of that polypeptide conformation.

Bradykinin was chosen for this experiment because of its biological importance and because it is a short, linear polypeptide in which problems of doubling back of segments would be minimized. The peptide sequence is

$$H_3N\text{-Arg-Pro-Pro-Gly-Phe-Ser-Pro-Phe-Arg-}CO_2.$$

The polypeptide was assembled from the residues in their calculated preferred conformations, see Figure 14. For simplicity in illustration, the lowest calculated energy conformation was chosen even when the minimum for some residues extended over a larger angle for the arbitrary 1 kcal range. Obviously, the calculated flexibility of glycine would permit a rotation of the first four residues through a 240° arc. Likewise, a 60° variation is calculated to be permitted at the serine.

It is interesting to note that the conformation shown in Figure 14 has no close interactions of side chains. This result falls out of the calculations of the individual residues without any *a priori* knowledge of where the adjacent residues are going to be in the assembled polypeptide.

We must emphasize that we do not claim to have necessarily calculated the conformation of bradykinin. Rather we have assembled the MO calculated residues, in their minimum energy conformation, into the same sequence as is found in bradykinin. The resulting structure passes one test of reasonableness in that there are no close interactions of side chains or side chains with the backbone structure. The final test will come when this calculated structure can be compared with experimental evidence.

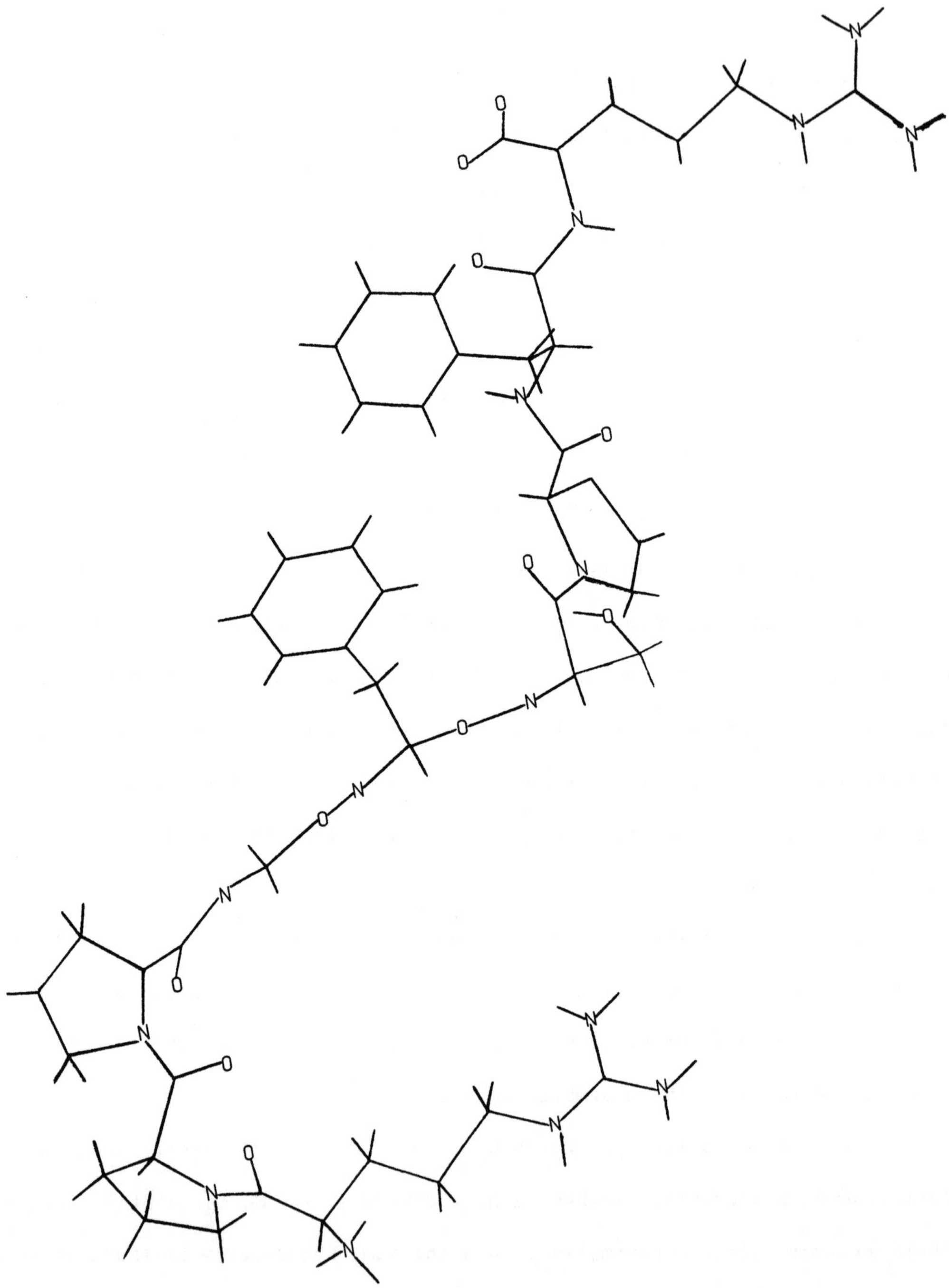

FIGURE 14. Conformation of the chain of residues corresponding to the amino acid sequence in bradykinin, from individual calculated residue conformations.

IV. ACKNOWLEDGMENTS

We wish to acknowledge the use of the computer facilities of Battelle Memorial Institute and the Ohio State University. This work was supported by National Institute of Health Grants GM-16312 and FR 5409. One of us (J.M.G.) is the recipient of a Public Health Service Research Career Development Award, Am 11519.

V. REFERENCES

[1] Flory, P. J., Chapter 14 in *Principles of Polymer Chemistry*, Cornell Univ. Press, Ithica, New York (1953).

[2] Kotelchuck, D., and Scheraga, H. A., *Proc. Nat. Acad. Sci. U. S.*, 61, 1163 (1968).

[3] Scott, R. A., and Scheraga, H. A., *J. Chem. Phys.*, 45, 2091 (1966).

[4] Ramachandran, G. N., Ramakrishnan, C., and Sasisekharan, V., *J. Mol. Biol.*, 7, 95 (1963).

[5] Brant, D. E., and Flory, P. J., *J. Am. Chem. Soc.*, 87, 663 (1965).

[6] DeSantis, P., Gilgio, E., Liquori, A. M., and Ripamonti, A., *J. Polym. Sci.*, 1, 1383 (1963).

[7] Hoffmann, R., *J. Chem. Phys.*, 39, 1397 (1963).

[8] Hoyland, J., this Symposium, Chapter 2.

[9] Kier, L. B., Chapter 2 in *Fundamental Concepts of Drug-Receptor Interaction*, edited by D. J. Triggle, Academic Press, New York (1969).

[10] Kier, L. B., and George, J. M., *Theoret. Chim. Acta*, 14, 258 (1969).

[11] Hoffmann, R., and Imamura, A., *Biopolymers*, 7, 207 (1969).

[12] Kier, L. B., *J. Med. Chem.*, 11, 441 (1968).

[13] Edsall, J., *Biopolymers*, 4, 121 (1966).

[14] Pauling, L., Corey, R., and Branson, H., *Proc. Nat. Acad. Sci. U. S.*, 37, 207 (1951).

[15] Ramachandran, G., and Sasiesekharan, V., *Adv. Prot. Chem.*, 23, 329 (1968).

[16] Bamford, C. H., Elliott, A., and Hanby, W. E., p. 445 in *Synthetic Polypeptides*, Academic Press, New York (1956).

[17] Edsall, J., Flory, P., Kendrew, J., Liquori, A., Nemethy, G., Ramachandran, G., and Scheraga, H., *J. Biol. Chem.*, 41, 1004 and 4167 (1966).

[18] Phillips, D. C., *Proc. Nat. Acad. Sci. U. S.*, 57, 484 (1967).

[19] Crick, F. H. C., and Rich, A., *Nature*, 176, 780 (1955).

[20] Kayama, Y., and Shimanouchi, T., *Biopolymers*, 6, 1037 (1968).

[21] Arnott, S., Dover, S., and Elliott, A., *J. Mol. Biol.*, 30, 201 (1967).

[22] Lotan, N., Berger, A., Katchalski, E., Ingwall, R., and Scheraga, H., *Biopolymers*, 4, 239 (1966).

[23] Sage, H., and Fassman, G., *Biochemistry*, 5, 286 (1966).

[24] Marsh, R., and Glusker, J., *Acta Cryst.*, 14, 1110 (1961).

[25] Leung, Y., and Marsh, R., *Acta Cryst.*, 11, 17 (1958).

[26] Fridrichsons, J., and Mathieson, A., *Acta Cryst.*, 15, 569 (1962).

[27] Cowan, P., and McGavin, S., *Nature*, 176, 501 (1955).

[28] Tooney, N., and Fassman, G., *J. Mol. Biol.*, 36, 355 (1968).

[29] Stern, A., Gibbons, W., and Craig, L. C., *Proc. Nat. Acad. Sci. U. S.*, 61, 734 (1968).

[30] Yang, J. T., amd Doty, P., *J. Am. Chem. Soc.*, 79, 761 (1957).

[31] Blout, E., and Shecter, E., *Biopolymers*, 1, 565 (1963).

[32] Epand, R. F., and Scheraga, H., *Biopolymers*, 6, 1551 (1968).

[33] Marsh, R., and Donohue, J., *Adv. in Protein Chem.*, 22, 252 (1967).

[34 Giordano, W., Hamann, J., Harkins, J., and Kaufman, J., *Mol. Pharmacol.*, 3, 307 (1967).

THE CORRELATION OF ELECTRONIC STRUCTURES OF INDOLE DERIVATIVES WITH THEIR BIOLOGICAL ACTIVITIES

by

Jack Peter Green*

and

Sungzong Kang*

I. INTRODUCTION

Much of our work to date has been focussed on indolealkylamines, and recently some calculations of hallucinogenic amphetamines have been made. Indoles were selected for several reasons. They have varied, potent, and important biological activities, and some, like 5-hydroxytryptamine (serotonin), are widely distributed in nature, including mammalian tissues. Many studies have been published quantitatively describing the actions of congeners on different

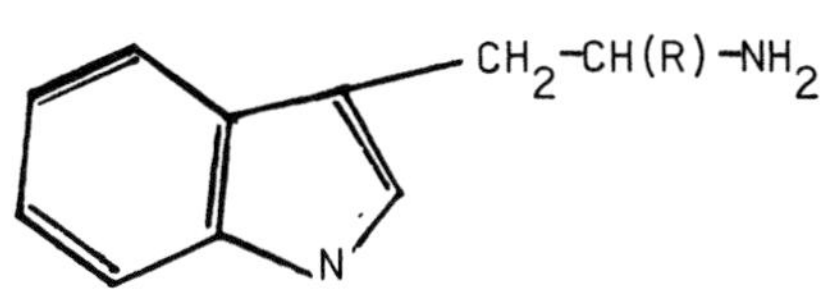

Indolealkylamine

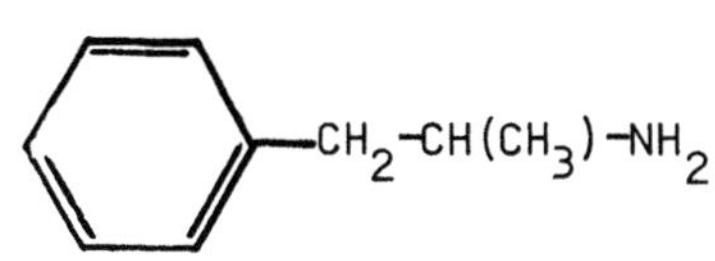

Amphetamine

*Department of Pharmacology, Mount Sinai School of Medicine, New York, New York

biological systems. Furthermore, enough information is available on the chemistry of indoles to test the reasonableness of the results of the calculations. In addition, being heterocycles and relatively large they typify many biochemicals and drugs, and as a planar ring system, they are more easily amenable to analysis. Finally, since molecular orbital methods have accounted for some of the chemical activities of indoles; it was hoped that a comparable approach could help to account for their biological activities. Amphetamines were studied for many of the same reasons including the fact that they have some of the same biological actions as do indoles and in some biological systems even act on the same receptors.

We selected four different biological systems for analysis, each representing increasing levels of complexity. First, indoleakylamines that had been studied as inhibitors of a soluble enzyme, 5-hydroxytryptophan decarboxylase [2]. Second, indolealkylamines that had been examined for their effects on the stomach strip of the rat suspended in an artificial medium in a closed system [3]. Third, indolealkylamines that were applied electrophoretically to the cat's lateral geniculate nucleus *in situ* [4]. Fourth, amphetamines that were examined for their hallucinogenic activity in man [5].

It would be expected that molecular orbital methods might be most successful with the least complicated system where the indoles are reacting in solution with, presumably, the active site of a soluble enzyme. In the second system, the effect of the indoles is attributable to a reaction with specific receptors in a complicated system containing a membrane barrier and many chemical components that are competing with the receptors for the indoles, including enzymes that catabolize the indoles. The pervasiveness of only one of these complications is clearly demonstrated in experiments showing that the relative activities of a congeneric series of indoles in contracting a muscle were different before and after inhibition of the catabolizing enzyme [3]. An additional complication is that the potency measured in this and similar systems may be composed of two independent variables, affinity and intrinsic activity [6].

The third system has all the complexities of the previous one in addition to others; for example, the tested substances can leave the open system. In the fourth system (a whole animal) the biological measurement, hallucinogenic activity, is not measured precisely. Even more important, the relative biological activity that is measured is the net result of a whole series of reactions between the tested compounds (*viz*, amphetamines) and biological sites. Some of the factors determining biological activity in these experiments are the rate of absorption of the drugs from the stomach, the extent of binding to plasma proteins and to tissues, the rate of catabolism by the liver and other organs, the rate of excretion by the kidney, the amount of drug that passes through the blood-brain barrier to enter the brain, and the amount that gets to the active site within the brain. There should be electronic correlates of each one of these determinants of biological activity, e.g. absorption through the stomach and passage into the brain are correlated with lipid solubility and hence often with ionization constant. Adsorption to plasma protein is an interaction that should have an electronic correlate(s) and so should the susceptibility of the amphetamines to enzymatic catabolism. In searching for the electronic correlate(s) of the hallucinogenic activity (or any other effect in the whole animal), we assume that the extent of the other interactions are about the same for each member of the congeneric series so that the relative potency as measured is close enough to truth. Thus, any correlation obtained in this fourth system is a net effect of many interactions, but since useful information about these interactions is not available for the amphetamines, we proceed with the assumption that the potency of the amphetamines in causing hallucinations is directly related to the gross effect that is measured.

Partial accounts of this work have appeared [7-9].

II. METHODS

Total valence electron calculations were carried out by the INDO method (Intermediate Neglect of Differential Overlap), devised by Pople, Beveridge and Dobosh [10]. We are grateful to Beveridge for providing the program and for advice during the course of this work. The INDO method gives good results in the calculation of dipole moments, molecular geometries, electron-nuclear hyperfine coupling constants, nuclear spin-spin coupling constants, and bending force constants [11-14].

We calculated charge density, frontier electron density, dipole moment, total energy and all energy levels.

For the Hückel method, the parameters of Pullman and Pullman [15] were used with the typographical corrections previously noted [16]. The nitrogen coulomb integral, which differs from that of Streitweiser, gave values of electron energy levels and electron distribution that correlate well with experimental findings on a series of anilines [17]. The π-frontier electron density (f^E) and superdelocalizability [(S^E), for an electron-donating reaction], were calculated as described [18]. These indexes, though based on a controversial theory, correlate well with chemical reactivities of many compounds [19].

Resonance constants were obtained from the table of Swain and Lupton [20].

All data were subjected to stepwise multiple regression analysis.

III. RESULTS

Inhibition of 5-hydroxytryptophan Decarboxylase by α-ethyltryptamines

The (weak) inhibitory activities on the decarboxylase [2] correlate with q_7 (charge at the 7-position) and S_7^E and S_2^E (Table 1), as calculated by the simple Hückel method. No electronic correlation could be made for monoamine oxidase inhibitory activity. The correlation between q_7 and S_7^E is not necessarily internal, for in another series of indoles in which comparable calculations were performed, charges and S^E did not consistently correlate [16]. Whether q_7, S_7^E or S_2^E is the meaningful correlate is impossible to say with any certainty. However, studies of the reactivities of indoles do not indicate that the 7-position is a site of attack of electrophilic species, whereas the 2-position is a preferred site for electrophilic attack.

The ambiguity and any inferences can be tested by designing laboratory experiments to see at which atomic sites the indoles interact with the enzyme. Another means of testing the inference and resolving the ambiguity is to synthesize and test compounds whose calculated electronic characteristics could permit one to infer which index or indexes matters.

TABLE 1. INHIBITORY ACTIVITY OF SOME α-ETHYLTRYPTAMINES ON 5-HYDROXYTRYPTOPHAN DECARBOXYLASE AND q_7, S_7^E, AND S_2^E CALCULATED BY THE SIMPLE HÜCKEL METHOD.

Derivative of α-ethyltryptamine	Inhibition, % at 10^{-2}M	q_7	S_7^E	S_2^E
6-NH_2	100	1.134	1.614	1.496
6-OCH_3	58	1.102	1.318	1.362
6-OH	58	1.100	1.296	1.352
1,2-$(CH_3)_2$	14	1.038	1.082	1.228
2-CH_3	13	1.039	1.030	1.228
5-OCH_3	7	1.034	1.078	1.242
2,7-$(CH_3)_2$	6	0.995	1.048	1.226
6-F	0	1.028	1.056	1.230
-	0	1.038	1.062	1.236
1-CH_3	0	1.037	1.082	1.236
7-CH_3	0	0.994	1.050	1.236
Correlation Coefficient		0.929	0.977	0.980

Table 2 shows that if q_7 is the important correlation, 4,6-dimethoxy-α-ethyltryptamine should be a more effective inhibitor than 6-amino-α-ethyltryptamine, the most effective compound yet tested in this series; and the 4-amino derivative would be less active than the 6-amino. If S_7^E is the important correlation, the 4,6-dimethyl derivative should be less active than the 6-amino derivative; and the 4-amino derivative would be as active as the 6-amino. If S_2^E is the important correlation, the inhibitory activity of the 4,6-dimethyl and 6-amino derivatives should be indistinguishable. Thus, the ambiguities may be resolved and a single inference may result by this approach, which is essentially extending the series.

TABLE 2. UNTESTED α-ethyltryptamines (HÜCKEL METHOD)

Derivative of α-ethyltryptamine	q_7	S_7^E	S_2^E
6-NH_2	1.134	1.614	1.496
4,6-$(OCH_3)_2$	<u>1.145</u>	0.936	1.498
4-NH_2	1.108	1.614	1.484

<u>Tryptamines on the Isolated Stomach Strip of the Rat</u>

The compounds were tested [3] on the stomach strip before and after inhibition of the enzyme, monamine oxidase, which destroys many of the tryptamines. The activities in causing contraction of the stomach strip were not related to partition coefficient or pK_a (Table 3). Activities were, however, correlated with

TABLE 3. PARTITION COEFFICIENTS (PC) AND IONIZATION CONSTANTS (pK_a) OF SOME TRYPTAMINES AND THEIR ACTIVITIES ON THE ISOLATED STOMACH STRIP OF THE RAT. PARTITION COEFFICIENT WAS MEASURED BETWEEN 1-OCTANOL AND 0.1 N PHOSPHATE BUFFER, pH 7.0.

Derivative of Tryptamine	Relative Biological Activity	PC	pK_a
5-OH	32	0.017	10.1
5-OCH_3	18.8	0.027	10.3
5-Cl	4.2	0.089	10.5
5-CH_3	3.6	0.202	10.2
--	1.0	0.095	10.2

the resonance contribution of the substituents to the indole ring [21], the biological activity of 5-substituted tryptamines and α-methyltryptamines increasing with decreasing resonance constant (Tables 4 and 5).

TABLE 4. THE RELATIONSHIP BETWEEN THE RESONANCE CONSTANT AND THE ACTIVITY OF SOME TRYPTAMINES ON THE ISOLATED STOMACH STRIP OF THE RAT BEFORE AND AFTER MONOAMINE OXIDASE INHIBITION. THE CORRELATION COEFFICIENTS ARE -0.984 AND -0.983 RESPECTIVELY.

Derivative of Tryptamine	Before MAO-inhibition		After MAO-inhibition		Resonance Constant
	E.M.R.[(a)]	$\log \frac{1}{E.M.R./32}$ [(b)]	E.M.R.[(a)]	$\log \frac{1}{E.M.R./32}$ [(b)]	
5-OH	1.0	1.505	1.0	1.505	-0.643
5-OCH_3	20.0	0.204	1.7	1.275	-0.500
5-Cl	100.0	-0.495	7.6	0.625	-0.161
5-CH_3	184.0	-0.760	9.0	0.551	-0.141
--	408.0	-1.105	32.0	0.000	0.0

(a) Equipotent molar ratio.

(b) The relative activity of tryptamine after MAO-inhibition was converted to unity, hence E.M.R. was divided by 32.

TABLE 5. THE RELATIONSHIP BETWEEN THE RESONANCE CONSTANT AND THE ACTIVITY OF SOME α-METHYLTRYPTAMINES ON THE ISOLATED STOMACH STRIP OF THE RAT. THE CORRELATION COEFFICIENTS ARE -0.999 BEFORE MAO-INHIBITION AND -0.989 AFTER.

Derivative of α-methyltryptamine	Before MAO-inhibition		After MAO-inhibition		Resonance Constant
	E.M.R.[(a)]	$\log \frac{1}{E.M.R./32}$ [(b)]	E.M.R.[(a)]	$\log \frac{1}{E.M.R./32}$ [(b)]	
5-OH	1.4	1.359	2.0	1.204	-0.643
5-OCH_3	2.9	1.043	2.5	1.107	-0.500
5-CH_3	14.0	0.359	16.0	0.301	-0.141
---	31.0	0.014	40.0	-0.097	0.0

(a) Equipotent molar ratio.

(b) The relative activity of tryptamine after MAO-inhibition was converted to unity, hence E.M.R. was divided by 32.

The resonance constant reflects the effect of the substituent on charge distribution in the π-electron system, and the high negative value of the activity constant implies that high electron density at the active site or sites may be associated with biological activity. Which atomic site(s) is involved is not revealed by this calculation. It is not the ring nitrogen because isosteres lacking this atom (*viz*, indenes and benzothiophenes) are active [22].

Both INDO and Hückel calculations showed that potency (after inhibition of monamine oxidase) was related to q_6, f_4^E, and f_5^E (Table 6). It is interesting that the simple Hückel calculation yielded correlation coefficients very nearly the same as those obtained with the INDO method. Both the 4- and 6-positions are known to react readily with electrophiles.

TABLE 6. THE RELATIONSHIP BETWEEN THE ACTIVITY OF SOME TRYPTAMINES ON THE ISOLATED STOMACH STRIP OF THE RAT AND THE CHARGE AT THE 6-POSITION (q_6), AND FRONTIER ELECTRON DENSITIES AT THE 4- AND 5-POSITIONS (f_4 and f_5) AS CALCULATED WITH THE INDO AND HÜCKEL METHODS.

Derivative of Tryptamine	Relative Biological Activity	INDO			Hückel		
		q_6	f_5	f_4	q_6	f_5	f_4
5-OH	32.0	−0.0302	0.1157	0.2123	−0.068	0.096	0.384
5-OCH_3	18.8	−0.0306	0.1120	0.2061	−0.069	0.106	0.398
4-OH	16.0	0.0611	0.0632	0.1461	−0.025	0.126	0.284
5-Cl	4.2	0.0227	0.0426	0.1876	−0.025	0.044	0.288
5-CH_3	3.6	0.0211	0.0364	0.1852	−0.044	0.058	0.314
--	1.0	0.0344	0.0151	0.1600	−0.031	0.026	0.288
5,6-$(OCH_3)_2$	0.21	0.1842	0.0147	0.0730	−0.0015	0.004	0.256
6-OH	0.06	0.2460	0.0092	0.0908	0.030	0.002	0.242
6-OCH_3	0.03	0.2423	0.0066	0.0952	0.028	0.002	0.232
Correlation Coefficient		−0.934	0.9677[a]	0.783	−0.920	0.919[a]	0.842

(a) Binomial correlation coefficient (the regression line is uniformly curved).

To delineate which of the three indexes is truly correlated with potency, we plan to synthesize and test a few congeners that have not been studied in this system. Table 7 shows that the 5,7-dihydroxy- and 5,7-dimethoxy-, 7-hydroxy- and 7-methoxy derivatives would be more potent than the most potent substance tested, 5-hydroxytryptamine (serotonin), if q_6 is the significant correlations. If f_4 is the significant correlation, only the aforementioned dihydroxy and dimethoxy derivatives would be more potent than serotonin. If f_5 is the significant one, then none of these would be more potent than serotonin. Synthesizing and testing the 5,7-dihydroxy- and the 7-hydroxy derivatives could indicate which of the reactivity indexes is correlated with gross potency.

TABLE 7. UNTESTED TRYPTAMINES (INDO METHOD)

Derivative of Tryptamine	q_6	f_5	f_4
5-OH	-0.0302	0.1157	0.2123
5-phenoxy	-0.0494	0.1060	0.1847
4-OCH_3	0.0601	0.0542	0.1368
7-OH	-0.0558	0.0377	0.2086
7-OCH_3	-0.0522	0.0411	0.2052
5,7-$(OH)_2$	-0.1216	0.0724	0.2508
5,7-$(OCH_3)_2$	-0.1187	0.0568	0.2334
5-NH_2	-0.0085	0.0930	0.2078
5-$N(CH_3)_2$	-0.0242	0.0994	0.1598
--	0.0344	0.0151	0.1600

The high value of q_6 in the 5-phenoxy derivative could suggest that if q_6 is the significant index then the 5-phenoxy derivative would be more potent than serotonin. However, as is often seen in studies of congeneric series, the addition of a bulky group can often confer on an agonist (serotonin, in this instance) the properties of an antagonist, i.e. a substance that blocks the action of serotonin (e.g., LSD-25). It is interesting that calculations of untested compounds with resonance constants suggested that the 5-amino and 5-phenoxy derivatives would be more active than serotonin. INDO calculations do not support this prediction for the 5-amino compound, although high activity is predicted.

One obvious consideration in the analysis of the results on untested compounds is that the correlation of potency with more than one index may not be adventitious, especially in this system where potency may be a function of at least two independent variables, affinity and intrinsic activity. In the small series that is available [6], affinity correlates with f_5 (Table 8) and intrinsic activity with f_4 (Table 9). It is possible that the most active compound will be the one where f_5 and f_4 are high. Of the compounds studied, only serotonin is high in both f_4 and f_5. In this context the 5-amino compound is also interesting (Table 7).

TABLE 8. RELATIVE AFFINITY OF SOME TRYPTAMINES FOR THE STOMACH STRIP AND q_6 AND f_5 CALCULATED BY THE INDO METHOD.

Derivative of Tryptamine	Affinity	q_6	f_5
5-OH	6.82	-0.0302	0.1157
4-OH	5.36	-0.0611	0.0632
--	4.71	0.0344	0.0151
6-OH	3.95	0.2460	0.0092

TABLE 9. RELATIVE INTRINSIC ACTIVITY OF SOME TRYPTAMINES ON THE STOMACH STRIP AND f_4 CALCULATED BY THE INDO METHOD.

Derivative of Tryptamine	Rel. Int. Activity	f_4
5-OH	1.0	0.2123
--	0.97	0.1600
4-OH	0.85	0.1461
6-OH	0.68	0.0908

Empirical studies have established that the side-chain amino group is necessary for activity [3], but the calculated charge on the aliphatic nitrogen did not reflect potency.

One impression that emerges from looking at the series [3] is that the molecular orbital calculations that we have made cannot account for the activities of all the derivatives. In a series of tryptamine derivatives with alkyl substituents on the primary amino group, the order of potency of the monoalkylamine derivatives is $CH_3 > CH_2{-}CH_3 > CH_2{-}CH_2{-}CH_3$; the order of potency of dialkyl derivatives is the opposite, *viz*, $(CH_2{-}CH_2{-}CH_3)_2 > (CH_2{-}CH_3)_2 > (CH_3)_2$. Our calculations do not account for these variations in potency. It is possible that measurements of partition coefficients or ionization constants or both could help to make sense of these observations. Even more befuddling is the observation that in the 5-hydroxytryptamine series, the order of potency is $(CH_2{-}CH_2{-}CH_3)_2 > (CH_3)_2 > (CH_2CH_3)_2$, different from the analogous tryptamine derivatives.

The Hypothetical Receptor for Tryptamines in the Rat Stomach

These molecular orbital calculations together with empirical studies stimulate speculation on the nature of the reactions of the indoles with the receptor and, by further inference, on the configuration of the receptor. Since the amino group, which is needed for activity, is protonated at physiological pH, it is reasonable to suggest that it forms either an electrostatic linkage with an acidic group or a hydrogen bond with an electron donor. The latter bond seems less likely because dialkyl substitution does not reduce the activity by much; the N,N-dipropyl derivatives of tryptamine is about as potent as tryptamine, and the corresponding analogue of 5-hydroxytryptamine is one-sixth as potent as 5-hydroxytryptamine [3].

The molecular orbital calculations suggest that the 4- or 5- or 6-position (or maybe more than one) reacts with an electrophile on the receptor. The reaction may be of the type $-XH{-}{-}\pi$ base, with the aforementioned position(s) on the indole ring contributing to the stabilization energy of the complex. XH could be any of a number of groups, e.g., hydroxyl, amide, imidazole, amono. Evidence for the binding of biogenic amines by hydrogen bonding to tissue components, including carbohydrates, has been reviewed [23,24].

A glycopolymer containing neuraminic acid is a likely candidate for a receptor. Many of these are found in membranes (where these tryptamines are acting) and they have a strong affinity for biogenic amines, due to the acidic carboxyl groups (the pK_a is about 3) and the hydroxyl groups. So strong is their affinity for biogenic amines that a neuraminic acid-containing polymer, even after extensive extraction and purification from brain, still retained measurable quantities of norepinephrine [25].

There is some evidence that a neuraminic acid polymer is the tryptamine receptor in the stomach [26-29; cf. 30). The polymer may be N-acetylneuraminyl-(2-8)-N-acetylneuraminyl-(2-3)-galactosyl-(1-4)-glucosyl-1-ceramide [27].

A molecular model of this compound shows a "hole" into which serotonin neatly fits, its primary amino group abutting against a carboxylate group of neuraminic acid and the 4-, 5-, and 6-positions of the indole against the sugar hydroxyl groups of the glucose. Both hypothetical interactions would be of low energy which is in accord with the ready reversibility of the biological effects.

Amphetamine, which acts on the tryptamine receptors in the stomach, also fits the hole and LSD-25, the antagonist of both compounds, can form the same kind of complex with additional sites of interaction.

The Activity of Tryptamines on Neurones of the Lateral Geniculate Nucleus

The activity of these derivatives in depressing excitation of the neurones [4] was poorly correlated with energy of the highest occupied molecular orbital (HOMO) as calculated by the INDO method (Table 10). The rank orders are parallel except for the 4-methoxy- and 6-hydroxy derivatives. It should be noted that the measurement of biological potency is here only grossly quantitative.

TABLE 10. THE ACTIVITY OF SOME TRYPTAMINES ON THE LATERAL GENICULATE NUCLEUS OF THE CAT AND THE ENERGY OF THE HIGHEST MOLECULAR ORBITAL CALCULATED BY THE INDO METHOD.

Derivative of Tryptamine	Potency	HOMO Energy (atomic units)
4-OH	18-24	-0.4582
7-OH	12-18	-0.4584
5-OH	12	-0.4735
$5\text{-}OCH_3$	6	-0.4787
$4\text{-}OCH_3$	6	-0.4566
6-OH	4-5	-0.4583
--	2-3	-0.4810

Hallucinogenic Activity of Some Amphetamines

Amphetamines and tryptamines share the same receptor in some biological systems. And like some indoles, amphetamine derivatives are psychotomimetic (hallucinogenic). The psychotomimetic activity of a series of amphetamines [5] correlated with HOMO (Table 11). Only one compound, the 2,4,5-trimethoxy derivative, was out of order. These results confirm and extend the Hückel calculations of Snyder and Merril [31].

It is hard to believe that HOMO is a biologically meaningful correlate of psychotomimetic activity, but surprisingly no other correlation could be obtained in this or in the series shown in Table 10.

IV. CONCLUSIONS

These beginnings suggest that molecular orbital methods may be valuable in studying the relationship between chemical structure and biological activity. In revealing relationships that were heretofore unnoticed, these methods emphasize that electronic as well as steric factors deserve consideration -- a seeming

TABLE 11. THE HALLUCINOGENIC ACTIVITY OF SOME AMPHETAMINES AND THE ENERGY OF THE HIGHEST OCCUPIED MOLECULAR ORBITAL CALCULATED BY THE INDO METHOD. THE CORRELATION COEFFICIENT IS 0.713.

Derivative of Amphetamine	Hallucinogenic Activity	HOMO Energy (atomic units)
2,5-$(OCH_3)_2$-4-CH_3	100	-0.4929
2,4,5-$(OCH_3)_3$	17	-0.5001
2,4,6-$(OCH_3)_3$	10	-0.5217
2,5-$(OCH_3)_2$	8	-0.5012
2,3,4,5-$(OCH_3)_4$	6	-0.5126
2,4-$(OCH_3)_2$	5	-0.5194
3,4,5-$(OCH_3)_3$	2	-0.5218
3,4-$(OCH_3)_2$	1	-0.5238
--	0	-0.5885

gratuity but not really, when one recalls that much of the biological data referred to here were analyzed solely in terms of stereochemistry.

At the beginning of this work it was hoped that the approach outlined here would help in the understanding of the forces determining the biological activity of molecules and that by inference we might gain insight into the nature of the receptor. It was also hoped that the information derived from a molecular orbital analysis of a congeneric series could not only test the inferences derived from a correlation but could lead to cogent suggestions of new derivatives worth making and testing. Further, it was hoped that the results of the calculations could lead us to design laboratory experiments to test the inferences, and we have made such designs. All in all, the work described here encourages us to pursue all these objectives. At the same time, the analysis shows that at this time a molecular orbital approach will often have to be combined with empirical studies, a clear appraisal of steric factors and reaction mechanisms, an understanding of the biological system, and a compulsive need to seek experimental verification of the findings, because analyses of this sort are a place to begin, not to end, experiments.

V. ACKNOWLEDGMENTS

This work was supported at various times by the National Institute of General Medical Sciences (GM-14278-02), the National Science Foundation (GB-6248) and the National Institute of Mental Health (MH-17489-01).

VI. REFERENCES

[1] Green, J. P., "The application of quantum mechanics to pharmacology: some substances active in the nervous system", p. 95 in *Molecular Basis of Some Aspects of Mental Activity*, (O. Walaas, ed.,) Vol. 2, Academic Press, New York (1967a).

[2] Hester, J. B., Greig, M. E., Anthony, W. C., Heinzelman, R. V., and Szmuszkovicz, J., *J. Med. Chem.*, 7, 274 (1964).

[3] Vane, J. R., *Brit. J. Pharmacol.*, 14, 87 (1959).

[4] Curtis, D. R., and Davis, R., *Brit. J. Pharmacol.*, 18, 217 (1962).

[5] Shulgin, A. T., Sargent, T., and Naranjo, C., *Nature*, 221, 537 (1969).

[6] Offermeier, J., and Ariëns, E. J., *Arch. Int. Pharmacol.*, 164, 216 (1966).

[7] Green, J. P., *Federation Proc.*, 26, 289 (1967b).

[8] Kang, S., Beveridge, D. L., and Green, J. P., *Federation Proc.*, 28, 794 (1969).

[9] Kang, S., Beveridge, D. L., and Green, J. P., *158th A.C.S. National Meeting, Div. of Med. Chem.*, (Sept. 8-12, 1969).

[10] Pople, J. A., Beveridge, D. L., and Dobosh, P. A., *J. Chem. Phys.*, 47, 2026 (1967).

[11] Beveridge, D. L., Dobosh, P. A., and Pople, J. A., *J. Chem. Phys.*, 48, 4802 (1968).

[12] Beveridge, D. L., and Dobosh, P. A., *J. Chem. Phys.*, 48, 5532 (1968).

[13] Pople, J. A., Beveridge, D. L., and Dobosh, P. A., *J. Am. Chem. Soc.*, 90, 4201 (1968).

[14] Pople, J. A., and Beveridge, D. L., *J. Chem. Phys.*, 49, 4725 (1968).

[15] Pullman, B., and Pullman, A., *Quantum Biochemistry*, New York, Interscience (1963).

[16] Green, J. P., and Malrieu, J. P., *Proc. Nat. Acad. Sci. U.S.*, 54, 659 (1965).

[17] Zweig, A., Lancaster, J. E., Neglia, M. T., and Jura, W. H., *J. Am. Chem. Soc.*, 86, 4130 (1964).

[18] Fukui, K., Yonezawa, T., and Nagata, C., *J. Chem. Phys.*, 27, 1247 (1957).

[19] Fukui, K., p. 513 in *Molecular Orbitals in Chemistry, Physics and Biology*, (P. O. Lowdin and B. Pullman, ed.), Academic Press, New York, (1964).

[20] Swain, C. G., and Lupton, E. C., Jr., *J. Am. Chem. Soc.*, 90, 4328 (1968).

[21] Kang, S., and Green, J. P., *Nature*, 222, 794 (1969).

[22] Winter, J. C., Gessner, P. K., and Godse, D. D., *J. Med. Chem.*, 10, 856 (1967).

[23] Green, J. P., *Adv. Pharmacol.*, 1, 349 (1962).

[24] Green, J. P., p. 125 in *Mechanisms of Release of Biogenic Amines*, (Euler, U.S. von Rosell, and Uvnäs, B., eds.), Pergamon, New York, (1965).

[25] Robinson, J. D., Carlini, E. A., and Green, J. P., *Biochem. Pharmacol.*, 12, 1219 (1963).

[26] Wooley, D. W., and Gommi, B. W., *Arch. Int. Pharmacodyn.*, 159, 8 (1966).

[27] W. Gielen, *Z. Naturforsch.*, 21 B, 1007 (1966).

[28] Wesemann, W., and Zilliken, F., *Biochem. Pharmacol.*, 17, 471 (1968).

[29] Vaccari, A., and Cugurra, F., *Biochem. Pharmacol.*, 17, 2399 (1968).

[30] Offermeier, J., and Ariëns, E. J., *Arch. Int. Pharmacodyn.*, 164, 192 (1966).

[31] Snyder, S. H., and Merril, C. R., *Proc. Nat. Acad. Sci. U.S.*, 54, 258 (1965).

THE APPLICATION OF HÜCKEL AND EXTENDED HÜCKEL MOLECULAR ORBITAL CALCULATIONS TO BIOCHEMICAL PROBLEMS

by

W. Brock Neely*

I. INTRODUCTION

Professor A. Szent-Györgyi, in writing of his research [1], said, "...my relations to the various sciences were very promiscuous and made me remain an amateur scientist but a professional poacher". A similar feeling arises from the complexity of the subject of structure activity analysis which requires the application of knowledge from all fields. In this endeavor, one quickly develops the ability to take the results and observations of other people in an effort to determine what is necessary for a chemical to be an active drug. The process leads to generalizations which, hopefully, will allow the design of better chemicals for specific end uses. One of the first generalizations discovered is that in this sort of study you cannot allow yourself the luxury of becoming too engrossed in any one discipline - you must maintain a proper perspective and attempt to keep all parameters in balance.

Of the two partners in a structure activity study, namely the drug and the biological system, the drug is comparatively simple. A place to start, therefore, is the study of chemicals and how they influence, in a selective manner, certain key reactions. Chemical reactions are usually enhanced by conditions which bring molecules into close proximity so that their electronic orbits overlap and facilitate the exchange of electrons. To bring about conditions in which sufficient overlapping occurs, it is sometimes necessary to put energy into the system before it will proceed spontaneously. This energy is known as the activation energy and is exemplified in many commonplace reactions. One way to achieve this is to bring reactants together in high concentration. In sub-atomic terms, this means that the

* Biochemical Research Laboratory, The Dow Chemical Company, Midland, Michigan.

orbits of the electrons on adjacent atoms are more likely to overlap. Another way of achieving the activation energy threshold is by the addition of heat to the system.

This type of activation (the concentration effect) is particularly important in living systems, since biochemical reactions in the absence of the physiological catalysts would require the input of heat to proceed spontaneously. It is highly likely that enzymes function by bringing the reactants together in high enough concentration so that the activation conditions are satisfied. Chemical reactions occur as a result of the interaction or sharing of electrons in the outer orbits of different atoms. Consequently, passage of electrons from one molecule to another is the key to our problem. What is needed, then, is a method to describe the distribution and the movement of electrons within molecules. Such a method is molecular orbital theory.

II. HÜCKEL THEORY

The simplest model is the Hückel LCAO approximation. Using this technique, remarkable success had been achieved in interpreting biochemical reactions [2,3]. In essence, the method considers each mobile or π electron as occupying a molecular orbital (MO) extending over the whole framework. This orbital is approximated by a linear combination of all available atomic π-orbitals φ_i.

$$\psi = \sum_i C_i \varphi_i \tag{1}$$

These MO's are eigenfunctions of an effective Hamiltonian operator $\underline{H}$ in the Schrödinger wave equation

$$\underline{H}\psi = E\psi \tag{2}$$

substituting (1) into (2) and making use of the variation principle generates the secular equation (3), where the i and j represent the ith MO and the jth atomic orbital. It is the solution of this equation which produces the various electronic characteristics of the molecule under consideration.

$$\sum_i C_i (H_{ij} - \varepsilon S_{ij}) = 0 \tag{3}$$

It is now necessary to make some approximations in order to achieve a solution of this equation, and as Streitwieser [3] says in his book, "At this point we now introduce some dillies". The various integrals, for the carbon aromatic system as represented by H_{ij} (bond integral), H_{ii} Coulomb integral) and S_{ij} (overlap integral) are given constant values of β, α, and 0 respectively. If the molecule contains heteroatoms, the integrals are modified by the inclusion of another set of parameters η and δ which modify the α and β's to bring the calculations into line with observable measurements. As may be seen, this method is insensitive to the geometry of the molecule. These assumptions dictate that the method is suitable for examining closely related members in a chemical family. If this aspect is accepted, countless examples show that the results obtained give excellent correlation of experimental observations. The absolute values are unimportant. What is important is the significance of the concepts which may be generated. For a thorough review of the application of the Hückel approach, the book by Pullman and

and Pullman [2] is recommended. In the following section examples are given from the author's work in this area.

Applications

Organophosphates

Such chemicals have been used for many years in the control of insects. Classically, the model that is used to depict this biological activity is shown in Figure 1 where the primary attack is the phosphorylation of the esteratic site in cholinesterase. From this model, it is deduced that those phosphates which are most susceptible to nucleophilic attack will be the most potent insecticides. The series of chemicals that we investigated were the phosphoramidates depicted by Structure I [4]. Since the only

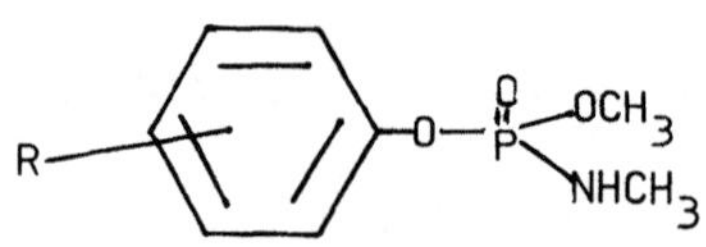

Structure I

substituents that were varied in this series were the substituents on the phenol, only the phenols were examined. Performing the Hückel calculations provides a measure of the relative election deficiency at the phenyl-C-O linkage. This is a measure of the stability of the phenoxy residue and hence is a measure of the ease with which the corresponding phosphate is subject to nucleophilic attack. Figure 2, demonstrates the correlation between the calculated density and the pK_a of the corresponding phenol. The latter is an experimental number which measures the same property. This correlation supports the conclusion that MO calculations can be used to measure which organophosphate in a given series will make the best enzyme inhibitor.

Imidazolines

The final example of the application of the simple Hückel calculations is illustrated with a series of substituted imidazolines (Structure II).

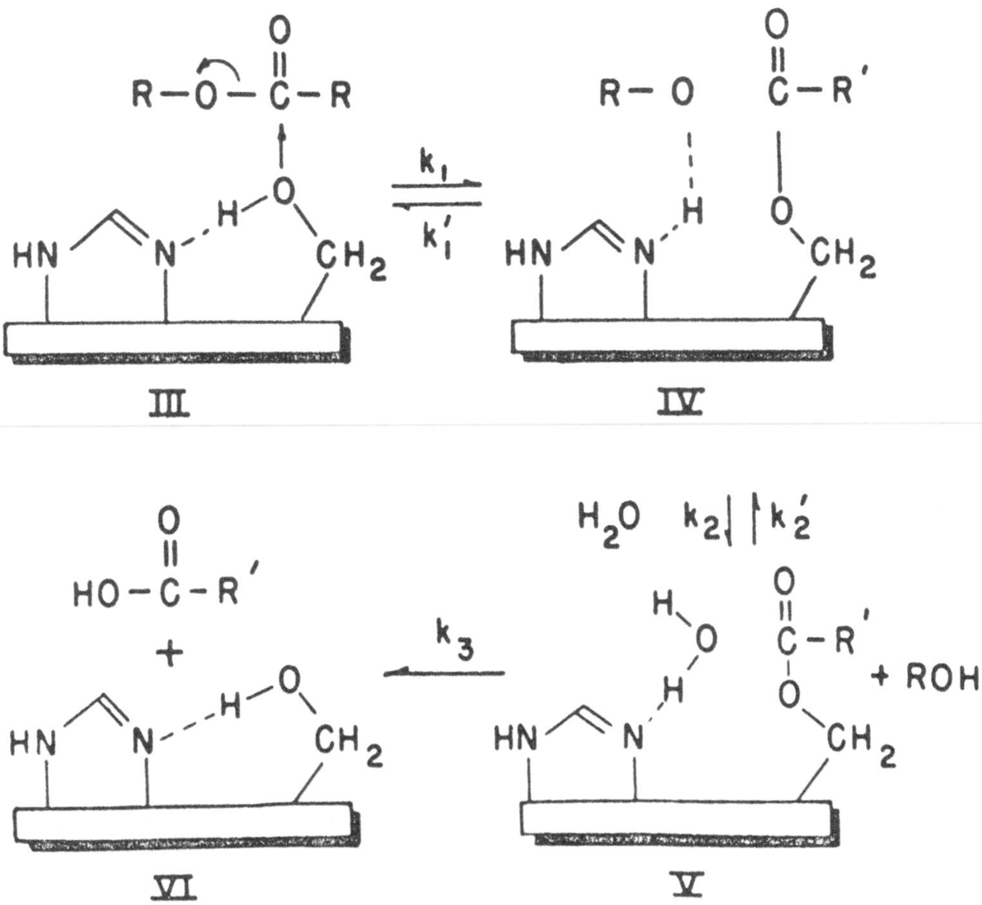

FIGURE 1. Possible model for the action of cholinesterase.

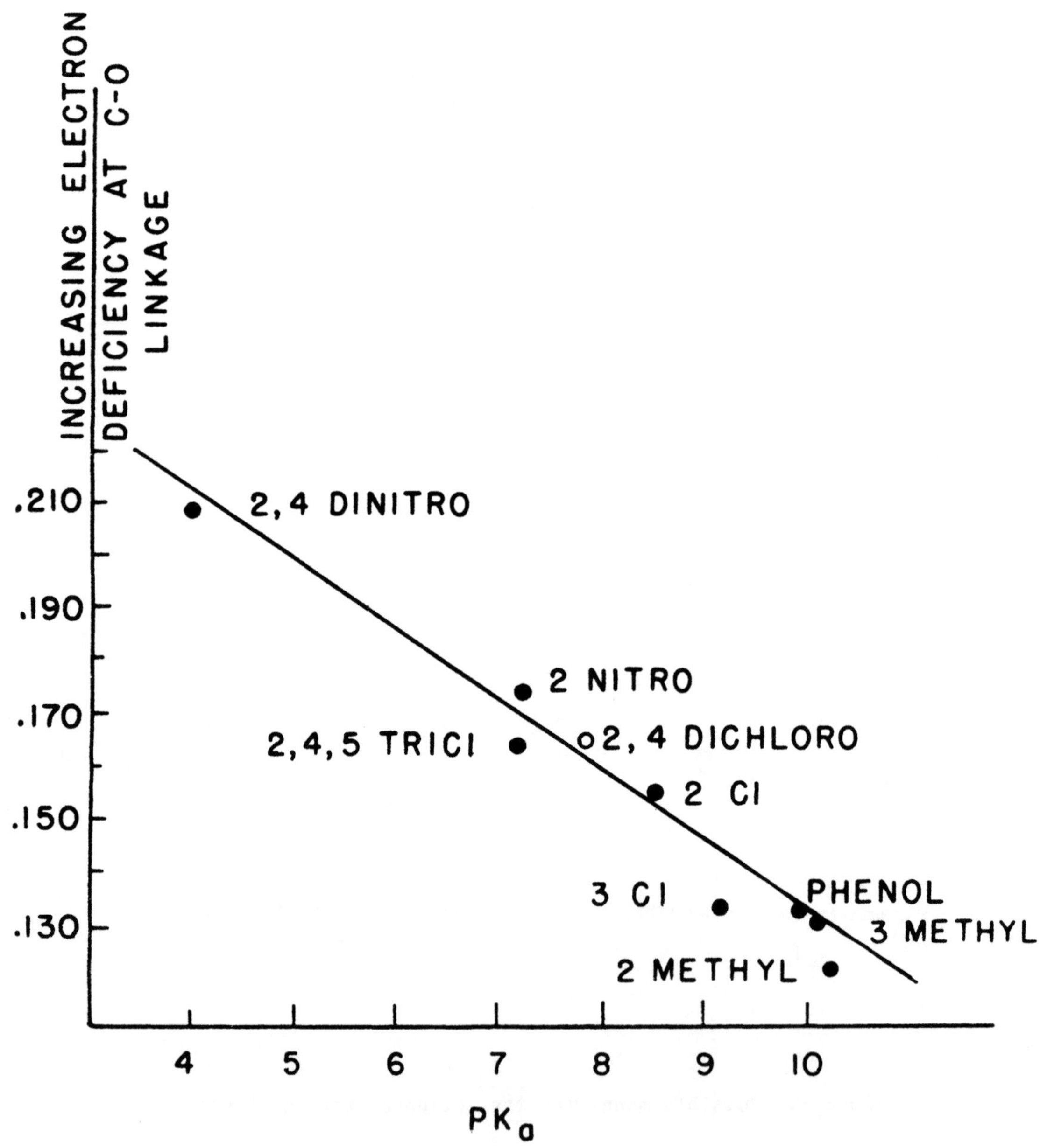

FIGURE 2. The correlation between the pK_a and the calculated electron deficiency at the C-O centers for various substituted phenols.

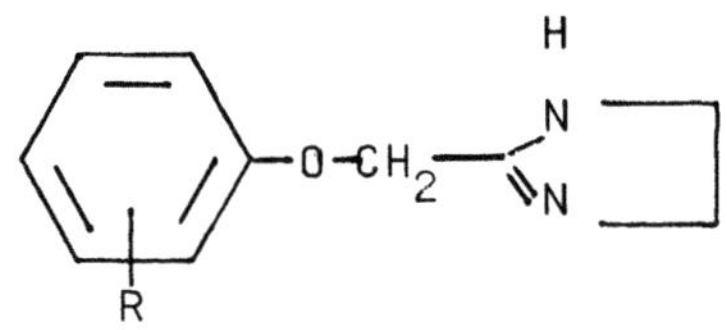

Structure II

that were prepared for their analgesic properties [5]. In a manner similar to the organophosphates described previously, only the substituted phenol was examined by means of MO calculations. In the present case the electronic index which appeared to be relevant was the energy level of the highest occupied molecular orbital (HOMO). This was calculated for the series of compounds represented in Table 1. This index is a measure of the ability of the electrons in the HOMO to be transferred to an acceptor molecule, i.e. a measure of the oxidation potential. Figure 3 shows the correlation that exists between the energy of the HOMO and the oxidation potential of the corresponding phenol. Combining the HOMO value with the partition coefficient as described by Hansch [6] it is possible to correlate the biological activity as a linear function of these two values. This model is based on the thesis that the amount of drug at the receptor site is a function of the partition coefficient. Once the drug has reached this critical location the reactivity of the molecule comes into play and elicits the biological response in question. This generates a relationship where the activity (in this case ED_{50}) is a function of the partition coefficient and the reactivity index. Multiple regression analysis can then be used to determine the coefficients. These statistics were performed on the above data and yielded Equation 4.

$$\text{Log } ED_{50} = 0.945\pi^2 - 1.80\pi + 7.90\,(\text{HOMO}) - 5.17 \qquad (4)$$

where 94% of the activity was explained. The surface generated by this equation is shown in Figure 4. While such an analysis does not give a molecular mechanism, it does suggest a model. The model that emerges consists of a receptor site which has the ability to accept electrons from an electron donating drug. The association is probably similar to a Michaelis-Menten type situation, hence the biological activity would have a short half life relative to a drug that forms a covalent linkage.

TABLE 1. BIOLOGICAL AND CHEMICAL PARAMETERS FOR A SERIES OF IMIDAZOLINE DERIVATIVES

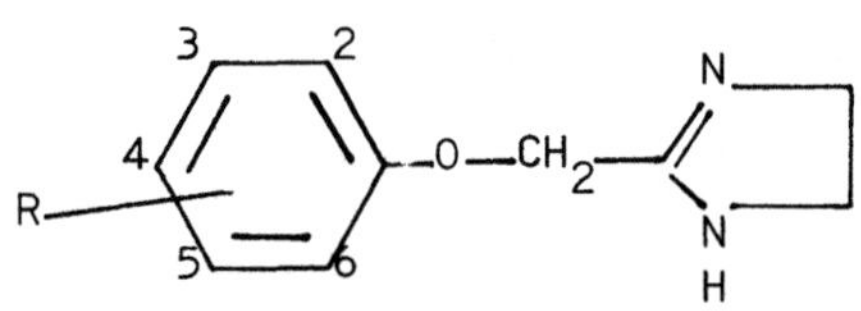

Substituent (R)	ED_{50} (a)	π (b)	HOMO (c)	Oxidation (d) Potential (Volts)
2,6-diCH3	0.6	1.36	0.716	0.469
2-Br, 6-Cl	2.0	1.34	0.802	0.642
2,6-di Br	3.2	1.50	0.797	0.634
2,6-di Cl	3.3	1.18	0.808	0.659
2,6-diCl, 3-CH_3	5.4 (e)	1.69	0.789	0.625
2,6-di OCH_3	25	-0.66	0.618	0.363

(a) Oral dose in mg/kilo (HCl induced rat writhing test for analgesics).

(b) Determined from Hansch's values [6].

(c) Energy of the highest occupied molecular orbital of the substituted phenol. The smaller the value, the greater the ease of electron donation.

(d) Oxidation potential of substituted phenol determined by means of a Leeds and Northrup Electro chromograph Type E.

(e) Estimated value derived from the value for a subcutaneous dose of this derivative compared to a similar type of injection of the other derivatives.

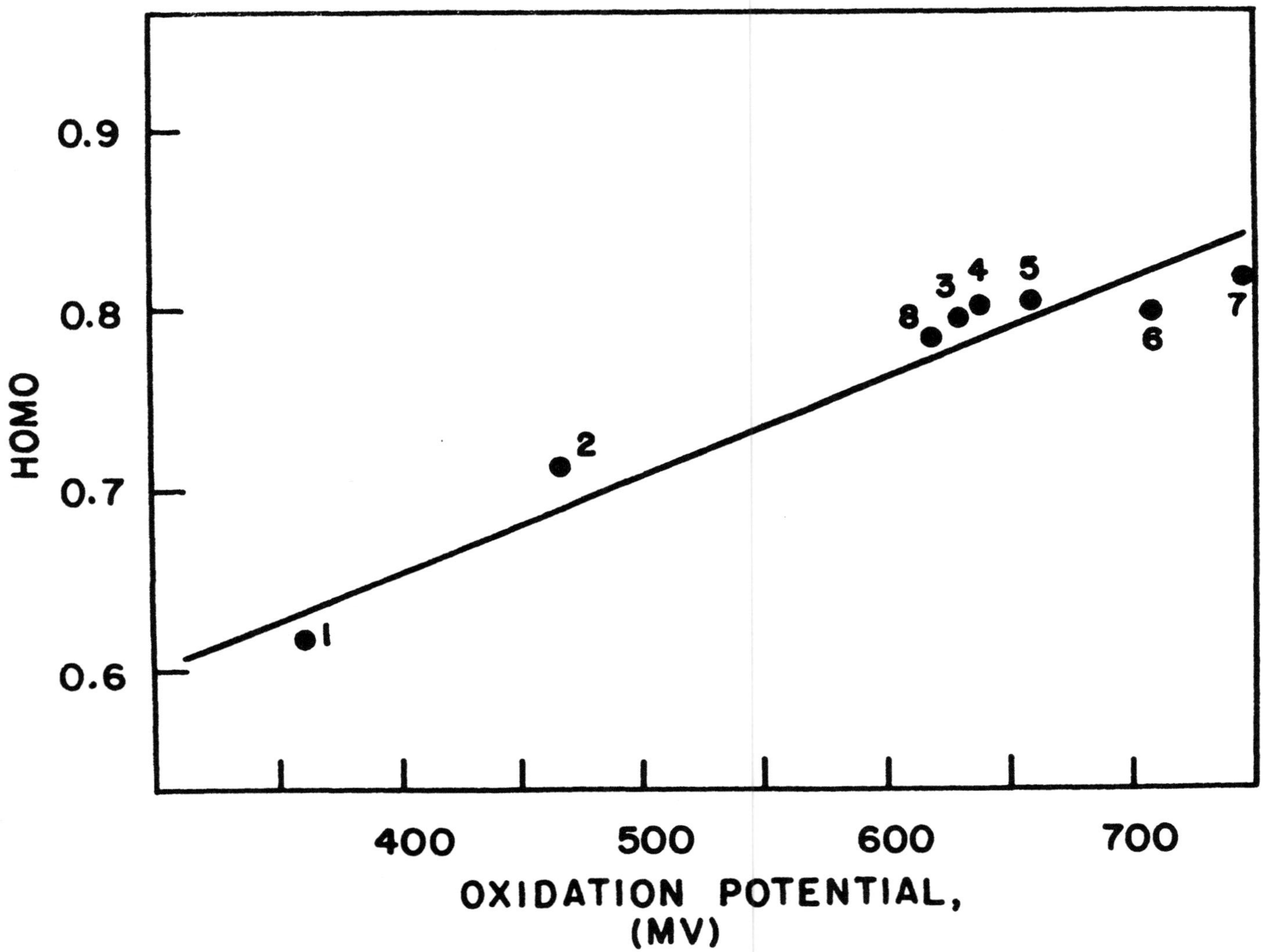

FIGURE 3. Plot of HOMO against the oxidation potential for a series of phenols. [5].

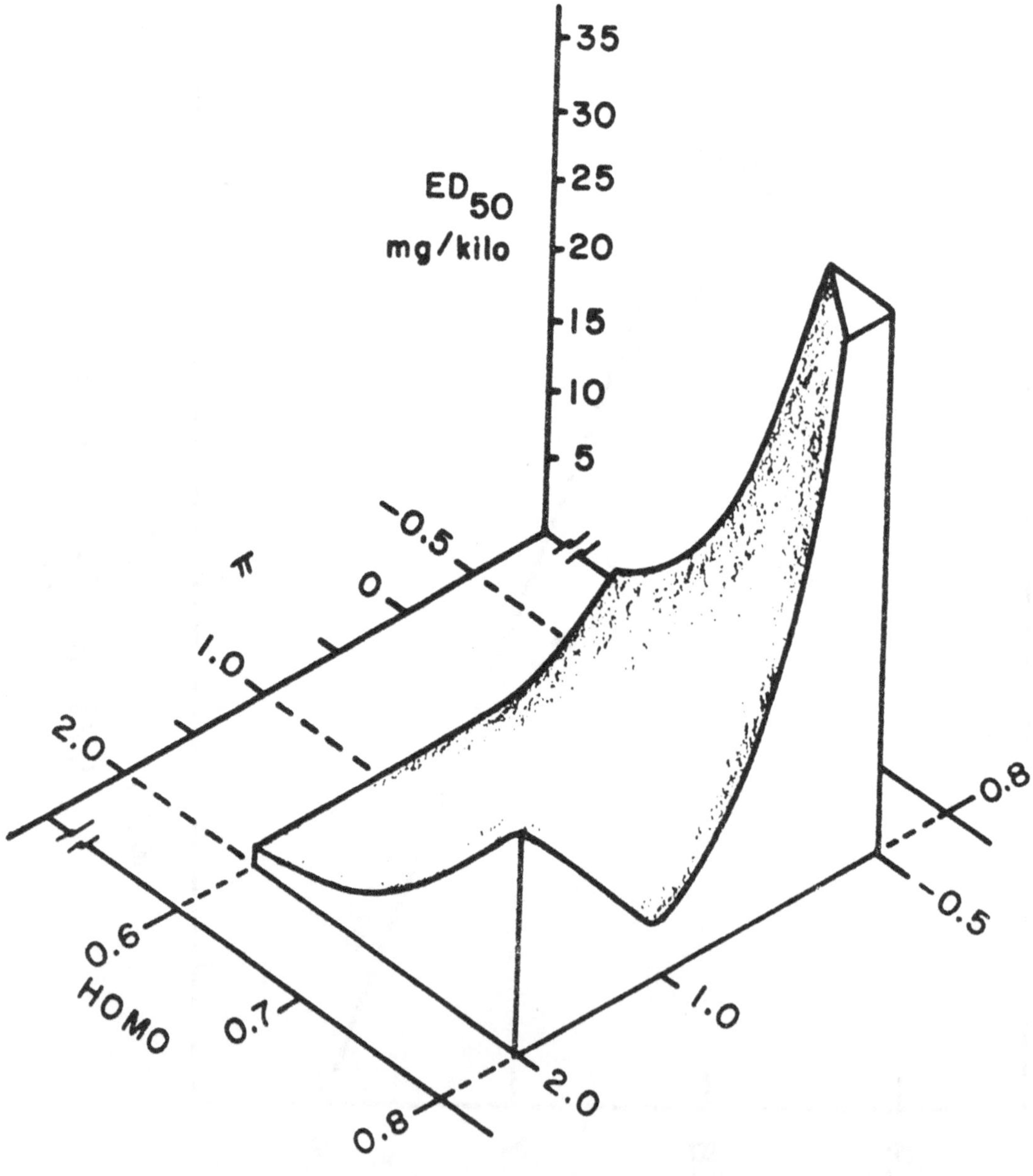

FIGURE 4. Structure activity surface generated by Equation (4). The most potent analgesic has the smallest ED_{50}.

III. EXTENDED HÜCKEL THEORY

As pointed out previously, the use of the Hückel technique must be confined to planar conjugated or aromatic systems. Hydrogens and heteroatoms are brought in by the use of parameters and the sigma pi separation has largely been ignored for non-planar compounds. It was just these considerations which led Hoffman [7] to develop the so-called extended Hückel theory (EHT). The method utilizes the secular Equation (3) derived previously. The calculations are performed for the valence electrons in the s and p orbitals using Slater orbitals as a basis set. The overlap integrals $S_{ij}(\int \varphi_i \varphi_j dT)$ are calculated. The matrix elements of the Hamiltonian are assigned values according to the following scheme: 1) H_{ii} are the valence state ionization potentials for the various orbitals while 2) H_{ij} is approximated as $0.5\,K(H_{ii} + H_{jj})S_{ij}$ (where K is given a value of 1.75). In addition to the above, the Cartesian coordinates for each atom must be included as input.

The solution of the eigenvalue problem yields a set of wave functions and energy levels. The total energy is considered to be the sum of the occupied energy levels. From this it is readily seen that the energy is a function of the assigned geometry.

The output of this program generates a number of items, only the relevant ones will be mentioned here.

(1) A distance matrix which is a useful check of the coordinate system used for the various atoms.

(2) Energy values for the occupied and unoccupied orbitals of the molecule. Since each filled orbital is doubly occupied, the total energy is $2\sum_i E_i$ (electron volts) where the summation is over the filled orbitals. By varying the geometry of the molecule and calculating the energy values, an indication of which conformation is the most stable may be determined. There have been many studies using this approach to conformational problems. The success of this technique is continually providing more confidence in the approach. A theoretical analysis by

Allen and Russell [8] has given even more credence to the use of this quantum mechanical treatment for predicting conformational energy.

(3) The Mulliken overlap population matrix is calculated. This latter matrix is useful for measuring relative bond order strength.

(4) A complete charge matrix is calculated. This gives an indication of the probability distribution of electrons in the molecule. For example, electrons in the highest filled MO have the greatest tendency to be donated to a receptor. An examination of the charge matrix will provide information as to which atom in the molecule has the highest density of these labile electrons.

(5) Finally, the total electron density for each atom is presented. This information may be useful in determining which centers will be subject to either nucleophilic or electrophilic attack.

Applications

There are numerous examples of the use of the EHT to problems relating to biologically active structures. Again, my intent is not to review the literature but merely to give an insight into the utility of the method.

Acetylcholine

This is taken from some work performed by L. B. Kier on the conformation of acetylcholine, muscarine and muscarone [9]. Dr. Kier studied the conformation of muscarine (Structure III).

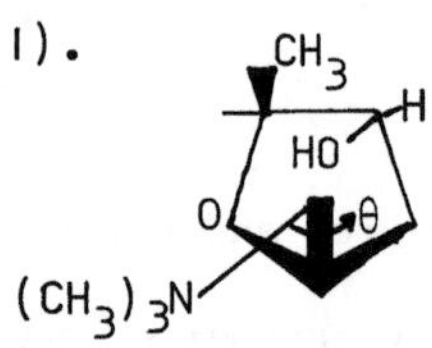

$\theta = 180^\circ$

Structure III

as a function of the angle θ. The zero angle being the eclipsing of the C–N bond with the ring C–C bond. The calculations revealed a definite energy minimum (hence, a stable conformation) at 180°. This was the same conformation reported by Jellinck on the basis of X-ray analysis [10].

Calculations were also performed on acetylcholine and muscarone. While these molecules exhibit greater flexibility than muscarine, the distance between the N and the two oxygens in the preferred conformation were similar to muscarine. These calculations are very gratifying especially in light of some recent work at the University of Iowa [11]. These investigators studied the cholinergic effects of the conformationally rigid analog of acetylcholine (Structure IV).

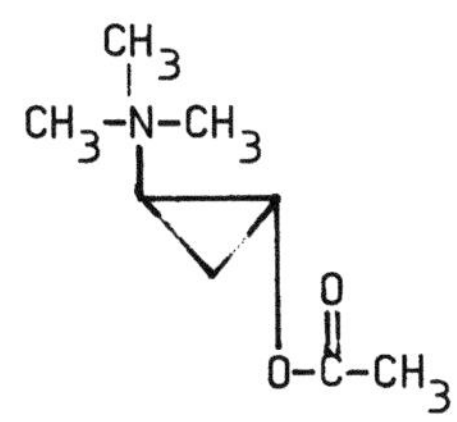

Structure IV (trans isomer)

They discovered that the trans isomer possessed high muscarine activity while the cis isomer was inactive. Crude measurements on wire models of the trans isomer gave a N to ester O of 3.5 Å - a value which is consistent with the calculations of Kier. This is a good example of the power of the MO technique in predicting useful quantities on biologically active molecules.

Glucopyranose

The various hexopyranoses are capable of existing in a great many different conformations. For example, glucopyranose can exist in eight different conformations, two chairs and six boats. Reeves [12] has analysed these conformers and made predictions as to which would be the most stable. Earlier this year, [13] Neely reported on the use of EHT as an additional technique in the analysis of this type of problem. The results of this study confirmed the results of Reeves and gave further support to the use of quantum mechanics in analyzing fairly complicated structures of biological interest. The structures analyzed are shown in Figure 5 and the results are in Table 2. The results of this study are summarized in Table 3 which compares this work with previous investigations.

Using the values for the interaction energies as discussed by Angyal [14] the non-bonded energies of the sugar conformations can be calculated (Table 3). Rao [15] has recently made use of the Buckingham potential energy function to calculate

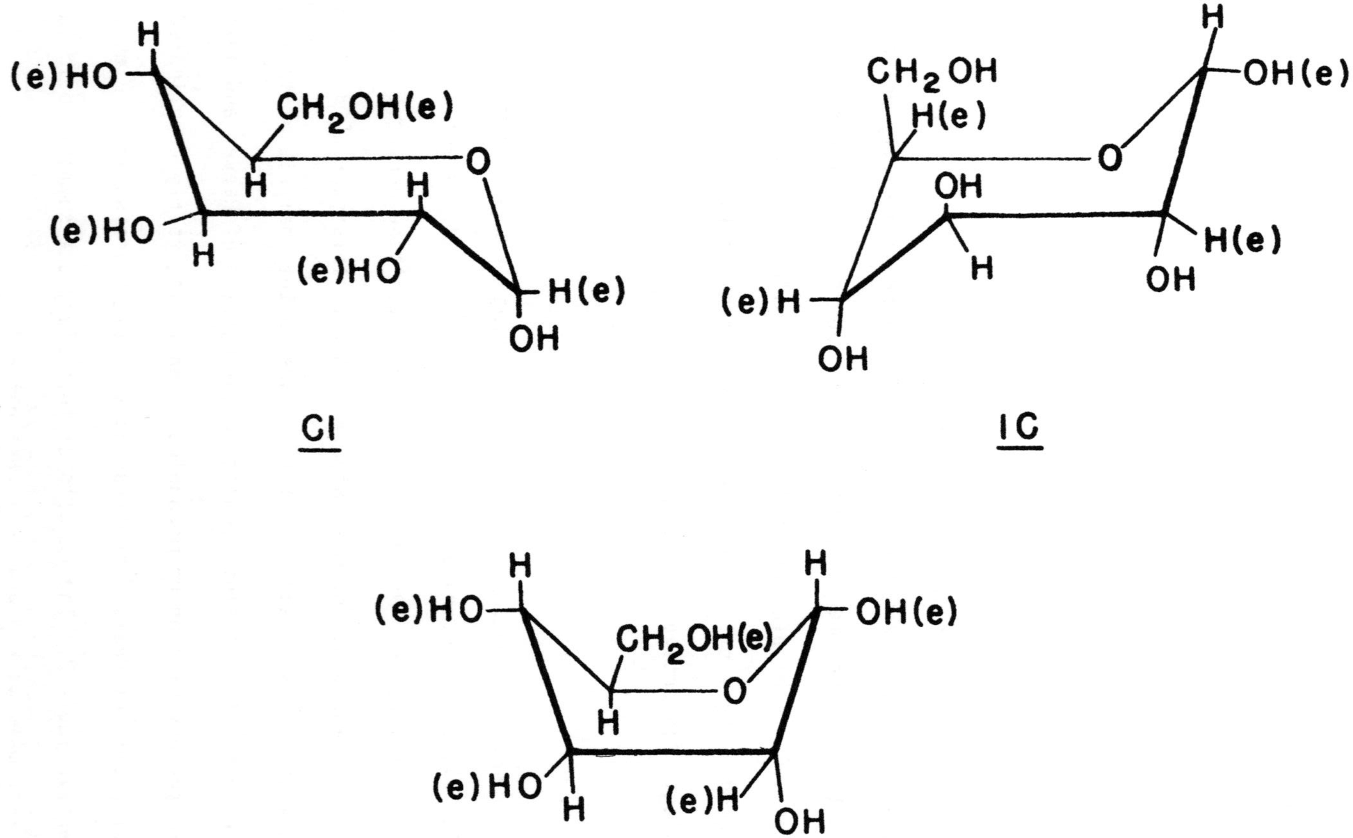

CI IC BI

FIGURE 5. The three conformations of α-D-glucopyranose that were studied.

TABLE 2. TOTAL ENERGY OF VARIOUS CONFORMATIONS OF GLUCOSE AND RELATED SUGARS

Sugar	Conformation	EHT	
		Energy (kcal)	Differences[a]
Glucopyranose	α-D-C1[b]	-34969	0
	β-D-C1	-34978	- 9
	α-D-1C	-34920	+48
	α-D-B1	-34963	+ 6
Galactopyranose	α-D-C1	-34958	+11

(a) This represents the difference in kcal between glucose in the α-D-C1 conformation and the other types. A negative difference indicates a structure that is energetically more stable.

(b) This is the designation used by Reeves [12] for the various chair and boat conformations.

non-bonded interactions. These results are shown in Table 3. It is interesting to note that all of these calculations agree in a relative way with each other. Again, it must be remembered that the absolute value is not important. What is important is the relative differences and the concepts that these relative differences translate into a quantitative language.

TABLE 3. TOTAL CALCULATED INTERACTION ENERGIES IN KCAL/MOLE OF THE SUGARS IN TABLE 2

Sugar	Conformation	Calculated Energies EHT [13]	I [14]	II [15]
Glucopyranose	α-D-C1	0	2.3	1.00
	β D-C1	- 9	1.95	
	α-D-1C	48	7.1	11.88
	α-D-B1	6	2.4	4.79
Galactopyranose	α-D-C1	11	3.2	

α(2,2,2-Trichloroethyl) Styrene

The structure III, α(2,2,2-trichloroethyl) styrene, has been found useful for controlling water grass in rice paddies [16]. We became interested in examining this chemical and related

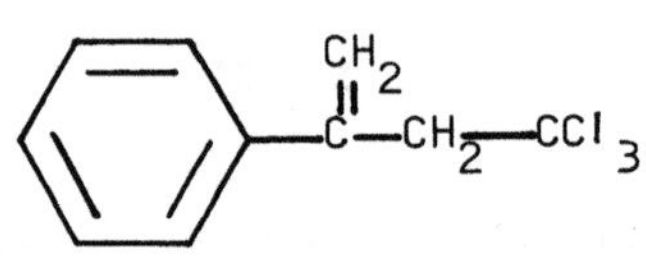

Structure III

methyl substituted analogs to determine what parameters were responsible for the activity. From an examination of models, there is an immediate question as to which conformation of this herbicide is the most stable. Is the vinyl group planar with the aromatic group or is it shifted out of the plane? For the purpose of this investigation, the trichloromethyl group was not included. Consequently, all of the calculations will involve α-methyl styrene. The phenyl ring was rotated around the phenyl-carbon bond and energy calculations were made at each angle. The results are shown in Figure 6 and Table 4. The most stable conformation from this type of analysis occurs when the vinyl group is out of the plane of the aromatic ring. While 60° is the calculated minimum, it is obvious that a stable conformation could exist over a wide range of angles centered at 60°. These stabilities agree in a qualitative manner with the observations of previous workers. Johnson

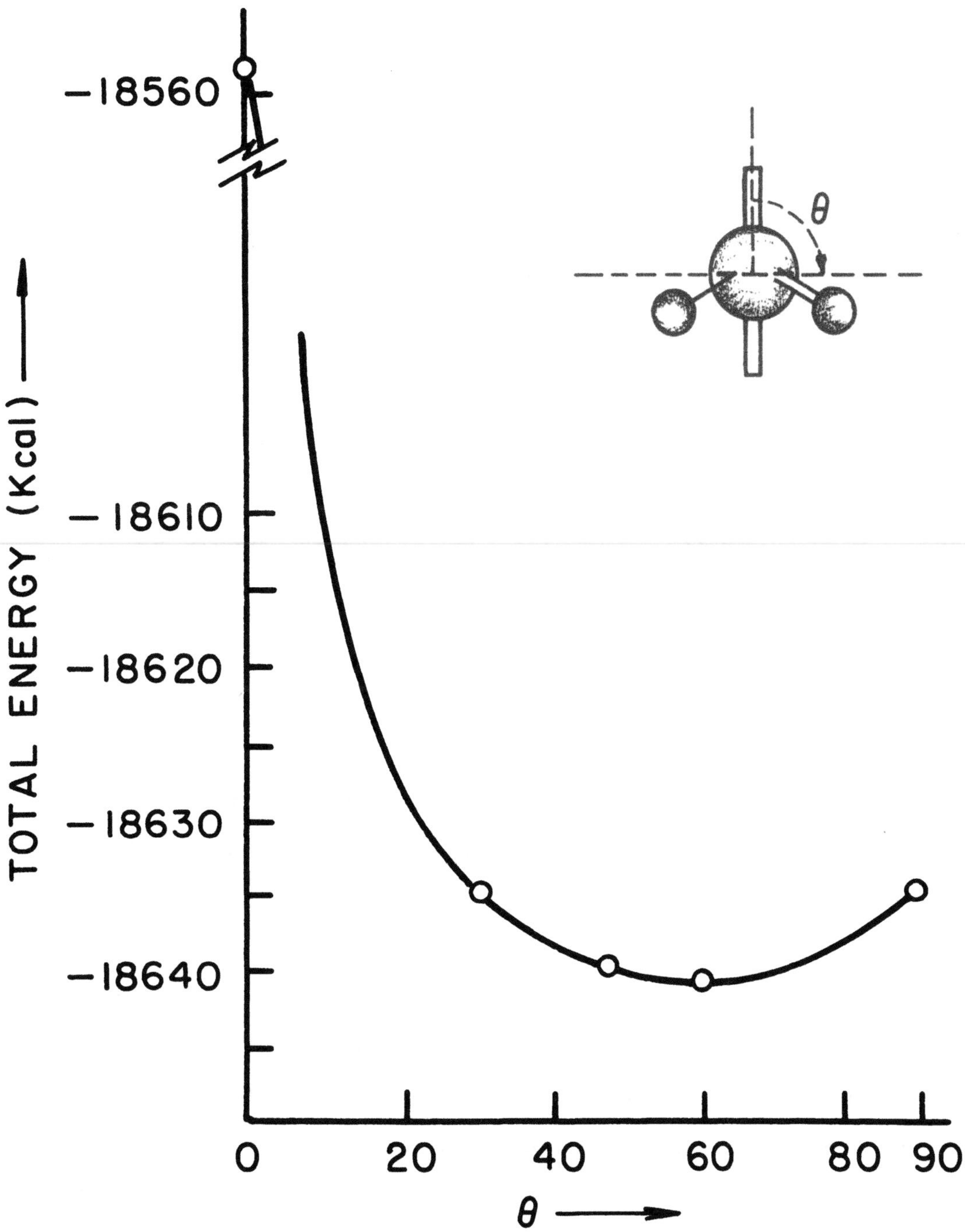

FIGURE 6. Total energy in kcal of α(2,2,2-trichloroethyl) styrene plotted against θ.

TABLE 4. RESULTS OF MOLECULAR ORBITAL CALCULATIONS ON THE CONFORMATIONS OF α-METHYL STYRENE

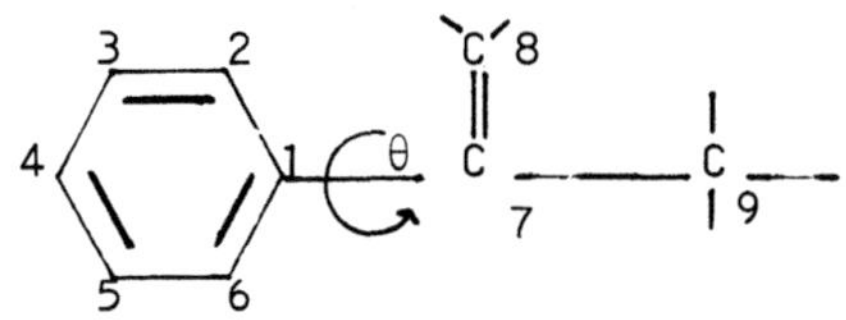

Conformation Angle = θ	Energy (V) (kcal)
0	-18558.0
30	-18636.6
45	-18639.9
60	-18641.2
90	-18635.0

[17] in his review of allylic strain suggested that non-bonded interaction between the phenyl ring and the α-methyl hydrogens would cause steric inhibition of resonance and result in a break of the coplanarity. Overberger [18] by measuring extinction coefficients came to a similar conclusion that steric inhibition or resonance must exist in α-methyl styrene.

Assuming a stable conformation where the angle = 60°, the question was raised as to what influence a methyl group substituted on the aromatic ring might have on the electron distribution. Calculations were performed on 2, 3 and 4-methyl substituted α-methyl styrene with the vinyl group 60° out of the plane of the aromatic ring. In addition, due to the steric hindrance of the 2-methyl group, calculations were carried out at 90° as well as 60° for this particular derivative. These results are shown in Table 5. The calculations indicate that the most stable conformation for the 2-methyl derivatives is 90°.

A word of explanation is needed for the column headed frontier orbital in Table 5. This is the term applied by Fukui et al. [19] to the orbital containing

TABLE 5. CALCULATIONS ON METHYL SUBSTITUTED α-METHYL STYRENE (θ = 60°) AND THE CORRESPONDING BIOLOGICAL ACTIVITY OF THE α(2,2,2-TRICHLOROETHYL) STYRENE DERIVATIVE

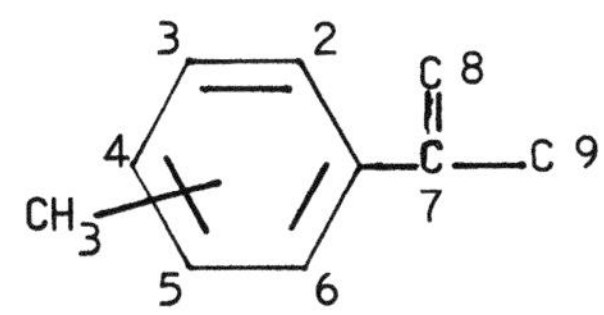

Compound	Energy (kcal)	Frontier Orbital Density at C 8	Biological Activity (a)
2-methyl (60°)	-21044.6	0.413	>50 ppm
2-methyl (90°)	-21049.6	0.197	>50 ppm
3-methyl	-21051.6	0.557	4 ppm
4-methyl	-21051.8	0.389	20 ppm
Unsubstituted		0.721	2 ppm

(a) Biological Activity is 50% growth inhibition of Japanese millet (*Echinochloa frumentaceal*). These tests were carried out in solution by Dr. T.W. Holmsen of the Biochemical Research Laboratory, the Dow Chemical Company, Midland, Michigan.

the pair of electrons in the highest MO in the ground state. These authors pointed out that this pair of electrons play a decisive role in various reactions. Consequently, density distribution becomes quite important. The value reported is for the atom containing the greatest density of these labile electrons. Since there are a maximum of two electrons in each orbital, the number listed for α-methyl styrene indicates a high probability of at least one electron being in the high energy level.

Using the frontier orbital density on carbon atom 8 as a measure of biological activity, the four compounds in Table 5 may be placed in the proper order of biological activity, i.e., α(2,2,2-trichloroethyl) styrene is greater than 3-methyl, greater than 4-methyl, and greater than 2-methyl substituted analogs which are the same order for the frontier orbital density of carbon 8. The distribution of electrons in the frontier orbital for each atom in these derivatives is given in Figure 7. Since the carbon 2p electron accounts for nearly 95% of the 2 electrons available for this molecular orbital, these are the only atomic orbitals listed in this figure.

Polypeptides

The problem of computing the stabilities of various conformations of polypeptides has been extensively studied by several laboratories (for a review see reference 15). Hoffmann and Imamura [20] used the EHT to study the conformations of glycyl and alanyl residues in the ground and excited states. The features generated by this study were similar to the potential surfaces calculated with the standard calculations. Besides allowing for an independent check of previous work, the EHT also provided an insight into the excited-state surface. These workers anticipate extending their studies to include solvation interactions as well as working with peptides of sufficient length to incorporate a single intramolecular hydrogen bond.

IV. FUTURE NEEDS

The Use of More Refined MO Procedures

The EHT method has achieved remarkable success in correlating calculated electronic indices with experimental observations. However, as pointed out by Boer et al. [21], a theoretical understanding has lagged behind the often spectacular achievements of its use. For example, Lipscomb et al. [22] demonstrated that the EHT method breaks down when the carbon 1s, core is included. These authors concluded that, since the method no longer works when an approximation is removed, the success depends on a fortuitous cancellation of errors. It was this observation that initiated a further study of Hoffmann's method. In 1966, a series of four papers were published in which Lipscomb and his associates generated a more theoretical approach to the problem [23]. In their treatment, the H_{ii} and K in the EHT procedure are based on values derived from self-consistent calculations for small molecules. Since the parameters are not fitted to experimental numbers, they

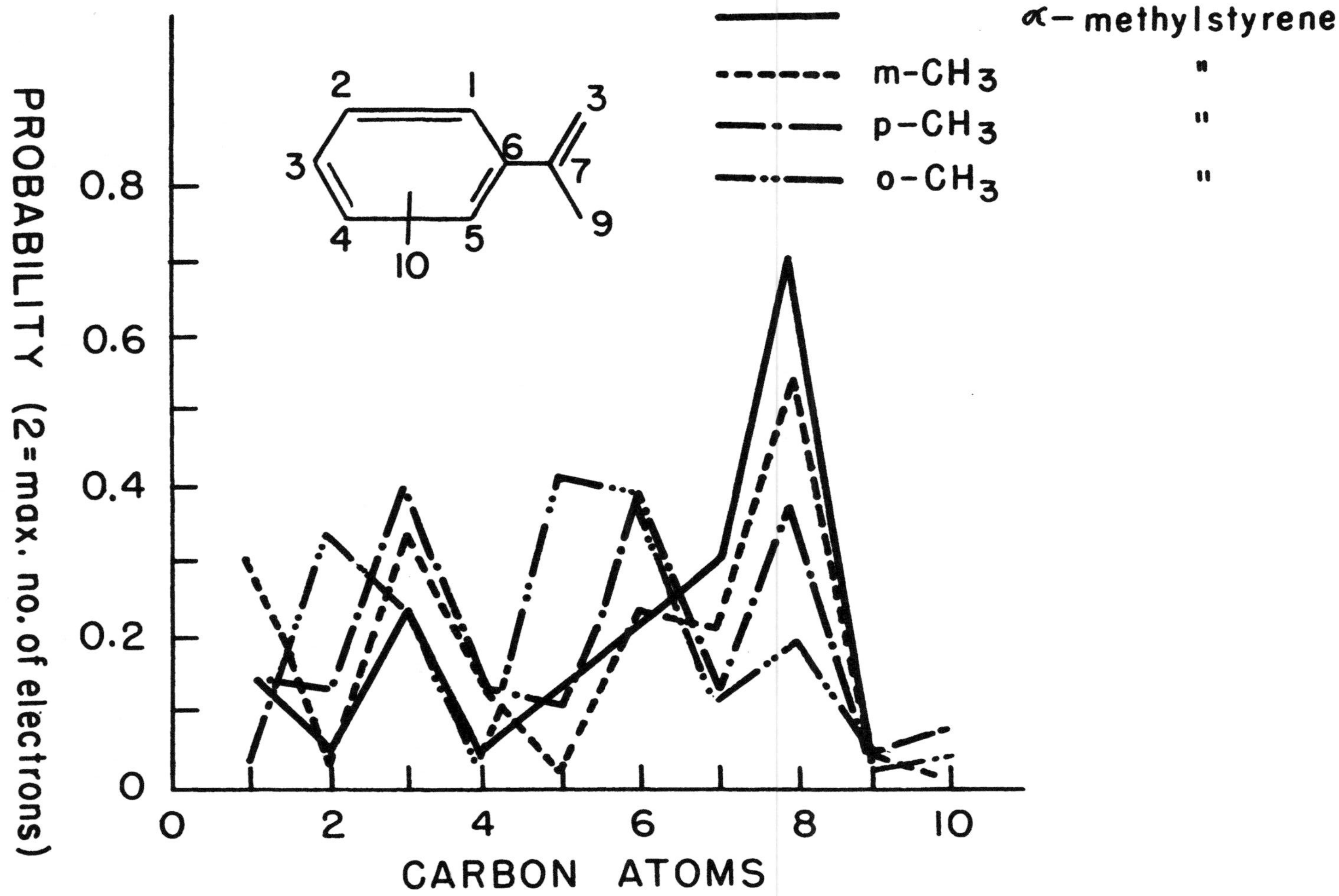

FIGURE 7. Probability distribution of electrons in the frontier orbital of α-methyl styrene and derivatives.

refer to their method as a non-empirical molecular orbital (NEMO) method. More recently, Boer and Lipscomb [24] have been including the d orbitals of sulfur.

Clearly, all of this activity suggests that a more accurate description of molecules will soon be available. With such a description, in hand, those who a are interested in structure *versus* biological activity will be in a better position to make correlations.

Solvent Interactions

The influence of solvation on drug receptor interactions is most important and, for the most part, has been largely ignored in many studies. Recently, Cammarata [25] has made use of some theoretical considerations of Klopman, et al. [26,27] in assessing the influence of desolvation.

Briefly, for a common receptor site, Cammarata has suggested that drug activity is related to the following functional equation

$$A = \sum_s (E_s + L_s + V_s) + k \qquad (5)$$

where

A = activity

E_s = electronic factor

L_s = desolvation component

V_s = steric effect

the summation is taken over all of the interacting atoms. The electronic factor E_s may be related to either q_s, the charge density of the respective atom, or C_s, the coefficient of the highest occupied MO, depending on the type of reaction being considered.

By application of the desolvation equations of Klopman [26,27] two cases were identified.

1) No charge transfer as in an ideal ionic interaction in which case $L_s = 0$ and the activity follows equation

$$A = \sum_s bq_s + C \quad . \qquad (6)$$

2) Where there is complete charge transfer between drug and receptor

$$L_s = (\frac{q \pm 1}{2R})^2(1 - \frac{1}{\varepsilon}) \quad . \tag{7}$$

In this equation, R is the effective radius of the atom and ε is the dielectric constant. For such a situation, the reaction is controlled by the frontier electrons and the activity follows equation

$$A = \sum_s (bC_s + \lambda q_s + \lambda^1 q_s^2) + C \quad . \tag{8}$$

Cammarata demonstrated some data for a series of sulfanilamides which followed this equation.

It can be confidently expected that as the theories become more refined, the equation relating biological activity to structure will become more sophisticated. We seem to be entering an era where the complete description of a biological reaction will be possible. Such a situation will allow more accurate predictions of structures with specified activity.

V. REFERENCES

[1] Szent-Györgi, A., p. 64 in *Current Aspects of Biochemical Energetics*, Academic Press, New York, (1966).

[2] Pullman B. and Pullman A., *Quantum Biochemistry* , Wiley (Interscience), New York, (1963).

[3] Streitweiser, A., Jr., *Molecular Orbital Theory for Organic Chemists* , Wiley, New York, (1961).

[4] Neely, W. B., Unger, I., Blair, E. H., Nyquist, R. A., *Biochemistry* 3, 1477, (1964); Neely, W. B., *Mol. Pharmacol.*, 1, 137, (1965).

[5] Neely, W. B., White, H. C., Rudzik, A., *J. Pharm. Sci.* 57, 1176, (1968).

[6] Fujita, T., Iwasa, J., Hansch, C., *J. Am. Chem. Soc.*, 86, 5175, (1964).

[7] Hoffmann, R., *J. Chem. Phys.*, 39, 1397, (1963).

[8] Allen, L. C. and Russell, J. D., *J. Chem. Phys.*, 46, 1029, (1967).

[9] Kier, L. B., *Mol. Pharmacol.*, 3, 487, (1967).

[10] Jellinek, F., *Acta. Cryst.* , 10, 277, (1957).

[11] Chiou, C. Y., Long, J. P., Cannon, J. G., Armstrong, P. D., *J. Pharmacol. Exp. Therap.*, 166, 243, (1969).

[12] Reeves, R. E., *Advan. Carbohydrate Chem.*, 6, 197, (1951).

[13] Neely, W. B., *J. Med. Chem.*, 12, 16, (1969).

[14] Eliel, E. L., Allinger, N. L., Angyal, S. J., Morrison, G. A., *Conformational Analysis*, Interscience, New York, (1965).

[15] Rao, V. S. R., Sundararajan, P. R., Ramakishnan, C., Ramachandran, G. N., p. 721, in *Conformation of Biopolymers*, 2, (G. N. Ramachandran, Ed.), Academic Press, New York, (1967).

[16] DeDatta, S. K., Bantilan, R. T., Park, J. K., *Nature*, 221, 64, (1969).

[17] Johnson, F., *Chem. Rev.*, 68, 375, (1968).

[18] Overberger, C. G. and Tanner, D., *J. Am. Chem. Soc.*, 77, 369, (1955).

[19] Fukui, K, Yonezawa, T., Shingu, H., *J. Chem. Phys.*, 20, 722, (1952).

[20] Hoffmann, R. and Imamura, A., *Biopolymers*, 7, 207, (1969).

[21] Boer, F. P., Newton, M. D., Lipscomb, W. N., *Ibid.*, 52, 890, (1964).

[22] Newton, M. D., Boer, F. P., Palke, W. E., Lipscomb, W. N., *Proc. Natl. Acad. Sci. U.S.*, 52, 890, (1964).

[23] Newton, M. D., Boer, F. P., Lipscomb, W. N., *J. Am. Chem. Soc.*, 88, 2353, (1966); Boer, F. P., Newton, M. D., Lipscomb, W. N., *Ibid.*, 88, 2361, (1966); Newton, M. D., Boer, F. P., Lipscomb, W. N., *Ibid.*, 88, 2367, (1966); Palke, W. E., Lipscomb, W. N., *Ibid.*, 88, 2384, (1966).

[24] Boer, F. P. and Lipscomb, W. N., *J. Chem. Phys.*, 50, 989, (1969).

[25] Cammarata, A., *J. Med. Chem.*, 11, 1111, (1968).

[26] Klopman, G. and Hudson, R. F., *Theoret. Chem. Acta*, 8, 165, (1967).

[27] Klopman, G., *J. Am. Chem. Soc.*, 90, 223, (1968).

QUANTITATIVE STRUCTURE-ACTIVITY RELATIONSHIPS AND MOLECULAR ORBITALS IN MEDICINAL CHEMISTRY

by

William P. Purcell*

and

John M. Clayton *‡

I. INTRODUCTION

Seeking to attain the ultimate goal of rational drug design and to aid in the postulation of drug-action mechanisms at the molecular level, investigators have employed two distinctly different techniques of particular interest to us. In the first technique, statistical methods have been applied to the correlation of biological activity data with either the arbitrary parameters of the mathematical models such as that reported by Free and Wilson [1] or linear free-energy-related physicochemical properties ascribed to portions of the molecule, such as the widely applied model of Hansch [2,3,4]. Although gradual changes in chemical structure and corresponding changes in biological activity have intrigued scientists for about 100 years [5], significant progress in quantitative correlation techniques has developed only in the past fifteen years or so [6,7,8].

In addition to the efforts to correlate changes in biological response with changes in structure and/or physicochemical properties, the advent of high-speed digital computers and labor-saving approximations to solutions of the Schrödinger equation have made it feasible for quantum biologists to calculate electronic indices of biologically important molecules [6,9], a second important technique. The purpose of performing such calculations (mostly on π-electron systems) has been associated primarily with attempted correlations between biological activity and electronic indices, such as HOMO, LEMO, charge density

* Department of Molecular and Quantum Biology, College of Pharmacy, University of Tennessee Medical Units.

*‡United States Public Health Services Fellow.

distribution, free valence, etc. Unfortunately, research associated with quantitative correlation techniques and that of "quantum biology" have proceeded along relatively independent lines, seldom meeting. These authors are of the opinion that real progress will be made when one can (1) characterize the molecules from a physicochemical point of view (nmr, infrared, dipole moments, etc.), (2) calculate important quantum mechanical properties, and (3) build models from the results from (1) and (2). Efforts along these lines are in progress in our laboratories.

II. EXAMPLE OF THE FREE-WILSON METHOD

One of the primary objectives of conducting regression analyses is to improve and streamline the selection of potentially useful molecules for synthesis and evaluation. For example, in 1965 we published the results of a regression analysis on 12 carbamoylpiperidines and their corresponding inhibitory potencies against butyrylcholinesterase [10]. Within this series, 36 of the homologs had not been synthesized and evaluated biologically; the Free-Wilson method was used to predict their inhibitory potencies. In this method, one assumes that the substituent group activities of an analogous series of compounds may be mathematically additive to the total biological response parameter [1]. For meaningful application of this method, the biological data should meet three basic prerequisites: (1) molecules in the series should be closely similar to increase the probability of a constant mechanism of action, (2) biological activity selected should be accurate, quantitative, and measured under uniform conditions for the series, and (3) the group contributions to the chosen activity parameters should be intrinsically additive [11]. It is also desirable for the data to have a high number of degrees of freedom since the greater the ratio of number of observations to number of unknowns, the more significant are the results. It should be emphasized that this method is proposed primarily to pinpoint the more active substituent groups and substituent positions. From a knowledge of the substituent group contributions, of course, one can calculate or predict activities of molecules within the series.

Using the Free-Wilson method, we predicted the pI_{50} value (the negative logarithm of the molarity of compound necessary to effect 50% inhibition of the enzyme) of 1-decyl-3-(N-ethyl-N-methylcarbamoyl) piperidine hydrobromide to be 4.99 [10]. Three years after our prediction of the activity, this compound was synthesized and evaluated against butyrylcholinesterase. The observed inhibitory potency was found to have a pI_{50} value of 5.01 ± 0.03 [12], which is in excellent agreement with the predicted value. The important point here is that the quantitative activity prediction for a single derivative, which preceded its synthesis by three years, agrees well with the observed value. It should be mentioned, however, that one may expect an activity for this particular compound in the range of $pI_{50} = 5.0$, but the significance of this result lies in the quantitative prediction rather than a qualitative estimate of the molecule's activity.

III. EXAMPLE OF THE HANSCH METHOD

The linear free-energy-related model of Hansch [2] has been suggested to relate certain physicochemical parameters (such as partition coefficients, Hammett constants, and steric parameters) of substituent groups in analogous series to a biological response parameter. In the generalized Hansch equation (Equation 1),

$$\log 1/C_X = -a\pi^2 + b\pi + \rho\sigma + c \qquad (1)$$

C_X is the concentration of compound necessary to elicit a defined response, such as the 50% inhibition of cholinesterase; a, b, ρ, and c are constants generated by the least squares solution. Pi is the free-energy-related substituent constant defined as the logarithm of the partition coefficient of the derivative minus the logarithm of the partition coefficient of the parent unsubstituted compound, and σ is the Hammett electronic constant for the substituent. If there is more than one substituent position in a series of compounds, each of these parameters would consist of the sums of the substituent parameters. We applied the Hansch method to six 1-decyl-3-carbamoylpiperidine hydrobromides from the same series studied by the Free-Wilson method [13]. Nine modifications of the Hansch equation were used (Equation 2-10)

$$pI_{50} = -a\pi^2 + b\pi + \rho\mu + c \tag{2}$$

$$pI_{50} = -a\pi^2 + b\pi + \rho m + c \tag{3}$$

$$pI_{50} = -a\pi^2 + b\pi + \rho\sigma^* + c \tag{4}$$

$$pI_{50} = b\pi + \rho\mu + c \tag{5}$$

$$pI_{50} = b\pi + \rho\sigma^* + c \tag{6}$$

$$pI_{50} = -a\pi^2 + \rho\mu + c \tag{7}$$

$$pI_{50} = b\pi + \rho m + c \tag{8}$$

$$pI_{50} = -a\pi^2 + b\pi + c \tag{9}$$

$$pI_{50} = b\pi + c \tag{10}$$

where μ is the electric dipole moment of the identically substituted nicotinamides [14], m is the amide group dipole moment [15], and σ^* is the Taft substituent constant which is dependent only upon the net polar effect of the substituent [16] and is analogous to the Hammett substituent constant [17]. Correlations between the observed and calculated pI_{50} values were all significant at greater than the 99% level of confidence with squares of the correlation coefficients greater than 0.94 (Table 1). Of the nine equations used, Equation 13 gave the best fit for the regression and a predicted pI_{50} value, 5.00, for 1-decyl-3-(N-ethyl-N-methylcarbamoyl) piperidine hydrobromide which is in excellent agreement with the observed value. It is of interest to calculate an ideal π value, π_0 [18], which is the π value giving maximum activity; π_0 from Equation 13 is 5.06.

IV. COMPARISON OF THE FREE-WILSON AND HANSCH METHODS

For some time we have been interested in making a side-by-side comparison of the results from a Free-Wilson and Hansch analysis on the same series of compounds; this work afforded an excellent opportunity to do so. The results of the two methods [13], along with the observed pI_{50} values, are given in Table 2. Again the reader's attention is called to 1-decyl-3-(N-ethyl-N-methylcarbamoyl)

TABLE 1. HANSCH ANALYSIS OF BUTYRYLCHOLINESTERASE INHIBITORY POTENCIES OF SOME 1-DECYL-3-CARBAMOYLPIPERIDINE HYDROBROMIDES[a]

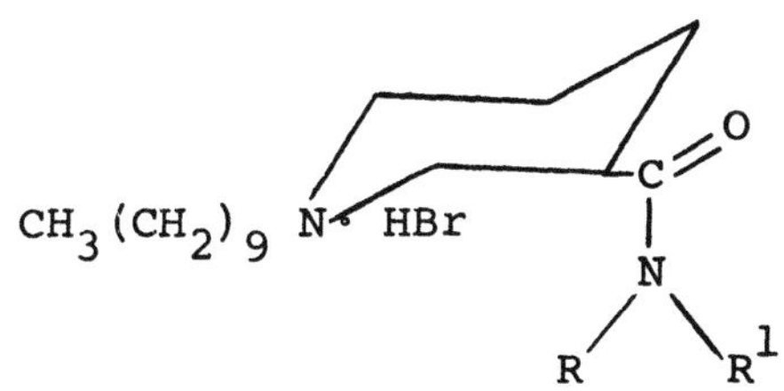

R =	H	H	H	CH_3	C_2H_5	C_3H_7
R^1 =	H	CH_3	C_2H_5	CH_3	C_2H_5	C_3H_7

Equation	Square of Correlation Coefficient r^2	F-ratio	
$pI_{50} = -0.058\pi^2 + 0.923\pi - 0.456\mu + 5.589$ ($\pi_o = 7.96$)	0.998	926.50	(11)
$pI_{50} = -0.060\pi^2 + 0.933\pi - 0.396m + 5.683$ ($\pi_o = 7.78$)	0.998	1194.50	(12)
$pI_{50} = -0.119\pi^2 + 1.205\pi + 0.687\sigma^* + 3.533$ ($\pi_o = 5.06$)	0.998	8984.10	(13)
$pI_{50} = 0.699\pi - 0.268\mu + 5.061$	0.994	274.30	(14)
$pI_{50} = 0.397\pi - 0.394\sigma^* + 4.566$	0.974	57.11	(15)
$pI_{50} = 0.132\pi^2 + 0.338\mu + 3.302$	0.943	24.71	(16)
$pI_{50} = 0.667\pi - 0.227m + 5.094$	0.994	269.08	(17)
$pI_{50} = 0.011\pi^2 + 0.535\pi + 4.203$	0.984	102.99	(18)
$pI_{50} = 0.570\pi + 4.187$	0.985	268.43	(19)

(a) Table 1 in Reference 13.

TABLE 2. OBSERVED AND CALCULATED BUTYRYLCHOLINESTERASE INHIBITORY POTENCIES OF SOME 1-DECYL-3-CARBAMOYLPIPERIDINE HYDROBROMIDES[(a)]

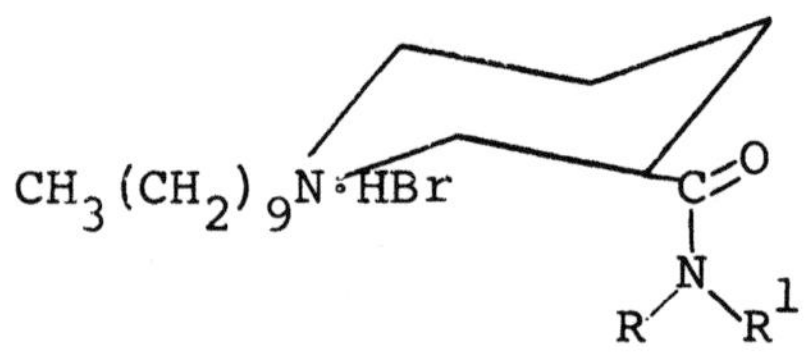

R	R^1	pI_{50}		
		Observed	Calculated	
			Free-Wilson	Hansch
H	H	4.21 ± 0.02	4.25	4.21
H	CH_3	4.46 ± 0.03	4.46	4.46
H	C_2H_5	4.86 ± 0.01	4.78	4.86
CH_3	CH_3	4.66 ± 0.04	4.66	4.66
CH_3	C_2H_5	5.01 ± 0.03	4.99	5.00
C_2H_5	C_2H_5	5.28 ± 0.02	5.32	5.29
C_3H_7	C_3H_7	5.98 ± 0.03	5.98	5.98

(a) Table 3 in Reference 13.

piperidine hydrobromide, which was not included in either regression analysis. Both predicted values, 5.00 by the Hansch method and 4.99 by the Free-Wilson analysis, for this derivative are within the experimental error of the observed pI_{50}, 5.01 ± 0.03. Although both methods give very good correlations, the calculated pI_{50} values from the Hansch analysis are all within the experimental error of the observed values. The calculated pI_{50} values from the Free-Wilson method, however, are within the experimental error of the observed values for only three of the six compounds, and one of these compounds, the dipropyl derivative, is forced to fit since it represents a single observation. One must conclude that both models fit these data quite well, although the Hansch method gives somewhat better quantitative results for this series.

V. MOLECULAR ORBITAL CALCULATIONS

For the past five years, we have been investigating the possibility of correlating electronic indices, from molecular orbital calculations, with antimalarial activity. This work is associated with the well publicized fight against drug-resistant strains of *Plasmodium falciparum* [19]. In an effort to categorize the "classical" antimalarials, the electronic structures of 34 of these drugs and related molecules were calculated by the Hückel molecular orbital method [20]. Comparison of the results of the antimalarial molecules quinine, chloroquine, primaquine, quinacrine, pyrimethamine, proguanil, cycloguanil, and 3-piperonylsydnone with those calculations on their appropriate parent or analogous molecules have elucidated the contributions of the substituents to the π-electron properties of the antimalarials [20]. Since so little is known about the mechanism of action of molecules against *Plasmodium falciparum* and since so few compounds have demonstrated significant activity, we have been unsuccessful thus far in our attempts to correlate physicochemical and quantum mechanical properties with antimalarial activity.

Another problem which has developed from our efforts to find a molecule effective against drug-resistant strains of malaria is that associated with the phototoxicity of the quinolinemethanol derivatives [21]. Derivatives of the quinolinemethanols of type I are reported to be both active against *Plasmodium berghei* in mice and phototoxic [22]. The 2-phenyl group is believed to contribute to the high activity by preventing oxidation to carbostyril [23]. The activity

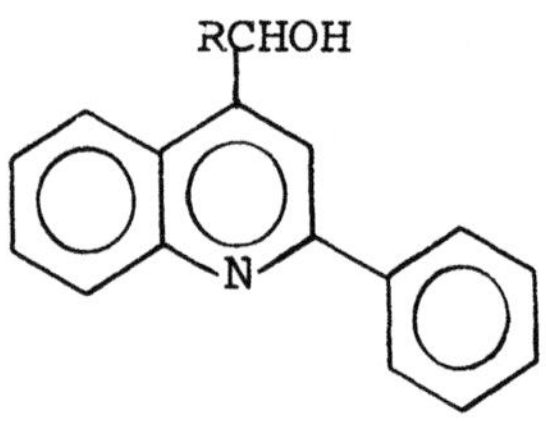

I

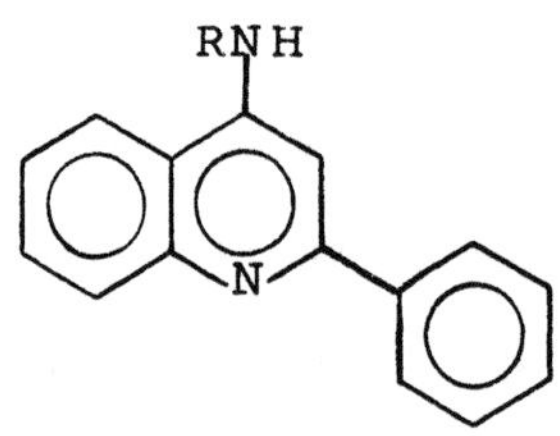

II

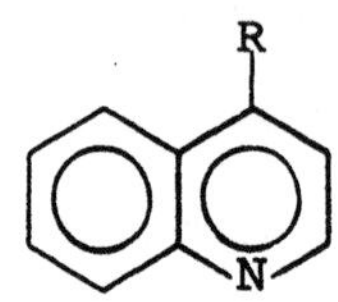

$R = R^1CHOH$ or R^1NH

III

decreases markedly and phototoxicity is not observed, however, when an >NH moiety replaces >CHOH (derivatives of type II) or if the 2-phenyl group is removed (derivatives of type III) [24]. Several laboratories, including ours, have as their target a molecular modification of quinolinemethanol which would preserve the high activity of the 2-phenyl derivatives and reduce the phototoxicity.

Chloroquine, IV, is also a derivative of quinoline and serves as an interesting compound for comparison. It undergoes metabolic attack on the amino side chain [25] rather than at the 2 position as is found in quinolinemethanols of

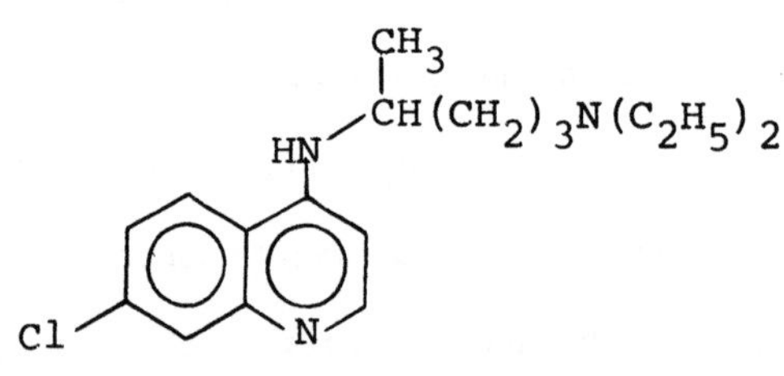

IV

type III. Also, since 2-phenyl anologs of chloroquine (type II) are not phototoxic [24], the phototoxicity of the quinolinemethanols of type I seems to depend on both the presence of a phenyl group at the 2 position and a methanol moiety at the 4 position.

With the idea that the electronic structures of these molecules are at least partially responsible for the activities and phototoxicities, Hückel molecular orbital calculations were performed on variations of the quinoline ring system. The aim was to use the results to assist in the rational design of molecules having maximum antimalarial activity and minimum phototoxicity. Unhappily, the results of the calculations of 16 molecules related to I, II, and III did not produce any clear-cut correlations between phototoxicity and electronic indices.

In view of the interest of sydnones as potential antimalarials [26], the Pariser-Parr-Pople-Brown-Heffernan molecular orbital method was applied to sydnone, sydnone imine, ψ-oxatriazole, and isosydnone rings [27]. The calculations suggest that, among the symbolism proposed for these mesoionic compounds, the one that best portrays the above deduction is the cyclic azo methine imine structure described by Stewart [28], V.

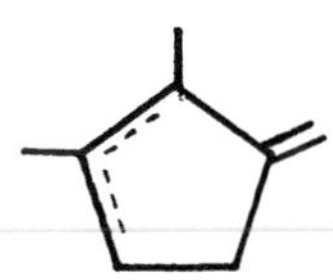

V

The net results of our various activities (application of the Free-Wilson method, application of the Hansch method, molecular orbital calculations of biologically important molecules, search for correlations between biological response and electronic indices and/or physicochemical parameters) are leading us to believe that regression analyses hold more immediate promise in drug design than do correlations between electronic indices or physicochemical parameters with biological response. This does not mean that most useful information has not come from molecular orbital calculations. To these authors, it simply indicates that the state of the art, particularly associated with the understanding of biological action at the molecular level, is, with a few exceptions, not at the level to expect clear-cut examples of useful correlations between quantum chemical indices and biological activities. We continue to anticipate that the quantum chemical indices may be most useful in the insertion of selected electronic parameters into equations which may then be subjected to regression analyses. In the meantime, however, it seems that many more examples of series of molecules with corresponding activity data will be better analyzed by the linear free-energy-related model of Hansch, or, perhaps, a mathematical model such as that proposed by Free and Wilson.

VI. ACKNOWLEDGMENT

The authors gratefully acknowledge support by the U. S. Army Medical Research and Development Command (DA-49-193-MD-2779), the National Science Foundation (GB-7383), the Cotton Producers Institute, the National Cotton Council of America, and a grant from Eli Lilly and Company during the period in which this manuscript was written. Computer facilities for the work reported were provided through Grant HE-09495 from the National Institutes of Health.

VII. REFERENCES

[1] Free, S. M., Jr., and Wilson, J. W., *J. Med. Chem.*, 7, 398 (1964).

[2] Hansch, C., and Fujita, T., *J. Am. Chem. Soc.*, 86, 1616 (1964).

[3] Hansch, C., pp. 141-167 in *Proceedings of the Third International Congress on Pharmacology, Sao Paulo, 1966*, Vol. 7, Pergamon Press, New York (1968).

[4] Hansch, C., in *Drug Design*, Vol. 1, (E. J. Ariëns, ed.) Academic Press, New York (in press).

[5] Brown, A. C., and Fraser, T., *Trans. Roy. Soc. Edinburgh*, 25, 151 (1869); through Ariëns, E. J., Simonis, A. M., and Van Rossum, J. M., "Drug-Receptor Interaction: Interaction of One or More Drugs with One Receptor System", Vol. 1, *Mol. Pharmacol.*, (E. J. Ariëns, ed.) Academic Press, New York (1964), p. 126.

[6] Purcell, W. P., Singer, J. A., Sundaram, K., and Parks, G. L., Chapter 10 in *Medicinal Chemistry*, 3rd Edition, (A. Burger, ed.) John Wiley and Sons, Inc., New York (in press), p. 164.

[7] Purcell, W. P., and Clayton, J. M., Chapter 28 in *Annual Reports in Medicinal Chemistry, 1968*, (C. K. Cain, ed.) Academic Press, New York (1969), p. 314.

[8] Cavallito, C., *Ann. Rev. Pharmacol.*, 8, 39 (1968).

[9] Pullman, B., and Pullman, A., *Quantum Biochemistry*, Interscience Publishers, New York (1963).

[10] Purcell, W. P., *Biochim. Biophys. Acta*, 105, 201 (1965).

[11] Purcell, W. P., and Clayton, J. M., *J. Med. Chem.*, 11, 199 (1968).

[12] Beasley, J. G., and Purcell, W. P., *Biochim. Biophys. Acta*, 178, 175 (1969).

[13] Clayton, J. M., and Purcell, W. P., *J. Med. Chem.*, 12, 1087 (1969).

[14] Purcell, W. P., and Singer, J. A., *J. Phys. Chem.*, 69, 4097 (1965).

[15] Purcell, W. P., *J. Phys. Chem.*, 68, 2666 (1964).

[16] Taft, R. W., Jr., Chapter 13 in *Steric Effects in Organic Chemistry*, (M. S. Newman, ed.) John Wiley and Sons, Inc., New York (1956).

[17] Hammett, L. P., *Chem. Rev.*, 17, 125 (1935).

[18] Hansch, C., Steward, A. R., Anderson, S. M., and Bentley, D., *J. Med. Chem.*, 11, 1 (1968).

[19] Tigertt, W. D., *Military Med., Suppl.*, 131, 853 (1966).

[20] Singer, J. A., and Purcell, W. P., *J. Med. Chem.*, 10, 754 (1967).

[21] Purcell, W. P., and Sundaram, K., *J. Med. Chem.*, 12, 18 (1969).

[22] Boykin, D. W., Jr., Patel, A. R., and Lutz, R. E., *J. Med. Chem.*, 11, 273 (1968).

[23] Pinder, R. M., and Burger, A., *J. Med. Chem.*, 11, 267 (1968).

[24] Rothe, W. E., and Jacobus, D. P., *J. Med. Chem.*, 11, 366 (1968).

[25] Williams, R. T., p. 652 in *Detoxication Mechanisms*, 2nd Edition, John Wiley and Sons, Inc., New York (1959).

[26] Nyberg, W. H., and Cheng, C. C., *J. Med. Chem.*, 8, 531 (1965).

[27] Sundaram, K., and Purcell, W. P., *Intern. J. Quantum Chem.*, 2, 145 (1968).

[28] Stewart, F. H. C., *Chem. Rev.*, 64, 129 (1964).

QUANTUM PERTURBATION THEORY AND LINEAR FREE ENERGY RELATIONSHIPS IN THE STUDY OF DRUG ACTION

by

Arthur Cammarata*

I. INTRODUCTION

Considerable emphasis is nowadays being placed on the development of available chemical theories for application in drug research. Impetus for these endeavors is provided by the possibility that these studies could lead to new approaches for predicting novel molecular structures having a desired biological effect. Until now the approach to the study and design of medicinal agents has centered primarily on the gross chemical structure of natural and synthetic compounds which have an established biological action. Variations of a basic structure are synthesized to arrive at structure-activity relations, and this compilation is used as a guide for the synthesis of other candidate compounds. This approach, it is estimated [1], leads to only one useful therapeutic agent out of every three to five thousand compounds synthesized.

Many persons working in drug research believe that physicochemical approaches will contribute little to our understanding of drug action and that these approaches do not seem to offer any advantage over classical methods in seeking new compounds. Mautner [2], for one, questions the physical significance of those correlations that have been obtained. These opinions are premature, for the modifications necessary to apply chemical theories to drug systems are just beginning to become known, and the operational limitations have yet to be defined. Even at this early stage, however, the statistical approaches implicit in quantum perturbation theory [3] are being applied with considerable success in mapping the

*Temple University, School of Pharmacy, Philadelphia, Pennsylvania.

electronic topography of certain drug receptors [4]. Linear free-energy methods are also being used effectively in predicting the biological potencies of compounds prior to their synthesis [5-7]. It seems proper, therefore, to reserve judgment on the worth of physicochemical approaches in the study of drug action until such time as their full potential can be realized.

II. THEORIES OF DRUG ACTION

Current theories of drug action liken the interaction of a drug with its receptor to the combination of a substrate with an enzyme. By this analogy, the elicitation of a pharmacological response is generalized in the Michaelis-Menten formalism as

$$S + R \underset{}{\overset{a}{\rightleftharpoons}} SR \xrightarrow{b} \text{response} \tag{1}$$

where S is a drug, R its receptor, and SR the drug-receptor complex leading to a given biological response. Once this formalism is accepted, the distinction between the current theories of drug action may be considered as corresponding to the choice of response (rate) determining step. Thus, in the kinetic theory of Paton [8], the association-dissociation of drug and receptor (Step a) is the response-determining step, while the occupation theory of Ariëns [9] places the response-determining step after the formation of the drug-receptor complex (Step b).

Extending this analogy further, it may be stated that in the absence of supplemental studies the number of steps preceding and following the response-determining step is largely unknown. In principle, any number of steps can lead to and follow the response-determining one. The actual steps that are taken, which if known would constitute the molecular mechanism of action for a drug, may be considered specific for a given type of drug and receptor. Hence, those theories of drug action which invoke a change in the structure [10] or function [11] of the receptor substance seem to provide mechanistic detail to the Paton and Ariëns theories and represent probable mechanisms of action, at the molecular level, for a given drug-receptor system.

The discussion which follows applies strictly to a single response (rate) limiting step in which only the nature of the drug (or substrate) is known. The relations deduced may apply to more complex situations provided that the apparent behavior of the drug is in accord with Equation (1). In this instance, however, a molecular interpretation becomes more difficult.

III. GENERAL CONSIDERATIONS

If it is assumed that drug activity is related to the free energy for the formation of the pharmacologically important drug-receptor complex, then a measure of drug activity, A, which suitably reflects the equilibrium or rate constant for the formation of the drug-receptor complex should be in accord with equations of the form

$$A = -\left(\frac{1}{RT}\right) \Delta G + d' \tag{2}$$

or if it is assumed that the entropy change is constant for a given series of drug-receptor interactions,

$$A = -\left(\frac{1}{RT}\right) \Delta E + d \quad . \tag{3}$$

IV. PARALLELISM BETWEEN QUANTUM AND LINEAR FREE-ENERGY APPROACHES

Equation (3) suggests that the formalisms arrived at by the application of quantum theory should be equally applicable in linear free-energy treatments of chemical interaction. Of course, the indices used differ in each approach, those arising from quantum theory being more soundly based; but quantum theory may be considered as providing a framework for the development of linear free-energy approaches.

In the usual quamtum chemical description of the energetics of chemical interactions, it is assumed initially that all factors influencing the interaction can be treated independently. With drug systems, electronic (e), solvation (d), steric (s), and conformational (p) energy changes may each be considered as contributing to varying degrees in the formation of a drug-receptor complex. Drug activity might, therefore, be discussed in terms of the relation

$$A = -\frac{1}{RT} (\Delta E^e + \Delta E^d + \Delta E^s + \Delta E^p) + d \quad , \tag{4}$$

where each component refers to the respective energy changes that could take place.

As will be indicated later, the use of free-energy changes in place of ground-state energy changes in Equation (4) leads to an extrathermodynamic relationship similar to one of those discussed by Leffler and Grunwald [12].

Many times one or more of the components in Equation (4) may be constant or negligible, but *a priori* there is usually no way to say with certainty which of the components can be eliminated in a specific application. The usual approach is to calculate first the electronic component, and if a satisfactory fit is found to the relation

$$A = -\frac{1}{RT}\Delta E^e + d \quad , \tag{5}$$

the other components are said to be constant or negligible. A poor fit to Equation (5) implies that one or more of the other components plays a role in the interaction under study. The solvation energy change is ordinarily the next term taken into account, and a fit is then sought to the relation

$$A = -\frac{1}{RT}(\Delta E^e + \Delta E^d) + d \quad . \tag{6}$$

With drug systems, if the conformation of the drug-receptor complex is not affected appreciably by the structure of the drug, data plotted according to Equation (6) should lead to dispersion when steric factors come into play. [13] Alternatively, if steric factors are taken into account in some manner, a fit is sought to the relation

$$A = -\frac{1}{RT}(\Delta E^e + \Delta E^d + \Delta E^S) + d \quad . \tag{7}$$

The procedure outlined is essentially the same as is followed by Hansch in his adaptation of the linear free-energy approach to biological systems. [14]

The parallelism between the quantum and the linear free-energy approaches becomes most evident when atom-for-atom or group-for-group interaction between drug and receptor is given by

$$A = -\frac{1}{RT}\sum_r\sum_s (E_{rs} + L_{rs} + V_{rs}) + d \quad . \tag{8}$$

Equation (8) is most readily applied when

a. each component is factorable

$$E_{rs} = E_r E_s ; \; L_{rs} = L_r L_s ; \; V_{rs} = V_r V_s \tag{9}$$

b. each component is additive

$$E_{rs} = \alpha E_r + \beta E_s ; \; L_{rs} = \mu L_r + \nu L_s ; \; V_{rs} = \tau V_r + \epsilon V_s \tag{10}$$

or if a combination of factorable and additive components pertain. Depending on the approach taken, s and r may be identified with properties of the substituents (or portions of a substituent) or of atoms associated with drug and receptor, respectively. Substitution of Equations (9) into Equation (8) leads to an expression equivalent to the result of the first-order interaction extrathermodynamic treatment given by Leffler and Grunwald [12]. Alternatively, quantum theory can be shown [3] to provide components of the form required by Equations (9) and (10). In each case, the equation takes the practical form

$$A = \sum_s (aE_s + bL_s + cV_s) + d \quad . \tag{11}$$

V. ADDITIVITY IN DRUG ACTIVITY

Before providing a quantum chemical development of Equations (8) and (11), it is suitable at this point to investigate the applicability of the relations developed previously to drug systems. Equation (4) suggests that drug activity, in at least some instances, should be interpretable in terms of independent physical components. More importantly, for those cases where Equation (4) does apply, it may be possible to show the additivity required by Equation (11). An interesting application of Equation (4), in extrathermodynamic terms, has been given by Belleau and Lacasse [15] in their studies of the conformational changes of the cholinergic receptor. [16,17] Cammarata and Yau [18] have demonstrated additivity for the same group of tetracyclines whose antibacterial effects have been correlated with quantum chemical indices [19].

In one treatment of enzyme-inhibitor interactions [20], the free-energy change accompanying the binding of an inhibitor to an enzyme is represented by

$$\Delta G = \Delta G_v + \Delta G_h + \Delta G_p \quad , \tag{12}$$

where the subscripts refer to independent contributions due to van der Waals forces (v), water-release or hydrophobic bonding (h), and conformational changes that the enzyme may undergo (p). With a conformationally related or an homologous series of compounds, the difference in binding noted between two members of a drug series may be given by

$$d(\Delta G) = d(\Delta G_v) + d(\Delta G_h) + d(\Delta G_p) \quad . \tag{13}$$

Consider the difference in the free energy of binding for the two competitive inhibitors of acetylcholinesterase (AChE) represented by Structures I and II in which a hydrogen atom of one of the inhibitors is substituted by a methyl group. The van der Waals and hydrophobic interactions a hydrogen sutstituent

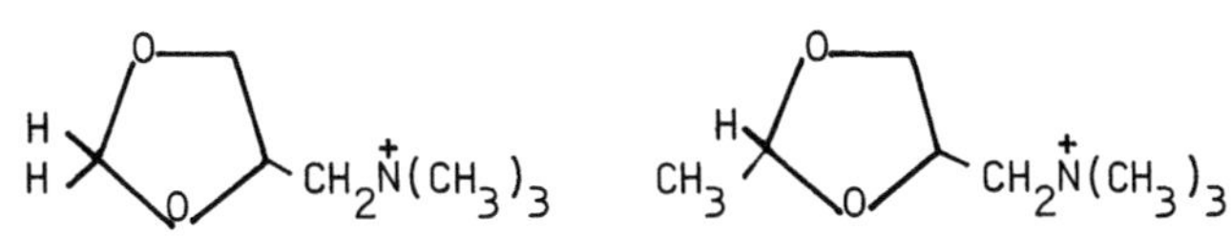

STRUCTURE I STRUCTURE II

may undergo with the receptor should be small relative to the corresponding interactions for a methyl substituent and may, therefore, be neglected. Hence, if conformational effects in the interaction between drug and receptor are constant or negligible, the observed difference in free energy (i.e., ΔpI_{50}, where I_{50} is one-half the concentration needed for maximum inhibition of AChE) should be related primarily to van der Waals and hydrophobic interactions attributed to the methyl group.

The free-energy change accompanying the loss of bound water from a methyl group is about -730 cal/mole [21] and the van der Waals energy for the interaction of a methyl group with another methyl or methylene group (which may be thought of as part of the enzyme) is about -600 cal/mole [22]. Thus, the maximum difference between the free energies of binding for Structures I and II should be near -1330 cal/mole. The experimentally determined value is -1355 cal/mole [15] which is in good agreement with expectations.

A general test of additivity within the observed activities of a series of drugs is provided by modifying Equation (11) to the form

$$A_n = \sum_g a_{ng} + \mu \tag{14}$$

where, for a series of N compounds, $n = 1, 2, \ldots, N$. Equation (14) may be recognized as the statistical model used by Free and Wilson [23] in correlating certain types of drug activity.

The regression technique followed by Free and Wilson in obtaining the activity contributions a_g for a specific system is a convenient one statistically [24], and others are adopting the same method [25-28]. There is now, however, a physical basis for Equation (14) and because of this, more attention should be given to the limiting conditions applied in the solution of this set of simultaneous equations. Insofar as it is possible, the limiting conditions should be defined so as to be compatible with the physical limitations imposed by the system under study. Singer and Purcell [29] have indicated the possible consequence of a parabolic behavior for a single component contained in a_g. In such instances, an equation similar in form to the statistical model used by Kopecky et al. [30-31] seems to result;

$$A = a_x + a_y + b_x b_y \quad . \tag{15}$$

One way to define conditions so as to apply Equation (14) is to set μ equal to the biological activity observed for a parent (unsubstituted) compound and to assign $(H)_g$ as zero for the biological effect of a hydrogen substituent. The group contributions presented in Table 1 are derived in this manner [8] using the *in vitro* bacteriostatic potencies observed [32] for the tetracyclines in Table 2. Since the antibiotics in Table 2 have only a single substituent on the aromatic D-ring (structure III), a test of additivity is provided by summing appropriate group contributions to attempt to predict the activities that should be observed for tetracyclines having multiple substitutions on the D-ring. Table 3 presents the calculated relative order of inhibition potencies that should be observed for some such tetracyclines with *Escherichia coli W* as the test organism. These are compared with the inhibition potencies observed [33] for the corresponding tetracyclines with *Staphylococcus aureus* as the test organism. Considering the difference in test organism and assay procedure, the general agreement, at least with respect to order, is satisfactory.

TABLE 1. GROUP PARAMETERS FOR TETRACYCLINES (*ESCHERICHIA COLI W* AS THE TEST ORGANISM)

Substituent[a]	Activity Contribution, a[b]	σ^2 [c]	σ_I [d]	r_v [e]
$(NO_2)_7$	0.899	1.613[f]		1.20[g]
$(OH)_6$	0.569		0.48	1.40
$(NH_2)_7$	0.284	0.436		1.20[g]
$(NH_2)_9$	0.186	0.436		1.55
$(Cl)_7$	0.170	0.051		1.20[g]
$(OH)_5$	-0.034		0.48	1.40
$(CH_3)_6$	-0.110		-0.04	2.00
$(Br)_7$	-0.261	0.054		1.20[g]
$(NO_2)_9$	-0.328	0.609		2.59
$(N(CH_3)_2)_9$	-0.601	0.360		3.11

(a) The subscript after the paecnthesis refers to the position of the substituent.

(b) Derived for the activities of Table 2 with $\mu = 1.975$ and $(H)_g = 0$.

(c) Hammett values from H. Jaffe, *Chem. Rev.*, 53, 191 (1953).

(d) From M. Charton, *J. Org. Chem.*, 29, 1222 (1964).

(e) From M. Charton, *J. Amer. Chem. Soc.*, 91, 615 (1969).

(f) Enhanced value.

(g) For 9-H.

TABLE 2. INHIBITION CONSTANTS FOR SOME TETRACYCLINES AGAINST *ESCHERICHIA COLI W*

Substituents(a)				Inhibition Constants(b)
R_5	R_6	R_7	R_9	log k_i
H	H	NO_2	H	2.874
H	OH	Cl	H	2.714
H	CH_3,OH	Cl	H	2.604
H	CH_3,OH	H	H	2.434
OH	CH_3,OH	H	H	2.400
H	H	NH_2	H	2.259
H	H	H	NH_2	2.161
H	H	H	H	1.975
H	H	Br	H	1.714
H	H	H	NO_2	1.647
H	H	H	$N(CH_3)_2$	1.374

(a) Positions indicated by subscript.

(b) Data of reference [32]. Derived using bacterial growth kinetics. The inhibition constant k_i is the slope in a plot of $k = k_0 - k_i(T)$ where T is the concentration of a given tetracycline.

TABLE 3. TETRACYCLINE ACTIVITIES CALCULATED FOR *ESCHERICHIA COLI W* AND OBSERVED WITH *STAPHYLOCOCCUS AUREUS* AS THE TEST ORGANISM

Substituents(a)			*In Vitro* Activities	
R_6	R_7	R_9	*E. Coli W*, calcd.(b)	*S. Aureus*, obsd.(c)
H	Cl	NH_2	2.331	525
H	Br	NH_2	1.900	320
H	NO_2	NH_2	1.833	275
CH_3	NO_2	NH_2	1.723	160
CH_3	Br	NH_2	1.790(d)	140(d)
H	NO_2	NO_2	2.546(d)	60(d)
H	Cl	NO_2	1.817(d)	21(d)
H	Br	NO_2	1.386	15

(a) Positions indicated by subscript.

(b) Based on the data contained in Table I.

(c) Data of Ref.[33] expressed as minimum inhibitory concentration (MIC) relative to tetracycline.

(d) Deleting these data points, the agreement is found to be

$$\log k_i(\text{calcd.}) = 0.50 \log \text{MIC(obsd.)} + 0.73 \quad \frac{n}{5} \quad \frac{s}{0.19} \quad \frac{r}{0.89}\ .$$

Two compounds, the 7,9-dinitro and the 7-chloro-9-nitro derivatives, have their place in the order of activities poorly predicted. With the dinitro derivative it may be postulated that the intramolecular hydrogen bond known to exist between the phenol and the adjacent 9-nitro group [34] is perturbed from its normal configuration by conjugation of the phenol with the 7-nitro substituent. Conversely, the conjugation of the 7-nitro group with the phenolic hydroxyl group is perturbed because of the intramolecular hydrogen bonding. Hence, it should not be unexpected that group contributions determined in the absence of these competing influences lead to poor predictabilities. A similar argument may not be suitable for the 7-chloro-9-nitro derivative, since a chloro substituent is not expected to be

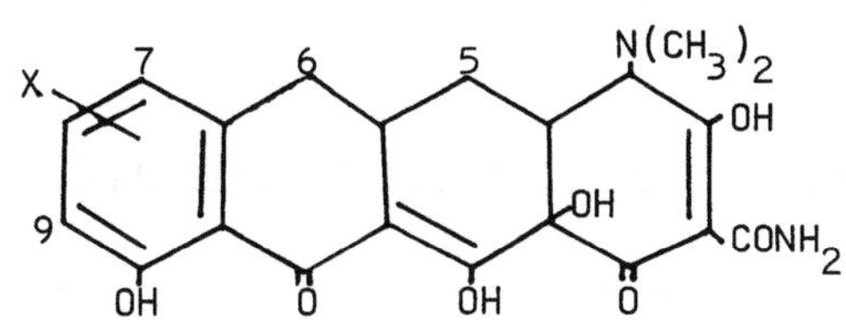

STRUCTURE III

as strongly conjugated as a nitro substituent. The origin of the apparent non-additivity in this instance is obscure at present.

If the group activities presented in Table 1 consist of additive physical components, as the theoretical development suggests, then it should be possible to show that this is indeed the case. Taking an extrathermodynamic perspective, Cammarata and Yau [7] have found that the group parameters referring to D-ring substitutions are correlated by the equation

$$a_{7\text{ or }9} = \underset{(\pm 0.18)}{0.87\,\sigma^2} - \underset{(\pm 0.16)}{0.57\,r_D} + 0.84 \qquad \frac{n}{7} \quad \frac{s}{0.22} \quad \frac{r}{0.93} \tag{16}$$

The standard deviations for each coefficient, indicated in parentheses, show each term in the equation to contribute significantly. A correlation is also found with group parameters associated with the aliphatic substituents, but there are too few substituent variations in this case to attach any great significance to the fits obtained.

According to Equation (16), electronic effects, as measured by the Hammett σ value, and steric effects, as are encompassed by the van der Waals contact distance r_v, both contribute importantly in determining the antibacterial potency of a tetracycline. Interestingly σ^2 appears in this correlation, indicating either the effect of a bound tetracycline on a second entering (or leaving) tetracycline, as might be observed for the reaction

$$MT + T \rightleftharpoons TMT$$

or the influence of two competing pathways for the binding of a tetracycline

$$M + T \longrightarrow MT$$
$$M' + T \longrightarrow M'T\ .$$

Both of these possibilities are under active investigation. It should be noted, however, that comparative studies of tetracycline effects on synchronously and non-synchronously growing cultures of *Escherichia coli* have led to the implication that there are not two competing mechanisms of action for the tetracyclines over the concentration range studied. [35-36].

VI. QUANTUM PERTURBATION THEORY AND DRUG ACTION

Two quantum chemical methods may be used to estimate the electronic energy change found in Equation (4). The first of these requires the ground-state electronic energy of drug, receptor and drug-receptor complex to be calculated by the variation method and a difference between the energies taken. For most drug systems, however, it is either impractical or impossible to calculate the electronic energy change in this way. The receptor substance is unknown ordinarily, and even if the receptor was known it would probably be too large a molecule to treat by present-day standards. A second method makes use of quantum perturbation theory. Here the electronic energy change is determined by applying perturbation theory to describe the mutual interaction of drug and receptor. A calculation based on the variation method is applied only to determine certain electronic characteristics of the drug molecules in this instance.

Dewar [36] was apparently the first to develop a perturbation method for calculating the energy change associated with the union of two π-conjugated species R and S to form the mesomeric system RS. A similar approach was taken by Fukui and co-workers [38-40] in their discussion of the formation of charge-transfer complexes and the reactivity of aromatic compounds towards electrophilic and nucleophilic agents. Inouye et al. [41] have used arguments paralleling those of the latter workers to justify the application of delocalizability indices [38-40] in pharmacological problems. It should be pointed out, however, that all such formulations are relatively gross approximations to reality.

Recently Klopman and Hudson have described a more general perturbation treatment [42,43] in which allowance is made for ionic interactions and which is not restricted to π-conjugated molecules as were the previous treatments. According to this method, the electronic energy change associated with the union of two molecules is given by the approximate expression

$$\Delta E^e = \sum_r \sum_s \left[\frac{\gamma_{rs}}{\epsilon_{rs}} Q_r Q_s + \sum_{\substack{m \\ \text{occ}}} \sum_{\substack{n \\ \text{unocc}}} \frac{2c_{mr}^2 c_{ns}^2}{E_m - E_n} \beta_{rs}^2 - \sum_{\substack{u \\ \text{unocc}}} \sum_{\substack{v \\ \text{occ}}} \frac{2c_{ur}^2 c_{vs}^2}{E_u - E_v} \beta_{rs}^2 \right] . \tag{17}$$

Equation (17) shows that the interaction between two molecules, the MO's for which are given by the LCAO's

$$\Psi_R = \sum_r c_r X_r \quad \text{and} \quad \Psi_S = \sum_s c_s X_s$$

is controlled by the net charges Q_r and Q_s and the energy difference between the occupied and unoccupied MO's. In the first term of Equation (17), γ_{rs} is the two-center repulsion integral $(rr|ss)$ and ϵ_{rs} is the local dielectric constant which modifies the interaction.

An immediate conclusion derivable from Equation (17) is the evident intimacy between interacting molecules. The electronic characteristics of one molecule in relation to the other determines the nature of the interaction that they may undergo. It is conceivable that Equation (17) might provide an electronic basis for drug specificity, the implication being that of the many possible binding sites available to a drug in a pharmacological system only one, or a very few, receptor molecules are complimentary with a given drug molecule and perform a function that can lead to a pharmacological effect.

The solvation energy change for the interaction of drug and receptor may be given by the Born equation [44,45]

$$\Delta E^d = \sum_r \sum_s \frac{Q_r Q_s}{2D_{rs}} \left(1 - \frac{1}{\epsilon_{rs}}\right) \tag{18}$$

or, tentatively, by the expression given by Klopman [46]

$$\Delta E^d = \sum_r \sum_s \left[\frac{(Q_s - 2b^2 c_{ns}^2 x)^2 - Q_s}{2D_{ss}} \left(1 - \frac{1}{\epsilon_{rs}}\right) + \frac{(Q_r - 2b^2 c_{mr}^2 x)^2 - Q_r^2}{2D_{rr}} \left(1 - \frac{1}{\epsilon_{rs}}\right) \right] \tag{19}$$

where D_{rs} is the distance between atom r and atom s and D_{rr}, D_{ss} represent the effective radii of the respective atoms. In addition, b is the variational parameter giving the contribution of Ψ_R to the perturbed MO Ψ_{RS} and, empirically, $x = Q - Q(Q - 1)K^{1/2}$ for $Q > 0$, K being a universal constant. Equation (19) bears most directly on the mutual effects of interacting species and will therefore be used in the subsequent discussion, although entropy effects may be important. It should be noted that each interacting atom contributes independently to the solvation energy change. Thus, each atom of a receptor should make an independent and constant contribution to the solvation energy change accompanying the interaction of a series of drugs with a common receptor.

The solvation energy change estimated by Equations (18) and (19) corresponds to a difference in the energy of solvation for the drug, the receptor and the drug-receptor complex. The energy of solvation is defined for a process where a molecule in the gas phase is introduced into a solvent. In contrast, hydrophobic bonding is represented by the process

$$R(W) + S(W) \rightleftharpoons RS(W) + jW(W)$$

where each species is indicated as solvated and the liberated solvent also has become solvated. It is an easy matter to show that the energy change for this process ΔE_h is related to the solvation energy change by the equation

$$\Delta E_h = \Delta E^d + \Delta_{solv} \qquad (20)$$

where Δ_{solv} is the energy of solvation for the solvent liberated. Thus, Equations (18) and (19) may be used directly to describe hydrophobic bonding in those instances where Δ_{solv} is the same essentially for a series of compounds. Conversely, when ΔE^d is negligible, Δ_{solv} takes on the same form as ΔE^d.

VII. OPERATIONAL RELATIONS

With drug systems it is not possible to apply Equations (17) and (19) because of the occurrence in them of properties belonging to the receptor substance. It is possible, however, to arrive at limiting forms for these equations which are well-suited to investigations of drug action. The limiting cases may then be used as initial model equations in a regression analysis. Only those terms indicated as significant in the statistical analysis are maintained in the final relations, and these may be said to indicate the atoms or properties most essential for a drug to lead to a pharmacological response.

Frontier-Controlled Case

Klopman and Hudson [42,43] have shown that when the energy differences in Equation (17) are considered in terms of the frontier orbitals, a degeneracy or near-degeneracy of the frontier orbitals for two interacting molecules causes the first term in Equation (21) to become relatively insignificant. The interaction could then be characterized as frontier-controlled. A first-order perturbation treatment then gives an approximate electronic energy change

$$\Delta E^{e} = \sum_{r}\sum_{s}\left[2c_{h'r}c_{\ell s}\beta - 2c_{\ell' r}c_{hs}\beta\right] \tag{21}$$

which, for practical purposes, can be written as

$$\Delta E^{e} = \sum_{s}(\alpha_s c_{\ell s} - \alpha'_s c_{hs}) \tag{22}$$

where the AO coefficients c_ℓ and c_h refer to the LEMO and the HOMO, respectively, of the drug. The quantities α and α' are approximately constant for a series of drugs which interact with a common receptor.

A frontier-controlled interaction accompanied by essentially complete charge-transfer has its solvation energy change given by [43]

$$\Delta E^{d} = \sum_{s}\frac{K(Q_s \pm 1)^2}{2D_{ss}}\left(1 - \frac{1}{\epsilon}\right) + d'' \tag{23}$$

where the components due to each atom r should be constant for a common receptor substance. Equation (23) may be applied either as a single-parameter equation

$$\Delta E^{d} = \sum_{s} z_s(Q_s \pm 1)^2 + d'' \tag{24}$$

or as a two-parameter equation

$$\Delta E^{d} = \sum_{s}(\lambda_s Q_s \pm \lambda'_s Q_s^2) + d'' \; . \tag{25}$$

Making use of Equations (22) and (25), the counterpart of Equation (6) may be written

$$A = -\frac{1}{RT}\sum_{s}(\alpha_s c_{\ell s} - \alpha'_s c_{hs} + \lambda_s Q_s \pm \lambda'_s Q_s^2) + I \; . \tag{26}$$

The pre-factor $1/RT$ is, of course, contained in each coefficient when a regression analysis is made using Equation (26) as the statistical model. In such an analysis, any of the coefficients can take on a value of zero. If all coefficients except λ are zero, it is not possible to distinguish between the frontier and the charge-controlled cases (see below).

Inouye et al. [41]have reported a correlation between the inhibition potencies of certain nicotinic acid derivatives (IV) towards AChE and the frontier orbital (LEMO) charge densities on the carbonyl carbon. The trend found

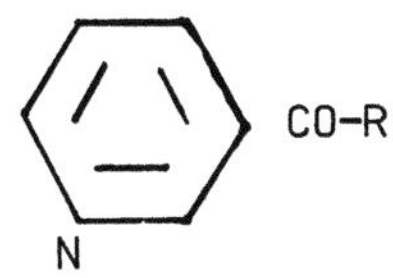

R = OH, NH_2, CH_3, OC_2H_5

STRUCTURE IV

for those compounds having a non-dissociable substituent is given in Figure 1.

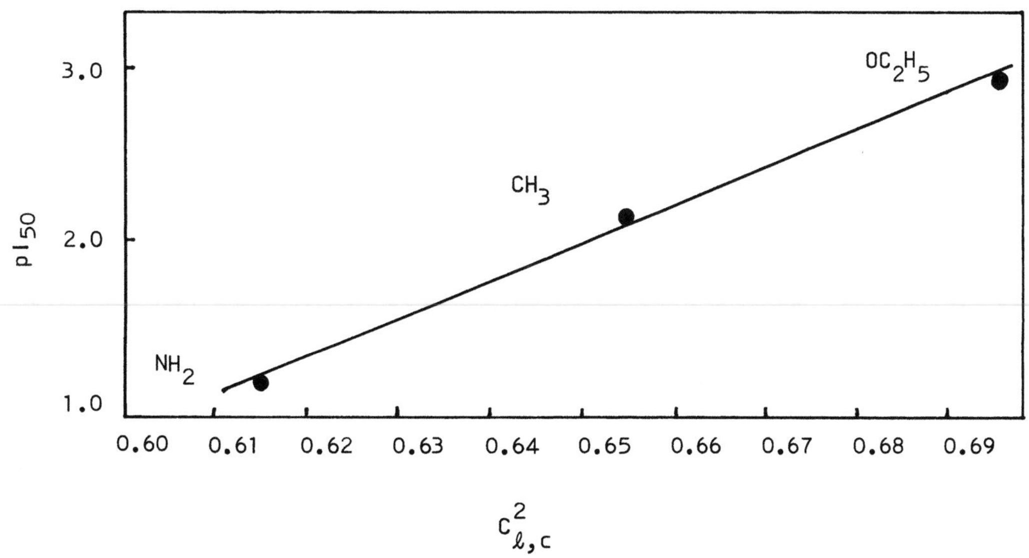

FIGURE 1. Correlation of the inhibition potencies of some nicotinic acid derivatives (3-COR pyridines) towards AChE with the frontier orbital (LEMO) charge density of the carbonyl carbon.

A regression analysis on the points illustrated leads to the equation

$$pI_{50} = 22.86\ c^2_{\ell,c} - 12.83 \quad \frac{n}{3} \quad \frac{s}{0.13} \quad \frac{r}{0.99}\ .$$

Including the point for nicotinic acid itself (not shown in Figure 1) leads to the relation

$$pI_{50} = 5.32\ c^2_{\ell,c} - 1.24 \quad \frac{n}{4} \quad \frac{s}{0.74} \quad \frac{r}{0.87}$$

The apparent lack of correlation in this very limited series may indicate that the inhibition of AChE by nicotinic acid includes a charge-controlled component.

The *in vitro* activities of at least two series of sulfanilamides towards *Escherichia coli* seems to also be dependent on a frontier-controlled interaction.[3] Minimum inhibitory concentrations (C_r) of some sulfonamides (Table 4) derived from substituted anilines are related to electronic properties calculated for the anilines by the equation

$$\log(1/C_r) = \underset{(\pm 0.73)}{1.70}\, c_{\ell,N} + \underset{(\pm 23.10)}{119.50}\, Q_N - \underset{(\pm 137.56)}{427.65}\, Q_N^2 - 2.94 \quad \frac{n}{6} \quad \frac{s}{0.05} \quad \frac{r}{0.99}\,.$$

Similarly, the activities observed for some sulfonamides derived from substituted benzamides can be related to electronic properties calculated for the benzamides

$$\log(1/C_r) = \underset{(\pm 3.22)}{8.84}\, c_{\ell,N} + \underset{(\pm 64.26)}{237.76}\, Q_N - \underset{(\pm 215.98)}{1670.92}\, Q_N^2 + 6.56 \quad \frac{n}{9} \quad \frac{s}{0.11} \quad \frac{r}{0.98}\,.$$

There is a large standard deviation associated with the determination of the coefficients in these equations, but nevertheless the trends do appear real. In no instance are the standard errors for the coefficients of greater range than the coefficients themselves.

Recently, Martin [47] has indicated that the two series of sulfonamides considered can have their activities fit to a single equation by including a dummy variable for the benzoyl series. The charge on the carbonyl carbon in this series is essentially constant and near 0.20. Use of this value for the carbonyl carbon in the benzamides and 0.00 for a corresponding value in the aniline series, which has no such group, leads to the regression equation

$$\log(1/C_r) = \underset{(\pm 2.39)}{8.76}\, c_{\ell,N} + \underset{(\pm 55.42)}{319.02}\, Q_N - \underset{(\pm 318.69)}{1731.54}\, Q_N^2 + \underset{(\pm 8.82)}{45.39}\, Q_C - 13.28 \quad \frac{n}{15} \quad \frac{s}{0.20} \quad \frac{r}{0.94}\,.$$

A comparison of this to the previous two regression equations shows that, in this instance, no substantial improvement is gained upon including a more physically realistic quantity for a dummy variable.

The magnitude of the coefficient for the Q^2 term indicates that solvation effects exert a greater influence in determining the activities of the benzamido sulfonamides than for the anilido sulfonamides. Bishop and Craig [48] have drawn attention to the possibility of counter-ions clustering in the vicinity of a charged site, and it may be that there is a greater amount of solvent (water) in the environment of the benzamido nitrogen than there is in the vicinity of the anilido nitrogen. Conceivably the loss of this charge-neutralizing arrangement of

TABLE 4. ELECTRONIC CHARACTERISTICS CALCULATED BY THE HÜCKEL METHOD FOR THE NITROGEN OF ANILINES AND BENZAMIDES AND THE *IN VITRO* ACTIVITIES OF THE CORRESPONDING SULFANILAMIDES

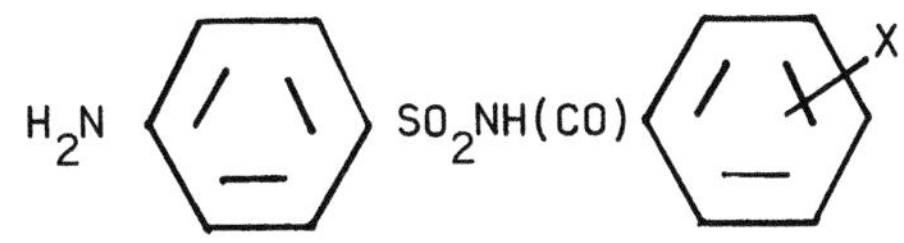

Substituent	$\log(1/C_r)^{(a,b)}$	$c_{\ell,N}$	Q_N	Q_N^2
		ANILINES		
4-NH_2	4.35	0.383	0.777	0.006
4-CH_3O	4.47	0.453	0.081	0.007
4-CH_3	4.57	0.453	0.081	0.007
H	4.80	0.477	0.083	0.007
4-Cl	4.80	0.459	0.082	0.007
4-NO_2	5.85	0.484	0.106	0.011
		BENZAMIDES		
3-CH_3,4-CH_3O	5.25	0.041	0.148	0.022
4-CH_3O(c)	5.40	0.035	0.148	0.022
3,4-CH_3	5.40	0.042	0.148	0.022
4-CH_3	5.40	0.036	0.148	0.022
3-CH_3	5.40	0.018	0.149	0.022
H	5.25	0.000	0.148	0.022
4-Cl(c)	5.10	0.027	0.148	0.022
4-CN(c)	4.05	0.000	0.151	0.023
4-NO_2(c)	4.50	0.000	0.153	0.023

(a) Minimum inhibitory concentration.

(b) Data of J. K. Seydel, *Mol. Pharmacol.*, 2:259 (1966); J. K. Seydel E. Wempe, *Arzneimittel-Forsch.*, 14:705 (1964).

(c) We gratefully acknowledge the testing of these compounds by J. K. Seydel.

solvent, as the molecule passes into a more lipophilic (less polar) solvent, could be a factor contributing to the increased Q^2 contribution in the case of the benzamido sulfonamides.

Charge-Controlled Case

When a primarily Coulombic interaction occurs with very little transfer of charge, the MO energy differences in Equation (17) will be great enough so that the small energy differences between the various molecular orbitals of each molecule can be neglected. [42,43] In this case the electronic energy change is given by

$$\Delta E^e = \sum_r \sum_s \Big[\frac{\gamma_{rs}}{\epsilon_{rs}} Q_r Q_s + \Big(\sum_{\substack{m \\ occ}} c_{mr}^2 \Big) \Big(\sum_{\substack{n \\ unocc}} \frac{2c_{ns}^2}{\bar{E}_m - E_n} \beta^2 \Big) - \Big(\sum_{\substack{u \\ unocc}} c_{ur}^2 \Big) \Big(\sum_{\substack{v \\ occ}} \frac{2c_{vs}^2}{\bar{E}_u - E_v} \beta^2 \Big) \Big] \qquad (27)$$

where $\bar{E}_m$ and $\bar{E}_u$ are average values for the occupied and unoccupied MO's of the receptor, respectively.

The last two terms of Equation (27) contain factors very closely related to Fukui's delocalizability indices, which are defined respectively by [38,39]

$$S^E = \sum_{\substack{v \\ occ}} \frac{2c_v^2}{k_v \beta_{cc}} \qquad S^N = \sum_{\substack{n \\ unocc}} \frac{2c_n^2}{k_n \beta_{cc}} \qquad (28)$$

where the energies are taken relative to the resonance integral of benzene β_{cc}. The use of these indices in Equation (27) provides an operational form of the equation for the charge-controlled case

$$\Delta E^e = \sum_s (\nu_s Q_s + \xi_s S_s^N + \zeta_s S_s^E) \,. \qquad (29)$$

The counterpart of Equation (6) therefore is

$$A = -\frac{1}{RT} \sum_s (\nu_s Q_s + \xi_s S_s^N + \zeta_s S_s^E) + \underline{I} \,. \qquad (30)$$

No term for the solvation energy change is needed, since in this case b^2 is zero and Equation (19) becomes [43]

$$\Delta E^d = 0 \,. \qquad (31)$$

An interesting, but not necessarily significant, pair of correlations can be given which indicate possible limitations on the application of Equation (30). Data reported by Waser [49] on the muscarinic activities of the compounds shown in Table 5 can be correlated[50] with charges calculated by the Berthod and Pullman procedure [51] a modification of that due to Del Re [52]. Assuming the active forms of muscarone and dehydromuscarone are the keto forms leads to the correlation

$$\log(1/C) = \underset{(\pm 1.16)}{5.63}\, Q_1^T + \underset{(\pm 0.74)}{3.62}\, Q_2^T + \underset{(\pm 0.52)}{1.85}\, Q_3^T + \underset{(\pm 1.67)}{13.52}\, Q_4^T + \underset{(\pm 1.28)}{8.85}\, Q_5^T + 2.86 \quad \frac{n}{7} \quad \frac{s}{0.11} \quad \frac{r}{0.99}\,.$$

in which the total of the σ and π net charges on all atoms are found to contribute to the biological activity observed. On the other hand, if the enol forms are assumed to be the active species, there is then obtained

$$\log(1/C) = \underset{(\pm 6.95)}{9.63}\, Q_1^T + \underset{(\pm 4.84)}{5.59}\, Q_2^T + \underset{(\pm 3.89)}{4.08}\, Q_3^T + \underset{(\pm 10.69)}{18.24}\, Q_4^T + \underset{(\pm 12.22)}{12.05}\, Q_5^T - 3.60 \quad \frac{n}{7} \quad \frac{s}{0.34} \quad \frac{r}{0.97}\,.$$

Here, the standard error of <u>each</u> coefficient is of greater range than the coefficient and no fit of the data is obtained.

A possible interpretation of these observations could have the keto forms of muscarone and dehydromuscarone the pharmacologically important species. However, no indication is provided by the correlation as to which are the most indispensable atoms in this drug series. Thus it cannot be said with certainty that the correlation reflects an actual drug-receptor interaction. Alternatively, it may be argued that this correlation is more properly considered an example of a frontier rather than a charge-controlled interaction. If this is the case, solvation energy changes are reflected by the correlation, which would be in general agreement with the views expressed by Belleau regarding the importance of water structure in cholinergic systems. [16,17] Clearly, additional studies are needed in this area.

A second cholinergic system is more definitely charge controlled. The competitive inhibitors of AChE shown in Table 6 have their inhibition potencies correlated by the equation [53]

$$pK_I = \underset{(\pm 487)}{-2571}\, Q^T - \underset{(\pm 42.90)}{283}\, S^E - 645 \quad \frac{n}{6} \quad \frac{s}{0.25} \quad \frac{r}{0.98}$$

This correlation is consistent with a hydrogen bonding interaction between the 3-OH group and the AChE receptor. [53]

TABLE 5. MUSCARINIC ACTIVITIES OF CYCLIC ANALOGS OF ACETYLCHOLINE AND CALCULATED NET CHARGES [50]

		$\log(1/C_r)$	Q_1	Q_2	Q_3	Q_4	Q_5
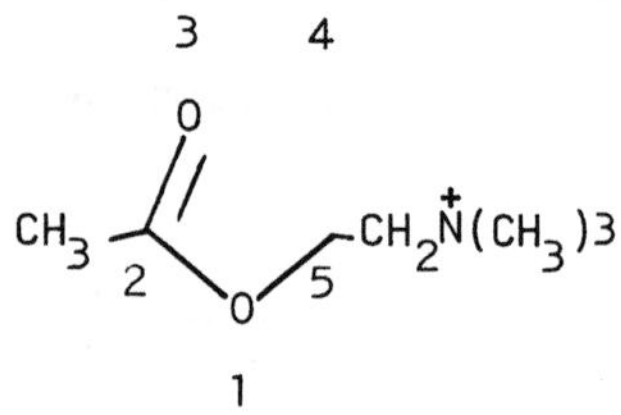		2.699	-0.193	0.335	-0.314	-----	0.032
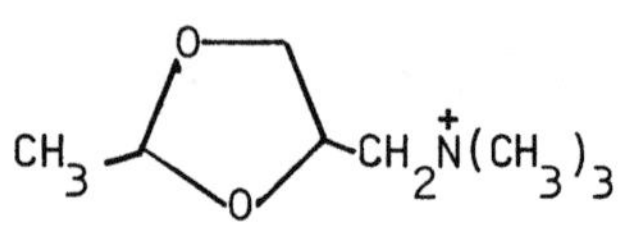		2.699	-0.266	0.167	-0.264	0.033	0.090
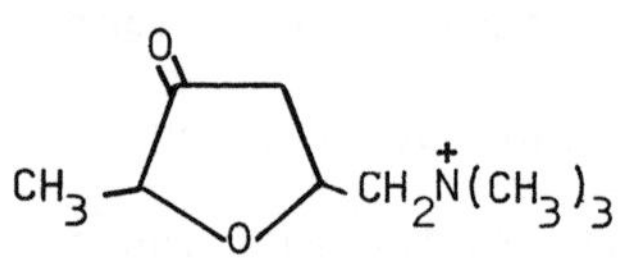	Keto:	2.000	-0.280	0.083	0.227	-0.048	0.079
	Enol:	2.000	-0.203	0.035	0.040	-0.041	0.081
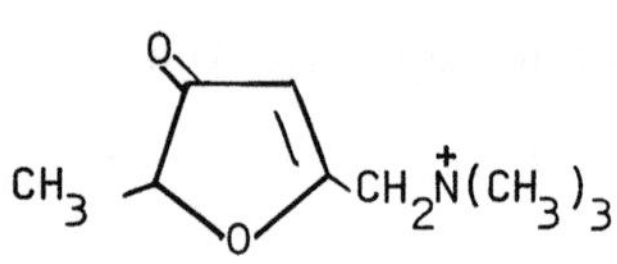	Keto:	2.000	-0.161	0.086	0.218	-0.213	0.247
	Enol:	2.000	-0.012	-0.007	0.078	-0.164	0.087
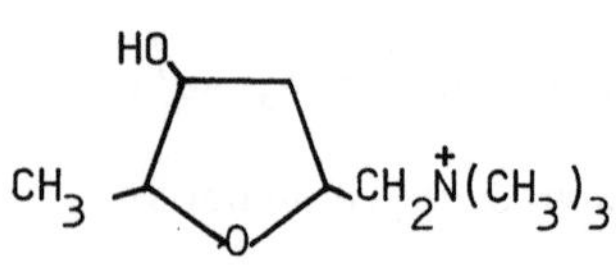		1.796	-0.281	0.079	0.091	-0.052	0.078
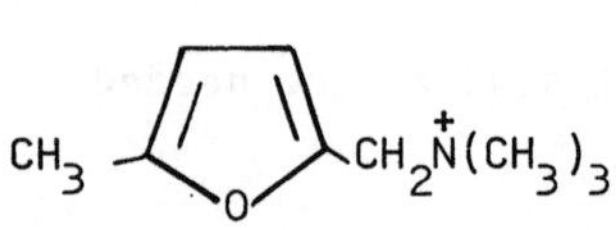		1.525	-0.004	0.072	-0.150	-0.149	0.081
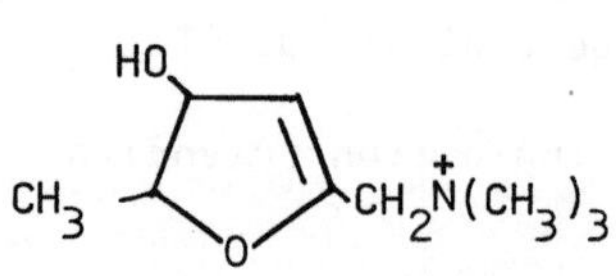		1.000	-0.177	0.082	0.104	-0.213	0.177

TABLE 6. INHIBITION CONSTANTS (pK_I), ACIDITY CONSTANTS (pK_a) AND CALCULATED ELECTRONIC PROPERTIES FOR SOME 3-HPTA DERIVATIVES

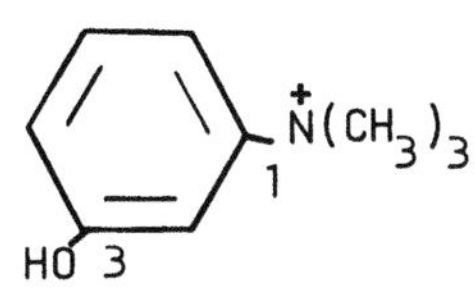

Substituent	pK_a (a)	pK_I (a)	For 3-OH(b) Q_0^T	S_0^E
4-CH_3	8.2	8.995	-0.3715	1.0628
6-CH_3	8.3	7.954	-0.3711	1.0624
5-CH_3	8.2	7.792	-0.3708	1.0610
6-CH_3O	8.6	7.716	-0.3716	1.0692
H	8.1	7.491	-0.3708	1.0610
4-CH_3O	8.0	6.068	-0.3738	1.0938

(a) From I. B. Wilson and C. Quan, *Arch. Biochem. Biophys.*, 73: 131 (1958).

(b) The reported [53] quantities are rounded-off and do not lead to correlation. Those figures given here are the properties on which the original correlation was based.

Peradejordi and Martin [19] have undertaken one of the most ambitious attempts to correlate biological potencies with calculated MO properties yet to be found. These workers employed the Del Re technique [52], as modified by Berthod and Pullman [51]; to calculate the electronic properties of 18 tetracyclines, eleven of which are found together with their *in vitro* bacteriostatic activities in Table 2. From a total of 356 possible regression formulas, the most significant statistically was the one arrived at initially

$$\begin{aligned}\log k_i = {} & 56.17\, Q^T_{O_{10}} + 16.91\, S^E_{O_{10}} \\ & + 48.79\, Q^T_{O_{11}} - 1.10\, S^E_{O_{11}} \\ & + 71.32\, Q^T_{O_{12}} + 18.36\, S^E_{O_{12}} \\ & + 3.38\, Q^T_6 + 18.39 \qquad \frac{n}{18} \quad \frac{s}{0.16} \quad \frac{r}{0.99}\end{aligned}$$

This result is consistent with a bacteriostatic mechanism in which the tetracyclines inhibit protein synthesis by binding with activated ribosomes, possibly mediated by chelation with a metal. [19]

VIII. A MO DESCRIPTION OF LIPOPHILICITY

The lipophilicity of a substance is defined ordinarily as the relative solubility of the compound in a non-polar and in a polar biophase. It is common practice to take as a measure of lipophilicity the partition coefficient for the distribution of the compound between a buffered solution and a common organic solvent. Since electronic properties should affect the solubility of at least small molecular weight compounds, it might be expected that lipophilicity should be capable of being correlated with MO indexes.

Consider the partitioning of a compound between a polar and a non-polar phase in terms of the cyclic process

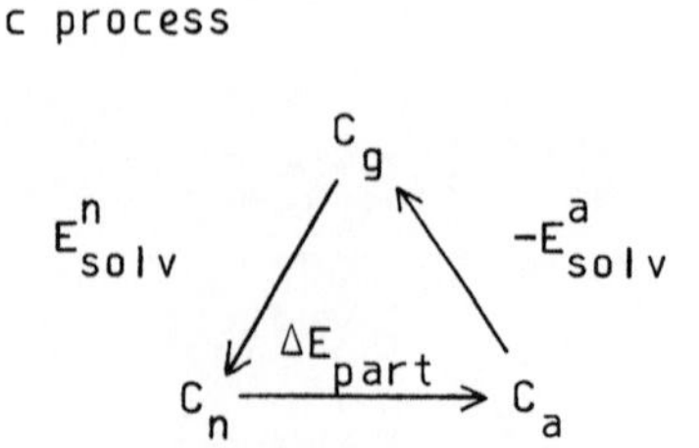

in which C_g, C_a and C_n is the compound as found in the gaseous, in an aqueous, and in an organic phase, respectively. In the first part of the cycle, the material is transferred from a gaseous to a solvated state in a non-polar solvent and the energy associated with the process is a solvation energy. In the second part of the cycle, the molecule is changed from one that is solvated with a non-polar solvent to one that is solvated with a polar, or aqueous, solvent. The energy change involved may be considered as the energy of partitioning. Finally, the compouns is stripped of its polar solvation shell and returned to the gaseous state. The energy for this process is a desolvation energy.

The energy change for the entire cycle may be represented by

$$\Delta E^o = E^n_{solv} - E^a_{solv} + \Delta E_{part} \quad , \tag{32}$$

but since no net energy change actually takes place ΔE^o is zero and hence

$$\Delta E_{part} = E^a_{solv} - E^n_{solv} \quad . \tag{33}$$

Substituting then leads to the expression

$$\ln K(o/w) = \frac{-1}{RT} (E^a_{solv} - E^n_{solv}) + d \quad . \tag{34}$$

Entropy changes are collected into d and assumed to be constant for members of a given series.

The solvation energies indicated in Equation (34) are ordinarily evaluated using the Born equation [44,45] or, alternatively, the expression due to Klopman [43, 44] (Equations (18) and (19), respectively). According to Klopman, however, solvation energies can arise optimally only in the case of frontier-controlled interactions (see Equations (23) and (31)). In this event, to consider the total set of interactions that a molecule may undergo upon being transferred from a gaseous to a solvated state, it would seem proper to take a sum similar to the combination of Equations (22) and (23). However, the use of frontier orbital coefficients implies charge-transfer and solvation is not necessarily accompanied by charge-transfer. Besides, the secondary interactions involved in solvation should be approximately additive, and there is little if any additivity with frontier orbital coefficients. To characterize a frontier controlled interaction that is not accompanied by a large transfer of charge, the delocalizability indices of Fukui [38,39] (Equation (28)) may be used in place of frontier orbital coefficients. This substitution should not introduce too great an error into the general development, since approximately 90 percent of the delocalizability indices result from the frontier orbitals. [38] As an added advantage, the use of the delocalizability indices ensure additivity, since they are a consequence of a second-order perturbation treatment. In this approximation, perturbation theory can lead only to additive properties. [54] From these considerations, and assuming only like atoms contribute predominantly, the solvation energy may be expressed in the form

$$E_{solv} = \bar{a} \sum_s Q_s^2 + \bar{b} \sum_s S_s^E + \bar{c} \sum_s S_s^N \qquad (35)$$

in which the bar over the coefficients designates that average atomic radii and dielectric constants should be used to effect the factorization.

Combining Equations (34) and (35) an expression is obtained that should relate observed partition coefficients to calculated MO properties

$$\ln K(o/w) = \frac{1}{RT}\left[(\bar{a} - \bar{a}') \sum_s Q_s^2 + (\bar{b} - \bar{b}') \sum_s S_s^E + (\bar{c} - \bar{c}') \sum_s S_s^N\right] + d\,. \qquad (36)$$

A primed coefficient in Equation (36) identifies terms associated with a polar or aqueous phase.

From the coefficients in Equation (36) it can be seen that, if in partitioning between an aqueous and an organic phase, the distribution of the compound in the aqueous phase is favored, then $\bar{a} < \bar{a}'$ and the first term should be negative. On the other hand, if distribution in the organic phase is favored, then $\bar{b} > \bar{b}'$ and $\bar{c} > \bar{c}'$ and the next two terms in Equation (36) should be positive. In the latter two instances the delocalizabilities are considered analogous to the abilities of a material to be polarized or to act as a polarizing substance, respectively.

Rogers and Cammarata [55,56] have reported correlations involving 30 aromatic molecules representing four chemical classes which are based on Equation (36). Each set of data, presented in Table 7, provides the equations

<u>Hydrocarbons (Table 7A)</u>

$$\ln K(o/w) = \underset{(\pm 2.96)}{-0.266} \sum_s |Q_s^T| + \underset{(\pm 0.28)}{0.758} \sum_s S_s^E + 0.116 \qquad \frac{n}{4} \quad \frac{s}{0.53} \quad \frac{r}{0.98}$$

Heteroatomic Aromatics (Table 7B)

$$\ln K(o/w) = \underset{(\pm 0.65)}{-2.279} \sum_s |Q_s^T| + \underset{(\pm 0.11)}{0.663} \sum_s S_s^E + 2.168 \quad \frac{n}{10} \quad \frac{s}{0.76} \quad \frac{r}{0.93} .$$

Substituted Indoles (Table 7C)

$$\ln K(o/w) = \underset{(\pm 0.58)}{-5.319} \sum_s |Q_s^T| + \underset{(\pm 0.14)}{0.566} \sum_s S_s^E + 7.974 \quad \frac{n}{9} \quad \frac{s}{0.38} \quad \frac{r}{0.97}$$

Substituted Benzenes (Table 7D)

$$\ln K(o/w) = \underset{(\pm 0.23)}{-2.639} \sum_s |Q_s^T| + \underset{(\pm 0.09)}{0.887} \sum_s S_s^E + 0.958 \quad \frac{n}{10} \quad \frac{s}{0.61} \quad \frac{r}{0.98} .$$

In these relations the absolute values of the net σ and π charges, calculated by the Berthod and Pullman method [51], are used.

Each correlation is acceptable on statistical grounds, with the possible exception of that obtained using the data of Table 7A. In this instance the correlation is compromised because of the limited number of data points. Nevertheless, the term analogous to induced polarization is indicated as most significant, which is in accord with what might be expected. Of greater importance, the signs to the coefficients in each correlation are as expected from the theoretical development. It is indeed gratifying that such a naive approach works so well.

The close correspondence between the coefficients of the respective correlations indicates that each structurally different set of compounds has their partition coefficients determined by common electronic effects. Hence, any property which correlates with partition coefficients should be essentially non-specific with respect to the structure of the aromatic compounds, at least. In the present case, all 30 compounds are correlated by

$$\ln K(o/w) = \underset{(\pm 0.23)}{-2.705} \sum_s |Q_s^T| + \underset{(\pm 0.06)}{0.708} \sum_s S_s^E + 2.467 \quad \frac{n}{30} \quad \frac{s}{0.73} \quad \frac{r}{0.94}$$

An MO description of lipophilicity, as embodied in Equation (36), does seem to relate well to reality and provides, now, a rationale for many properties of partition coefficients previously arrived at on an empirical basis. Hansch et al. [57] found partition coefficients to be additive and constitutive properties

TABLE 7. PARTITION COEFFICIENTS AND CALCULATED MO INDICES

Compound	ln K(o/w)[(a)]	ΣQ^T	ΣS^E
A. HYDROCARBONS			
Biphenyl	7.272	1.076	10.292
Naphthalene	6.932	0.866	8.874
Indene	6.430	1.084	8.464
Benzene	3.584	0.636	4.998
B. HETEROATOMIC AROMATICS			
Carbazole	7.576	1.799	12.177
Thianaphthene	7.113	1.812	14.698
Indole	5.182	1.438	9.114
Quinoline	4.754	1.487	8.333
Benzothiazole	4.673	2.299	12.000
Indazole	4.190	1.245	8.881
Benzoxazole	3.664	1.817	8.114
Benzimidazole	2.773	2.177	8.443
Oxindole	2.639	2.206	8.843
Quinoxaline	1.946	2.352	7.954
C. SUBSTITUTED INDOLES			
5-Bromo	6.906	1.488	11.481
1,2-Dimethyl	6.498	1.538	12.051
5-Chloro	6.269	1.492	11.343
5-Methyl	6.180	1.546	10.427
3-Methyl	5.984	1.433	10.691
5-Fluoro	5.268	1.638	9.973
H	5.182	1.438	9.114
5-Methoxy	4.754	1.855	11.883
5-Hydroxy	2.434	2.136	10.524
D. SUBSTITUTED BENZENES			
Anilyl	7.427	1.873	12.302
Phenyl	7.272	1.076	10.292
Dimethylamine	6.026	1.198	10.266
Methyl	4.852	0.826	6.253
Methoxy	4.700	1.169	7.674
H	3.584	0.636	4.998
Hydroxy	3.277	1.457	6.335
1-Hydroxy, 2-amino	2.542	2.343	8.274
Amino	1.775	1.636	6.804
1-Hydroxy, 2-Carboxy	-1.514	3.716	8.468

(a) Determined for distribution between n-octanol: aqueous Na_2PO_4 buffer, pH 7.4.

similar to parachor or molecular refractivity. These authors used this property in calculating expected partition coefficients which were then related to the biological activities of the respective compounds. The results of the correlations based on Equation (36) suggest that, while partition coefficients will vary from system to system (the regression coefficients vary), the variance in partition coefficient between systems is not great (the regression coefficients vary only slightly).

Because of the additivity of Equation (36), an indication of the nature of π may be gained. In effect, π is defined [58,59] by

$$\delta \log K(o/w) = \log K(o/w)_X - \log K(o/w)_0 = \pi \qquad (37)$$

where $K(o/w)_0$ is the partition coefficient of a parent (usually unsubstituted) member of a series and $K(o/w)_X$ is a derivative containing the substituent X. Substitution of Equation (36) into Equation (37) shows that π provides a measure of the lipophilicity in terms of the relative change in Q^2 and S^N, S^E <u>taken over all atoms of the respective molecules</u>. The usual identification of π with a substituent property is correct only insofar as the total electronic properties of the respective compounds do vary with the nature of the substituent.

IX. QUASI-EMPIRICAL RELATIONSHIPS

If the MO approach to studies of drug action can be considered as based on a theoretical framework, and the linear free-energy approach is taken as essentially empirical in origin, then those attempts to relate biological activities to linear combinations of MO and free-energy derived indices may be termed a quasi-empirical approach. The implication associated with the use of this term is that the initial empirical indices are found eventually to relate to accepted theory. Usually the free-energy derived index in these correlative attempts is π, since the more common indices derived by MO methods often do not provide a good fit of the data when used alone in a regression equation. [14,60,61] Occasionally π and π^2 are used to take account of a parabolic dependence of biological activity on lipophilicity. Such parabolic fits to biological data will not be considered here. Their use is a practical convenience which, it may be argued, is intended to take account of two competing processes each of which is proportional to π but which differs in sign. Leffler and Grunwald [12] give the features essential to this argument.

Some quasi-empirical correlations have appeared in the literature. [14,60, 61] Many of these may be considered as consisting of a linear combination of the charge and frontier-controlled cases [62] generalized by the equations

$$A = -\frac{1}{RT}\left[\sum_s (\nu_s Q_s + \xi_s S_s^N + \zeta S_s^E) + h \log K(o/w)\right] + \underline{I}\,, \tag{38}$$

or

$$A = -\frac{1}{RT}\left[\sum_s (\nu_s Q_s + \xi_s S_s^N + \zeta S_s^E) + h\pi)\right] + \underline{I}'\,. \tag{39}$$

The activity of the parent compound and the summation appropriate to this compound are part of the terminal constant in Equation (39).

As an example, the rate of acylation of aromatic amines by pigeon liver acetyl transferase [63] is correlated by the equation [60]

$$\log k_a = \underset{(\pm 2.20)}{-18.16}\, Q_N + \underset{(\pm 0.02)}{0.29}\, \pi + 2.51 \qquad \frac{n}{6} \quad \frac{s}{0.04} \quad \frac{r}{0.99}\,.$$

Net charge densities, calculated using the simple Hückel method by Perault and Pullman [64], were used in deriving this relation.

X. A MO PERSPECTIVE ON THE LINEAR FREE-ENERGY APPROACH

The evidence presented suggests that Equation (38) could be used to provide a link between the MO and the linear free-energy approaches in the study of drug action. Of primary concern is the bearing of Equation (27) on substituent parameters intended to provide a measure of electronic effects.

The first term of Equation (27) can be written

$$\Delta E_1^e = \sum_s \left(\sum_r \frac{Q_r \gamma_{rs}}{\epsilon_{rs}}\right) Q_s \tag{40}$$

or, expressing the two-center repulsion integral by Pople's Approximation [65],

$$\Delta E_1^e = \sum_s \left(\sum_r \frac{Q_r e}{\epsilon_{rs} D_{rs}}\right) Q_s \tag{41}$$

where e is a unit reference charge. Equation (41) may be compared to the relation given by Sixma [66] for the effect of a substituent on the localization energy E_L of a reaction

$$E_L = \sum_s \left(\sum_p \frac{Q_p e}{\varepsilon D_{ps}}\right) Q_s^0 \tag{42}$$

in which the p atoms are those of the substituent and Q^0 is the net charge on an aromatic nucleus prior to conjugation with a substituent. Equation (42) gives the perturbing influence of a substituent on an aromatic nucleus, and Equation (40) gives the perturbing influence of a drug-receptor on a drug molecule.

Sixma demonstrated convincingly that the localization energy E_L is related to the Hammett σ constant [12] by an equation of the form

$$\sigma = fE_L \ . \tag{43}$$

By analogy, it may be expected that a constant characteristic of a drug-receptor interaction is given by

$$A' = f'\Delta E_1^e \ . \tag{44}$$

According to the present treatment, the observed biological activity characterizes the drug-receptor interaction. If a drug-receptor interaction affects the localization energy by modifying the charge on the drug substituent, then a relation should exist between Equation (43) and (44). For a receptor of essentially constant conformation with respect to a series of drugs, only a fixed proportion of the receptor charge can affect the charge on a substituent. In this case, Equations (43) and (44) are linearly related

$$A' = \rho\sigma \ . \tag{45}$$

For the next two terms of Equation (27), there is no reported linear free-energy counterpart. A possible measure to define these parameters might be provided by suitable donor-acceptor pairs whose charge-transfer characteristics correlate only with S^E or S^N for atoms *ortho*, *meta*, and *para* to a given substituent. Alternatively, the results of MO calculations on a standard series of molecules might be used to provide these indices. Work along these lines is in progress. If these desired parameters are found to be sufficiently general, a very convenient working hypothesis is provided by the equation

$$A = -\frac{1}{RT}\left(\rho\sigma + k'C^N + k''C^E + h\pi\right) + d \tag{46}$$

in which C^N and C^E are defined in a manner similar to that of Equation (37).

There is a formal similarity between the definition of S^E (Equation (28)) and the quantum mechanical expression for induced polarization. The similarity arises because each index is derived by the application of perturbation theory, and does not necessarily reflect any fundamental interrelation between the two. For lack of a better measure for C^E, molar refractivities of substituted phenols were calculated from available index of refraction measurements and were used to define a substituent constant γ_{ar} such as is done in Equation (37). [67] These substituent constants were then fit to corresponding values for aliphatic substituents calculated from tabulations of bond refractivities. [68] The correlation is given by

$$\gamma_{ar} = 0.023\ \gamma_{al} + 0.175\ \gamma_{al}^2 + 0.0168 \qquad \frac{n}{12} \quad \frac{s}{0.018} \quad \frac{r}{0.98}$$

The use of this parameter led to considerable improvement in the correlation of a limited number of AChE hydrolysis rates of <u>para</u>-substituted benzoylcholine esters [69]

$$\log K_m = 1.521\ \sigma - 6.442\ \gamma_{aro} + 0.266 \qquad \frac{n}{5} \quad \frac{s}{0.151} \quad \frac{r}{0.972}$$

$$\log v_m = 1.544\ \sigma - 5.731\ \gamma_{aro} + 0.380 \qquad 5 \quad 0.123 \quad 0.965\ .$$

A linear free-energy analogy to Equation (7) can be gained by introducing the van der Waals radius r_v into Equation (46). The overall model, which assumes conformational changes of the receptor substance are constant or negligible, then becomes given by

$$A = -\frac{1}{RT}\,(\rho\sigma + k'C^N + k''C^E + h\pi + tr_v) + d\ . \qquad (47)$$

It is evident that Equation (47) contains two more terms C^N and C^E than are used in the model equation proposed by Hansch [14]. In a rough sense these new terms may be viewed as representing the ability of a drug to act as a polarizing substance (C^N) or to be polarized (C^E) in the interaction with the receptor substance. [53,62]

XI. THE FUTURE APPLICATIONS OF MO METHODS

Second-order perturbation theory, as applied by Klopman and Hudson, seems to treat qualitatively at least some of the elements needed for a description of drug-receptor interactions. To strengthen this view, and to define limiting conditions for its application, additional MO studies may take the approach of comparing the results of a quantum chemical and a linear free-energy treatment of biological activity data. For a given system, a physically significant pair of correlations should complement one another.

Assuming the model equations afforded by quantum theory are adequate for a description of drug action, their modification to conform to already established statistical models [24,70] should greatly extend the types of molecular structures whose activities may be compared. There is overlap between the statistical models that may be employed [7] and the major difficulty seems to be the proper solution of each model to maintain this equivalence. As has been indicated previously, a convenient statistical treatment of a set of data may impose conditions which are physically unrealistic.

Many drugs are capable of assuming a number of possible conformations [71], and there is presently no way of telling which of these conformations is the more important pharmacologically. The synthesis of model compounds of rigid sterochemistry provides some indication, but there is no assurance that the models behave in a manner fully equivalent to their conformationally mobile parent in leading to the observed response. MO calculations can provide an indication of the preferred conformations of a drug molecule, but the conformation calculated as preferred in the unrestricted state does not necessarily conform to the conformation of the drug bound to the drug-receptor. Thus, in this area it seems reasonable to expect that future work will attempt to define possible preferred conformation for the bound drug. An analysis of drug activity may then take the form

$$A = x_1 a_1 + x_2 a_2 + \cdots + x_j a_j \tag{48}$$

where x is the fraction of drug in a given conformation and a is the biological activity for the drug in this conformation. If the individual activities a can be obtained from the overall observed biological activity A for a drug, these may be used in studies attempting to define the nature of the drug-receptor interaction.

XII. ACKNOWLEDGMENT

The author sincerely thanks the Medical College of Virginia, Virginia Commonwealth University, Richmond, Virginia, for the encouragement and support provided for much of this work while he was a member of their faculty. Added thanks are due to NIH whose grant (AI-09199) made possible the development of the work reviewed.

XIII. REFERENCES

[1] Schnaare, R. S., and Martin, A. N., *J. Pharm. Sci.*, 54, 1707 (1965).

[2] Mautner, H. G., *Pharmacol. Rev.*, 19, 107 (1967).

[3] Cammarata, A., *J. Med. Chem.*, 11, 1111 (1968).

[4] Wohl, A., this symposium.

[5] Fuller, R. W., Marsh, M. M., and Mills, J., *J. Med. Chem.*, 11, 397 (1968).

[6] Beasley, J. G., and Purcell, W. P., *Biochim. Biophys. Acta*, 178, 175 (1969).

[7] Cammarata, A., and Yau, S. J., submitted.

[8] Paton, W. D. M., *Proc. Roy. Soc. (London)*, B154, 21 (1961).

[9] Ariëns, E. J., Simonis, A. M., and van Rossum, J. M., p. 119 in *Molecular Pharmacology*, edited by E. J. Ariëns, Academic, New York (1964).

[10] Belleau, B., *J. Med. Chem.*, 7, 778 (1964).

[11] Bloom, B. M., and Goldman, I. M., p. 121 in *Advan. Drug Res.*, Vol. 3, Academic, New York (1966).

[12] Leffler, J. E., and Grunwald, E. G., *Rates and Equilibria of Organic Reactions*, Wiley, New York (1963).

[13] Peradejordi, F., *Cahiers Phys.*, 158-159, 1 (1963).

[14] Hansch, C., p. 347 in *Ann. Repts. of Med. Chem.*, edited by C. K. Cain, Academic, New York (1966).

[15] Belleau, B., and Lacasse, G., *J. Med. Chem.*, 7, 768 (1964).

[16] Belleau, B., *Ann. N. Y. Acad. Sci.*, 144, 705 (1967).

[17] Belleau, B., p. 89 in *Advan. Drug Res.*, Vol. 2, edited by N. J. Harper and A. B. Simmonds, Academic, New York (1965).

[18] Cammarata, A., and Yau., S. J., submitted.

[19] Peradejordi, F., and Martin, A. N., submitted.

[20] Cammarata, A., and Martin, A. N., in *Medicinal Chemistry*, edited by A. Burger, Wiley, New York (1969).

[21] Cohn, E. J., and Edsall, J. T., *Proteins, Amino Acids and Peptides*, Harper, New York (1943).

[22] Salem, A., *Can. J. Biochem. Physiol.*, 40, 1287 (1962).

[23] Free, S. M., and Wilson, J. W., *J. Med. Chem.*, 7, 395 (1964).

[24] Anderson, R. L., and Bancroft, T. A., *Statistical Theory in Research*, McGraw-Hill, New York (1952).

[25] Smithfield, W. R., and Purcell, W. P., *J. Pharm. Sci.*, 56, 577 (1967).

[26] Purcell, W. P., and Clayton, J. M., *J. Med. Chem.*, 11, 199 (1968).

[27] Purcell, W. P., *Biochem. Biophys. Acta*, 105, 201 (1965).

[28] Ban, T., and Fujita, T., *J. Med. Chem.*, 12, 353 (1969).

[29] Singer, J., and Purcell, W. P., *J. Med. Chem.*, 10, 1000 (1967).

[30] Boček, K., Kopecký, J., Krivucová, M., and Vlachová, D., *Experientia*, 20, 667 (1964).

[31] Kopecký, J., Boček, K., and Vlachová, D., *Nature*, 207, 981 (1965).

[32] Miller, G. H., Khalil, S., and Martin, A. N., *J. Pharm. Sci.*, accepted.

[33] Spencer, J. L., Hlavka, J. J., Petisi, J., Krazinski, H. M., and Boothe, J. H., *J. Med. Chem.*, 6, 405 (1963).

[34] Beereboom, J. J., Ursprung, J. J., Rennhard, H. H., and Stephens, C. R., *J. Amer. Chem. Soc.*, 82, 1003 (1960).

[35] Collett, J. H., Collett, C., Martin, A. N., and Cammarata, A., submitted.

[36] Cammarata, A., Yau, S. J., Martin, A. N., and Collett, J. H., submitted.

[37] Dewar, M. J. S., *J. Amer. Chem. Soc.*, 74, 3341 (1952).

[38] Fukui, K., Yonezawa, T., and Nagata, C., *Bull. Chem. Soc. Japan*, 27, 423 (1954).

[39] Fukui, K., Yonezawa, T., and Nagata, C., *J. Chem. Phys.*, 27, 1247 (1957).

[40] Morokuma, H., Kato, H., and Fukui, K., *Bull. Chem. Soc. Japan*, 36, 541 (1963).

[41] Inouye, A., Shinagawa, Y., and Takaishi, Y., *Arch. Intern. Pharmacodyn.*, 144, 319 (1963).

[42] Klopman, G., and Hudson, R. F., *Theoret. Chim. Acta*, 8, 165 (1967).

[43] Klopman, G., *J. Amer. Chem. Soc.*, 90, 223 (1968).

[44] Born, M., *Z. Physik*, 1, 45 (1920).

[45] Hoijtink, G. J., De Boer, E., van der Meij, P. M., and Weijland, W. P., *Rec. Trav. Chim.*, 75, 487 (1956).

[46] Klopman, G., *Chem. Phys. Letters*, 1, 5 (1967).

[47] Martin, Y. C., private communication.

[48] Bishop, D. M., and Craig, D. P., *Mol. Phys.*, 6, 139 (1963).

[49] Waser, P. G., *Pharmacol. Rev.*, 13, 465 (1961).

[50] Cammarata, A., and Kier, L. B., unpublished.

[51] Berthod, H., and Pullman, A., *J. Chim. Phys.*, 942 (1965).

[52] Del Re, G., *J. Chem. Soc.*, 4031 (1958).

[53] Cammarata, A., and Stein, R. L., *J. Med. Chem.*, 11, 829 (1968).

[54] Morgenau, H., *Rev. Mod. Phys.*, 11, 1 (1939).

[55] Rogers, K. S., and Cammarata, A., *J. Med. Chem.*, 12, 692 (1969).

[56] Rogers, K. S., and Cammarata, A., *Biochem. Biophys. Acta*, accepted.

[57] Hansch, C., *Proceedings of the 3rd International Pharmacological Meeting, Sao Palo, 1966*, Vol. 7, Pergamon, (1968).

[58] Hansch, C., and Fujita, T., *J. Amer. Chem. Soc.*, 86, 1624 (1964).

[59] Fujita, T., Iwasa, J., and Hansch, C., *J. Amer. Chem. Soc.*, 86, 5175 (1964).

[60] Hansch, C., Deutsch, E. W., and Smith, R. N., *J. Amer. Chem. Soc.*, 87, 2738 (1965).

[61] Hansch, C., in *Drug Design*, edited by E. J. Ariëns, Wiley, New York (1969).

[62] Cammarata, A., *J. Med. Chem.*, 12, 314 (1969).

[63] Jacobson, K. B., *J. Biol. Chem.*, 236, 343 (1961).

[64] Perault, A., and Pullman, B., *Biochim. Biophys. Acta*, 66, 86 (1963).

[65] Pople, J. A., *Trans. Faraday Soc.*, 49 1375 (1953).

[66] Sixma, F. L. J., *Rec. Trav. Chim.*, 72, 673 (1953).

[67] Cammarata, A., and Yau, S. J., in preparation.

[68] Vogel, A. I., *Elementary Practical Organic Chemistry, Part 2: Qualitative Organic Analysis*, 2nd ed., Wiley, New York (1966).

[69] Zimmerman, J. J., and Goyan, J. E., submitted.

[70] Draper, N. R., and Smith, H., *Applied Regression Analysis*, Wiley, New York (1966).

[71] Kier, L. B., this symposium.

POSSIBLE INTERACTIONS IN THE PRIMITIVE TRANSLATION PROCESS

by

Robert Rein*, Marc S. Rendell** and J. P. Harlos*

I. INTRODUCTION

In the present study we wish to consider one particular aspect of the general problem of the genetic code and its evolution. This aspect is concerned with the nature of physical interaction involved in the recognition process. Broadly speaking we can consider two fundamental mechanisms operating in biological molecular recognition processes [1,2]. The first mechanism, which we can refer to as an electronic template mechanism, involves direct physical interactions between the molecules or between a molecule and part of a macromolecule. These interactions are often mainly electrostatic in nature, with some contribution from dispersion, polarization and overlap forces. The electrostatic components are often controlled by the charges of single atoms of interacting species or, at least, by the charge distribution in a limited region or domain of the molecules. A very good example of this type of interaction is hydrogen bonding; the role of hydrogen bonding in the recognition process between nucleotide bases necessary for replication and transcription is well understood.

The other mechanism by which molecular recognition can occur can be referred to as the steric template mechanism. This mechanism requires steric complementarity, that is, a "close steric" fit of a substrate molecule into a cavity defined by a complicated macromolecule [3]. This mechanism is assumed to be operative in enzyme substrate interactions. It is apparent that the requirements

*Department of Experimental Pathology, Roswell Park Memorial Institute, Buffalo, New York, and Center for Theoretical Biology, SUNY/B.

**Downstate Medical Center, summer research associate, Center for Theoretical Biology, SUNY/B.

for the operation of the first mechanism are far simpler than those of the second. The first can operate even with inorganic surfaces and certainly with the nucleotide sequences.

On the other hand, the requirements for the second mechanism are much more involved requiring a complicated macromolecule with a complex secondary and tertiary structure. This is usually fulfilled by an ordered polypeptide chain molecule. From the evolutionary point of view it is far simpler to assume the first mechanism occurs in processes under prebiotic conditions rather than the second.

In the contemporary view of the operation of the translation system the involvement of both these mechanisms has been suggested [1,2]. Let us briefly consider what is involved in the operation of this system. The minimum requirements are the presence of transfer RNA (t-RNA) which carries the anticodon complement to the messenger RNA (m-RNA) codon, an enzyme, the aminoacyl transferase, the amino acid to be "loaded" and ATP. The currently more popular view attributes the recognition of both the amino acid and t-RNA particular to that amino acid to the enzyme. Thus this enzyme must be a highly sophisticated one which performs a three-fold function: the recognition of the t-RNA, or the amino acid and catalysis of the attachment of the amino acid onto the terminal site of the t-RNA. A second view attributes some importance to a direct interaction of the amino acid with some part of the t-RNA. In this case the enzyme need only support this process.

However, irrespective of what the details of the contemporary mechanism are, it is difficult to envision that the first process would be operative in the primitive code. The sophisticated enzyme required could not have evolved without an already existing translation mechanism.

This apparently leaves, for the primitive transcription mechanism, only the one suggested by Orgel, [4] namely the direct physical interaction and recognition of the codon by a complementary amino acid. Such an assumption has the additional attractive features that it leads to a determinalistic model and can also explain the universality of the genetic code. The difficulty with this model is that there is apparently no experimental support for it. In fact, dialysis experiments involving the combination of amino acids and t-RNA and then dialysied give negative results. However, as will be pointed out later, due to the nature of the forces involved, these negative experiments may not be conclusive. It is, therefore, of some interest to examine the problem from a theoretical point of view. Such calculations would not only indicate the feasibility of the model but might also direct attention to appropriate experimental conditions required to demonstrate the interaction.

II. METHOD

In order to approximate the amount of molecular interaction between two molecules some knowledge is required of the non-interacting molecules. For our calculation the most important quantities were the charge distributions of the molecules. Since the electrostatic energy to the total interaction energy will be the largest contribution, it is vital that reasonable charge distributions are used. While many semi-empirical molecular orbital calculations will yield charge distributions, many of these methods tend to overestimate or exaggerate the relative charge distribution. Some methods, such as the iterative extended Hückel theory (IEHT) method, yield reasonable charge distributions. The IEHT results do not tend to exaggerate charge at hetero atoms and are therefore appropriate for biologically important molecules. Also required were estimates of the molecular ionization potential also obtained from the IEHT method. The details of the computational procedures used in the IEHT method have been detailed elsewhere [5].

Iterative extended Hückel calculations were performed on four nucleotide bases; guanine, cytosine, adenine and uracil. These bases were calculated with a methyl substituent at the sugar substituted position in order to more closely approximate the structure in RNA. The resulting charge distributions were similar to those of the hydrogen substituted homologues [6]. Similar calculations were also performed on glycine which is treated as the dipolar ion, since this is the predominant form at cellular pH. Furthermore, the calculations were performed with glycine in a planar configuration, that is, all atoms but two amino hydrogen and the α carbon hydrogens were assumed to be coplanar.

The interaction energies were then assumed to be given as the sum of the electrostatic dispersion and polarization energies. Overlap interactions were ignored since the closest approach of two atoms was approximately 2 angstroms. The electrostatic contributions are then given as [7]

$$E_{electrostatic} = \sum_{i=1}^{n_1} \sum_{j=1}^{n_2} \frac{q_i q_j}{r_{ij}}$$

where the summation extended over the n_1 atom of molecule 1 and the n_2 atoms of molecule 2. q_i and q_j are the atom charges and r_{ij} the interatomic distance.

The dispersion interaction energy is given by [7]

$$E_{disp.} = -\frac{1}{4}\frac{I_1 I_2}{I_1 + I_2} \sum_{i=j}^{b_1} \sum_{j=1}^{b_2} \frac{1}{r_{ij}^6} [6\alpha_i^T\alpha_j^T + \alpha_i^T\delta_j \{3(\bar{\alpha}_j^L \cdot \bar{r}_{ij})^2 + 1\}$$
$$+ \alpha_j^T\delta_i \{3(\bar{\alpha}_i^L \cdot \bar{r}_{ij})^2 + 1\} + \delta_i\delta_j \{3(\bar{\alpha}_i^L \cdot \bar{r}_{ij})(\bar{\alpha}_j^L \cdot \bar{r}_{ij})$$
$$- (\bar{\alpha}_i^L \cdot \bar{\alpha}_j^L)\}^2] \quad .$$

Here the summations extend over the number of bonds in molecule 1, b_1, and the b_2 bonds in molecule 2. I_1 and I_2 are the molecular ionization potentials. α_i^T and α_i^L are the transverse and longitudinal polarizabilities of the i^{TH} bond and r_{ij} distance separating the midpoints of the i^{TH} and j^{TH} bond. $\bar{\alpha}_i^L$ and $\bar{r}_{ij}$ are unit vectors pointing respectively along the i^{TH} bond and the line joining the midpoints of the i^{TH} and j^{TH} bonds. Furthermore, $\delta = \alpha^L - \alpha^T$.

The polarization energy resulting from the net charge located on the atoms of molecular 1 perturbing the bonds of molecule 2 is given as [7]

$$E_{pol}^{1\to 2} = -\frac{1}{2} \sum_{k=1}^{b_2} [\alpha_k^T(\bar{\mathcal{E}}_k \cdot \bar{\mathcal{E}}_k) + \delta_k(\bar{\mathcal{E}}_k \cdot \bar{\alpha}_k^L)^2]$$
$$\bar{\mathcal{E}}_k = \sum_{\beta=1}^{n_1} \frac{q_\beta}{R_{\beta k}^3} \bar{R}_{\beta k} \quad .$$

The symbols have the same meaning as above, except for $\overline{R}_{k\beta}$ which is the vector connecting the atom β with the midpoint of the k^{TH} bond. $R_{\beta k}$ is then the magnitude of this vector. A similar expression exists for the polarization of the bonds of molecule 1 by the atom net charges of molecule 2, $E_{pol}^{2\rightarrow 1}$. The total polarization energy is then given as the sum of the two components.

$$E_{pol} = E_{pol}^{1\rightarrow 2} + E_{pol}^{2\rightarrow 1}$$

The energies and orientation of the base-glycine complex were ascertained by performing a scan of a constrained configurational space. The constraint applied here was to limit the interaction to a two dimensional plane containing the two molecules. Furthermore, both molecules were to lie in this plane. Keeping the base in a fixed position, the glycine molecule was translated along both x and y axes in 0.2 Å units and rotated around the new axes in 5° increments. At each position the electrostatic energy was calculated. The resulting scan developed an electrostatic energy surface. At those points where the electrostatic interaction was greatest, a further scan was carried out with reduced increments. Here the translational movement was made in 0.1 Å units and the rotational movement in 2.5°. In this second scan the dispersion and polarization interaction energies were calculated and added to the electrostatic energies and the configuration of greatest interaction noted.

III. RESULTS AND DISCUSSION

The results of these calculations may be summarized as indicating that glycine interacts in a specific manner with each of the nucleotide bases. The details of this interaction will now be discussed.

Figure 1 depicts the results of the IEHT calculations on glycine and indicates the resulting charge distribution of the dipolar ion. The salient features are the negative charge localized at the carboxyl group and positive charge at the amino group.

Figures 2-5 contain the geometric configurations that yielded the greatest amount of interaction. The pertinent atom net charges in the nucleotide

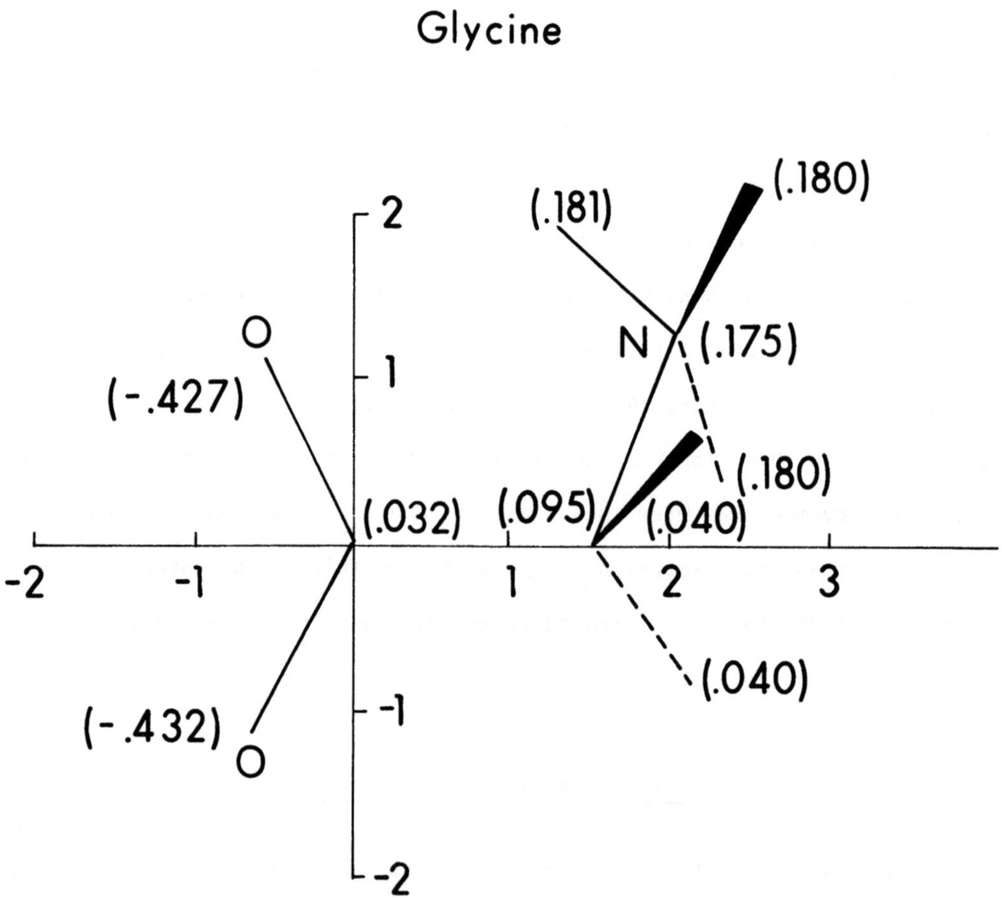

FIGURE 1. Glycine - IEHT net atom charges.

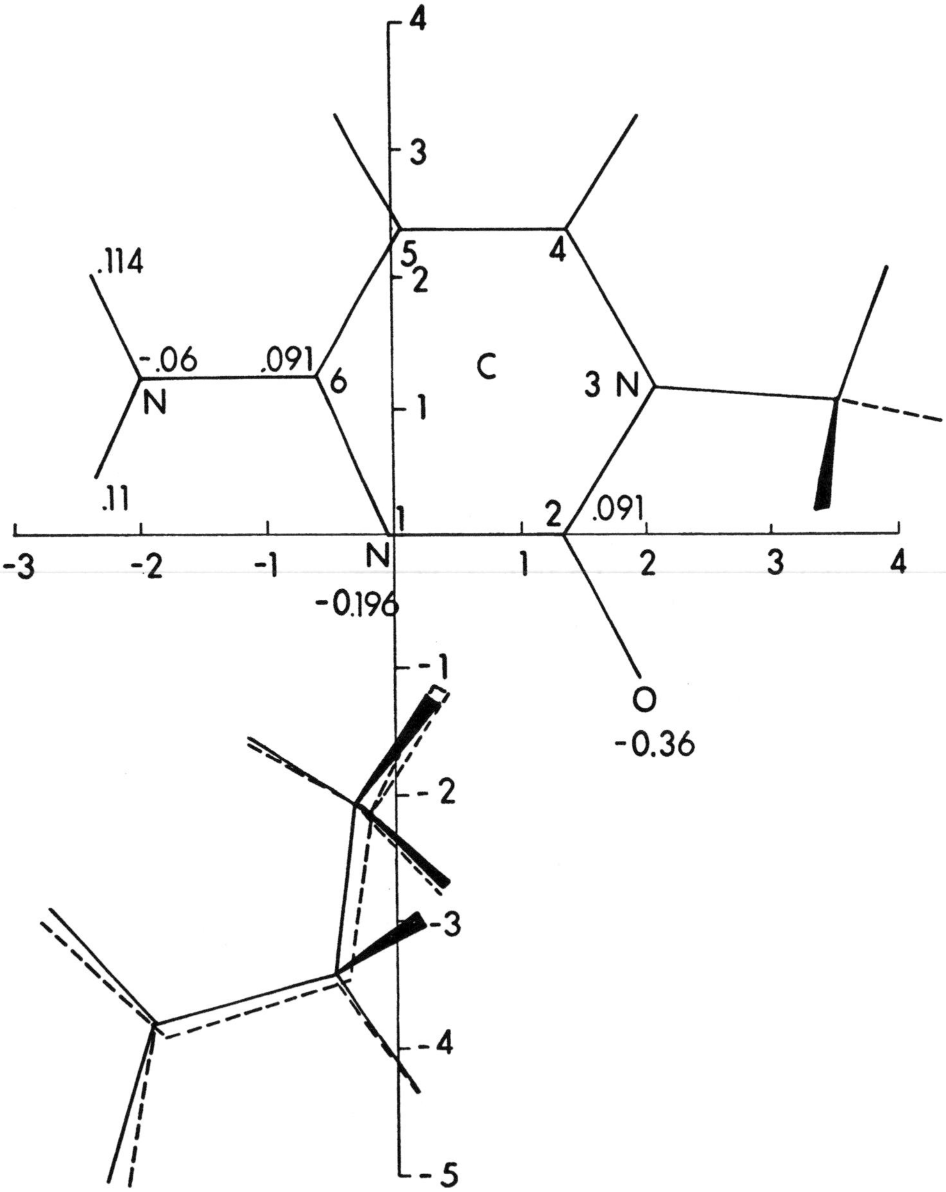

FIGURE 2. Cytosine-Glycine-relative orientation
dotted glycine - total interaction energy
solid glycine - electrostatic interaction energy.

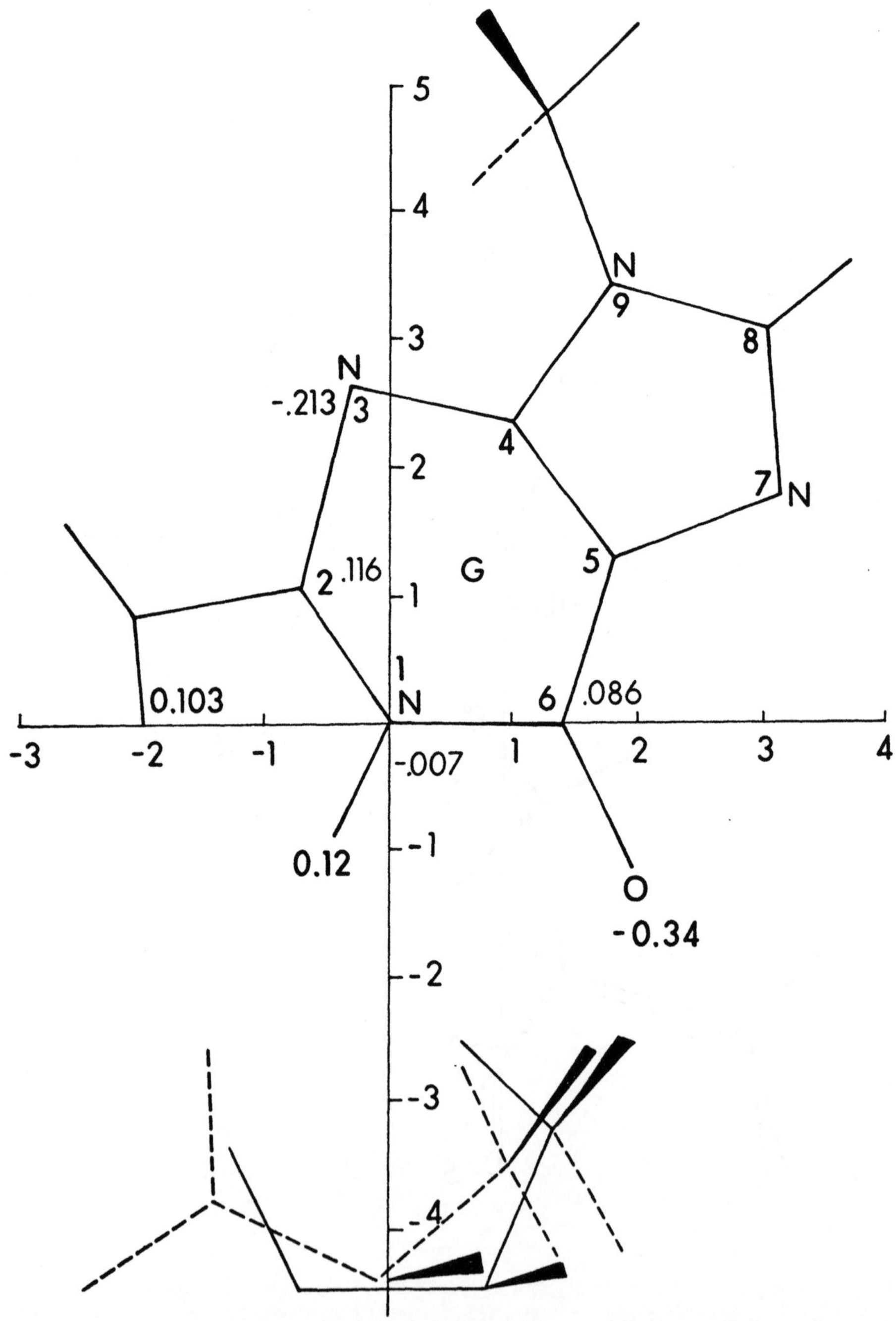

FIGURE 3. Guanine-Glycine-relative orientation
dotted glycine - total interaction energy
solid glycine - electrostatic interaction energy.

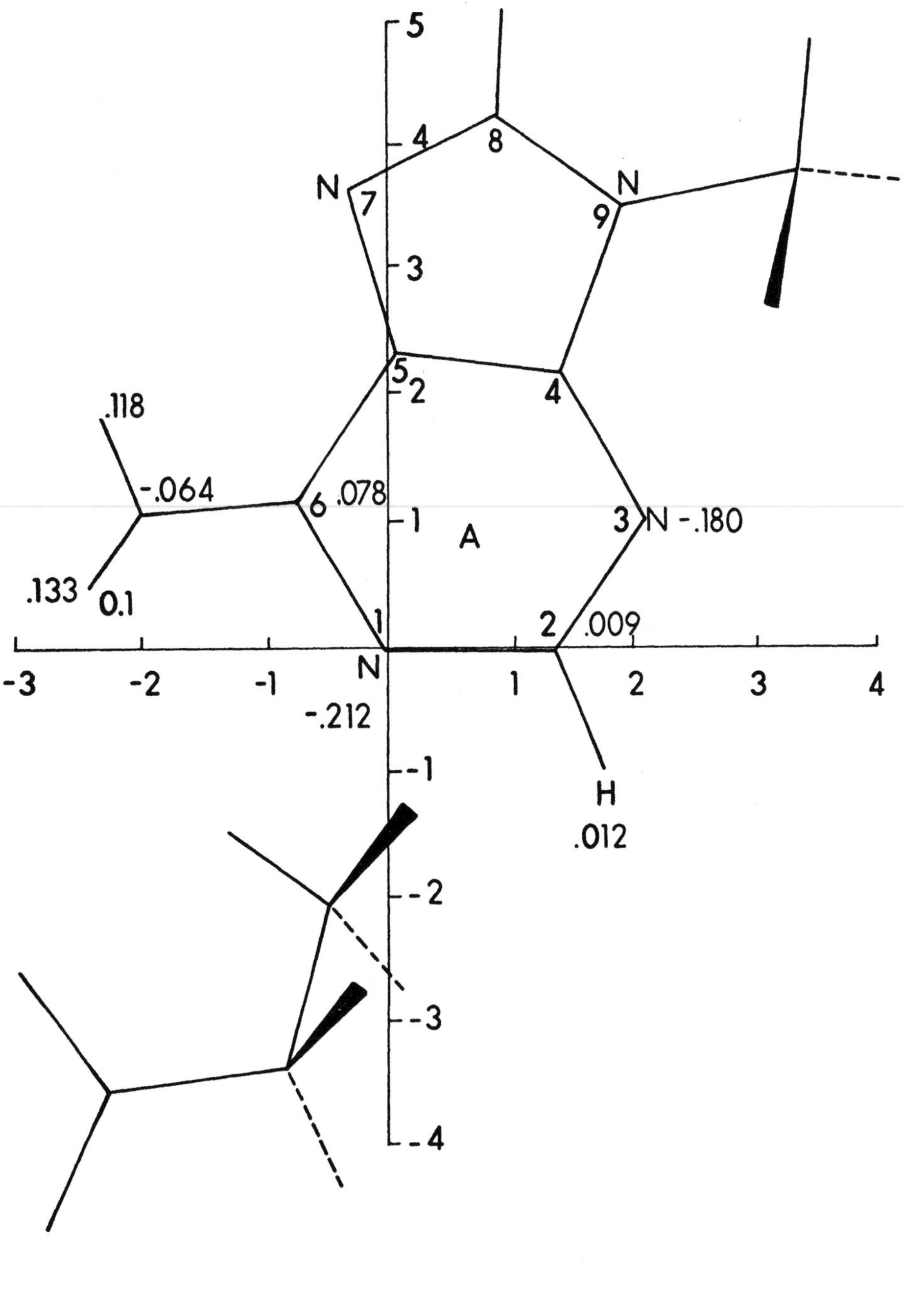

FIGURE 4. Adenine – Glycine – relative orientation.

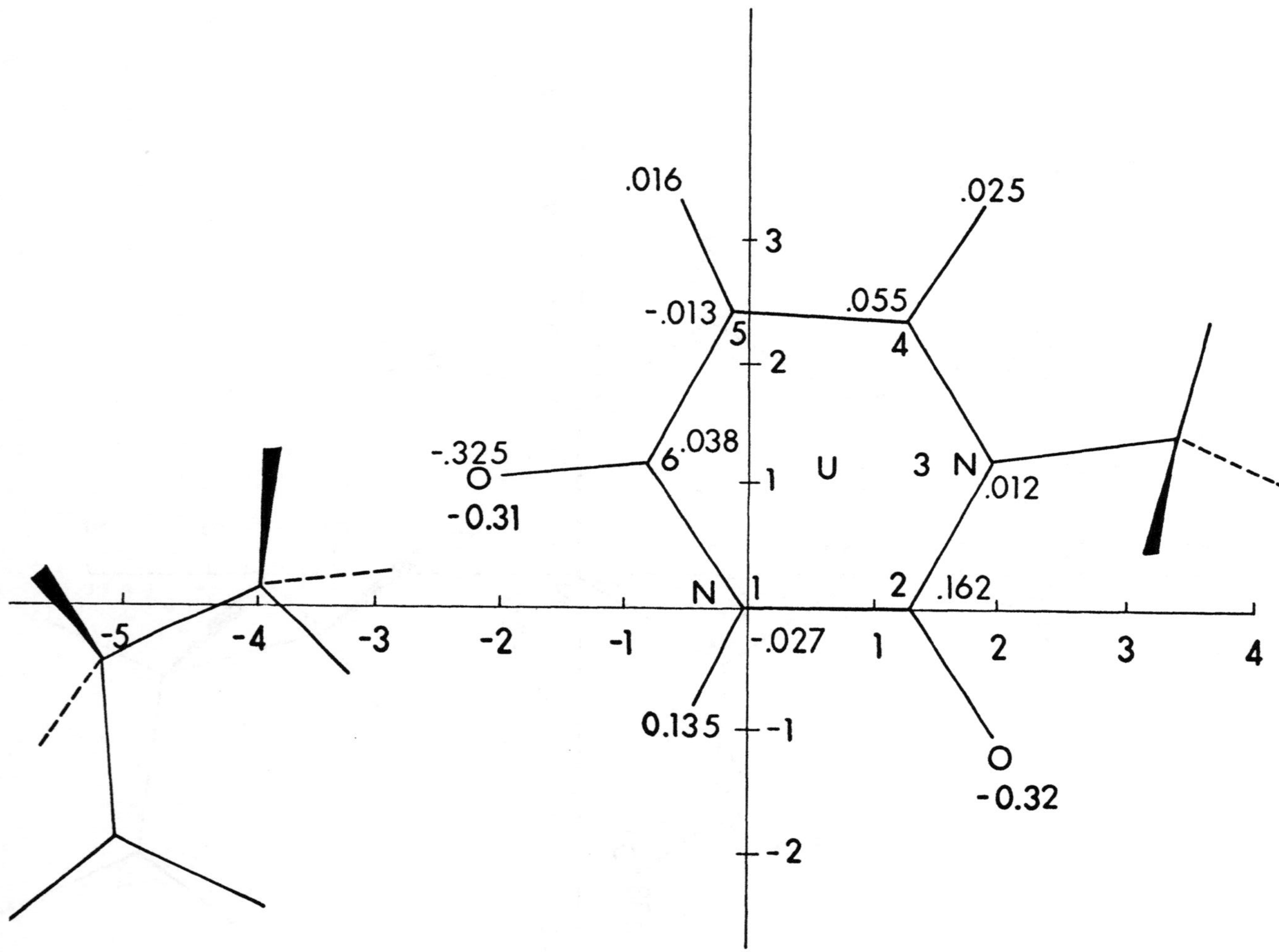

FIGURE 5. Uracil - Glycine - relative orientation.

base are also given in these figures. It should be noted that the glycine orients itself in a specific manner which depends upon the charge distribution in the base. Thus the bonding is directional with the positive ammonium group of the glycine interacting with the negative region of the coding face.

In the cases of cytosine and adenine, these negative regions are the nitrogens while for guanine and uracil the negative regions are the keto oxygens. In all cases except for uracil, the orientation of the glycine is further determined by the interaction between the negatively charged carboxyl group of the glycine and the relatively positive charge located on the amino hydrogens of the base.

In the case of guanine, there is another configuration depicted in Figure 6, involving the non-coding face of the base. This form will be discussed later.

Figure 7 summarizes the electrostatic interaction energy and shows numerically the dependence upon the charge distribution. The relative order of stability is cytosine followed by guanine, uracil and adenine. While the interaction between the non-coding face of guanine is apparently stronger than that of cytosine, we believe that this is a result of neglecting the sugar-phosphate backbone of t-RNA. It is our opinion that the inclusion of the backbone would give rise to steric blocking of this position.

Figure 8 contains the electrostatic, dispersion, polarization of total interaction energies. It is apparent that the total interaction energy between cytosine and glycine is far greater than any of the other bases. We again neglect the non-coding face interaction for the reasons given above.

The resulting order is then, cytosine (-41.4 kcal), followed by guanine (-28.5 kcal), adenine (-27.8 kcal) and uracil (-22.1 kcal). It is of interest to note that the secondary interaction effects, the dispersion and polarization interactions, were capable of reversing the order of adenine and uracil from that obtained using only electrostatic interactions. It does appear that the glycine-cytosine interaction is favored energetically over any of the other possible combinations.

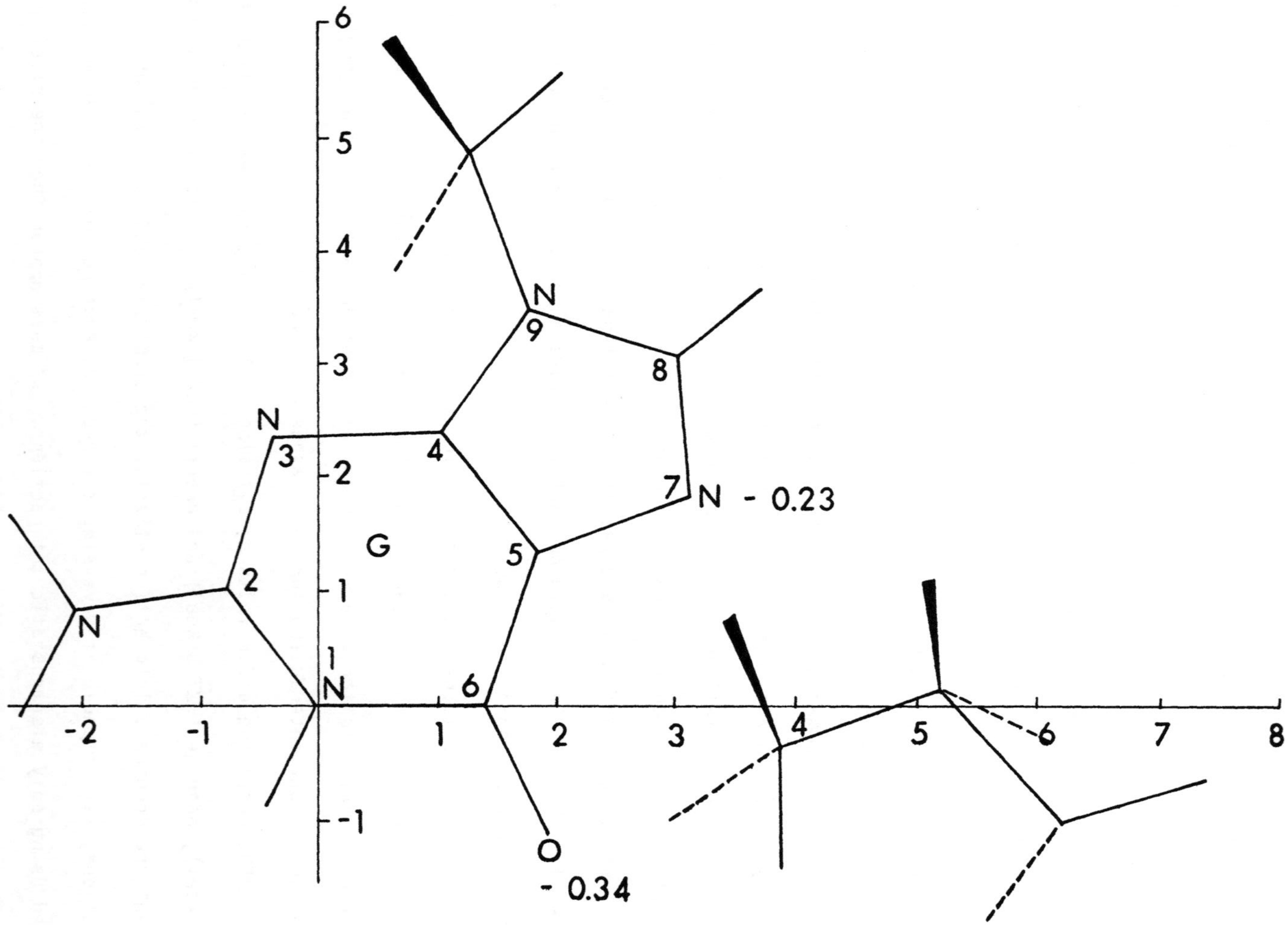

FIGURE 6. Guanine - Glycine - relative orientation, non-coding face.

	$E_{el. st.}$	Net Atomic charge in the coding face		
Cytosine	-22.6	$H_{6'}$ = 0.1;	N_1 = - 0.20*;	$O_{2'}$ = -0.36
Guanine	-20.2	$H_{2'}$ = 0.10	H_1 = 0.12	*$O_{6'}$ = -0.34
Uracil	-14.8	$O_{6'}$ = -0.33*	H_1 = 0.14	$O_{2'}$ = -0.32
Adenine	-12.6	$H_{6'}$ = 0.13;	N_1 =* - 0.21	$H_{2'}$ = 0.01
Guanine* (side)	-24.4	$O_{6'}$ = -0.34	*	N_4 = -0.2

FIGURE 7. Electrostatic energies and relevant atom charges for nucleotide bases, in kcal.

	$E_{electrostatic}$	$E_{disp.}$	E_{polar}	E_{total}
Cytosine	-22.6	-8.3	-10.5	-41.4
Guanine*	-20.2	-2.7	-5.6	-28.5
Adenine	-12.6	-6.8	-8.4	-27.8
Uracil	-14.8	-2.4	-4.9	-22.1
Guanine+	-24.4	-10.2	-11.3	-45.9

* Coding face
+ Non-coding face

FIGURE 8. Interaction energies for nucleotide bases in kcal.

We may further speculate that the use of amino acids other than glycine, with side chains and additional polar groups may cause the involvement of adjacent bases. Such a model, with the further increase in interaction energies, may improve the sensitivity of the interactions for other bases. This remains to be examined in further studies.

Finally, we would like to comment on the possible experimental demonstration of this effect. In view of the large part that electrostatic forces play in holding the complex together, it is not surprising that dialysis experiments are negative. In a media of low dielectric the electrostatic forces would be sufficient to ensure bonding, however in an aqueous media these forces may be overcome by hydration effects. Furthermore, it is clear that the micro environment of the amino acid base interaction in the primitive transcription process must have been anhydrous. Thus, in any attempt to experimentally demonstrate this direct physical complementarity of amino acids with nucleotide bases must involve an anhydrous media and may then be successful.

IV. CONCLUSION

In the present study we have demonstrated the feasibility of a direct physical interaction between an amino acid and a nucleotide base. For the case of glycine interacting with the nucleotide bases, we have shown that there are specific orientations of the two molecules. Furthermore, the magnitudes of the energies of interaction suggest that glycine is most strongly attracted to cytosine.

V. ACKNOWLEDGMENT

We gratefully acknowledge support for this investigation from NASA Grant NGR 33-015-016. Further we appreciate support given these studies by the Computer Center of the State University of New York at Buffalo.

VI. REFERENCES

[1] Crick, F. H. C., *J. Mol. Biol.*, 38, 367 (1968).

[2] Woese, C. R., *The Genetic Code*, New York:Harper & Row (1967).

[3] Pelc, S. R., and Welton, M. G. E., *Nature*, 209, 868 (1966).

[4] Orgel, L. E., *J. Mol. Biol.*, 38, 381 (1968).

[5] Rein, R., Fukuda, N., Win, H., Clarke, G. A., and Harris, F. E., *J. Chem. Phys.*, 45, 4743 (1966).

[6] Rein, R., Fukuda, N., Clarke, G. A., and Harris, F. E., *J. Theoret. Biol.*, 21, 88 (1968).

[7] Rein, R., Claverie, P., and Pollak, M., *Intern. J. Quantum Chem.*, 2, 129 (1968).

THEORETICAL STUDY OF PHOTODIMERIZATION OF THYMINE

by

Robert M. Sayre*, J. P. Harlos* and Robert Rein*

I. INTRODUCTION

Thymine has great biological importance, because it is a constituent of the DNA of all living organisms. Any photochemical event affecting thymine, before or after its incorporation into DNA, has the potential, not only to affect the present cell, but all future progeny of that cell.

The photochemistry of thymine has been explored to the extent that many possible photo reactions involving it have been postulated, isolated and detected. Figure 1 indicates the numbering system used throughout this study. Thymine has

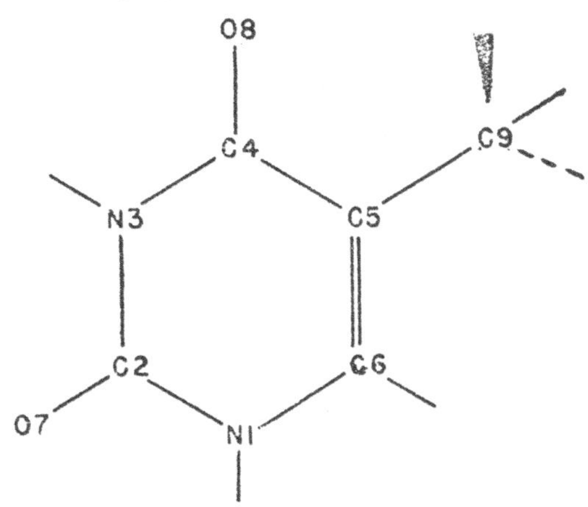

FIGURE 1. Thymine Monomer (numbering indicates that used throughout paper.

been shown to form an isomeric series of photodimers (see Figure 2), photohydrates, mixed dimers formed from one molecule of thymine with another of uracil or cytosine, and at times to decompose into smaller photoproducts [1-4]. In addition, recently

* Department of Experimental Pathology, Roswell Park Memorial Institute, Buffalo, New York, and Center for Theoretical Biology and The Department of Biophysical Sciences, State University of New York at Buffalo.

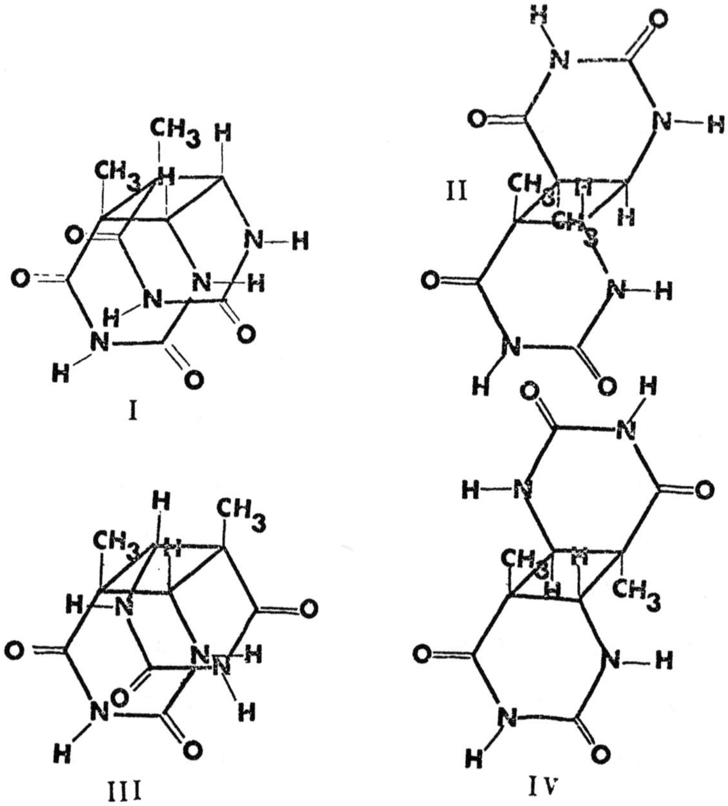

FIGURE 2. Thymine Dimer Isomers
I *cis* (head-to-head)
II *trans* (head-to-head)
III *cis* (head-to-tail)
IV *trans* (head-to-tail)

several new products, whose exact structure and composition are undetermined, have been formed from poly-thymidine [5,2,3,6]. Most studies have dealt with the problems of isolation and detection of the thymine photoproducts, either in aqueous or frozen solutions or *in vivo* and *in vitro* in DNA. A good review of the photochemistry of thymine and of DNA is found in Smith and Hanawalt's recent monograph [7].

The theoretical studies on thymine dimerization have for the most part compared ground state properties to those of the singlet and triplet excited states [8-11]. These studies involve only the examination of the π-electron system. All studies tend to indicate that in the ground state the 5-6 bond has almost double bond character - a high bond order. While in an excited state, the 5-6 bond order greatly decreases in strength [8-11]. Such lessening in bond order suggests that the bond is more prone to attack. The monomer studies further indicate that upon excitation the free valence on the 5 and 6 carbon atoms increases [9,11]. When the triplet state of thymine has been studied, these investigators report that both on the 5 and 6 carbon atoms there appears proportionally large spin densities [8-11]. The reports vary concerning changes in charge density on atoms 5 and 6 during excitation. Denis and Pullman [9] find that the net charge on atom 6 increases on excitation, but Danilov [8] finds that there is a decrease in this same charge in the singlet state. Finally Pullman [11] has compared the decrease in bond order on excitation for a series of thymine analogues to their ability to dimerize. In general his comparison shows that the greater the decrease in bond order for the 5-6 double bond, the greater the possibility of the formation of a dimer.

Jordan and Pullman [12] have performed an extended Hückel calculation on the ground state properties for thymine and uracil photodimers. Their calculations have particularly compared the total orbital electronic energies for the various thymine dimer conformations, including some in which the planar thymine bases have been replaced with the "best" half chair bases. They determine that for thymine the *cis* (head-to-tail) and *trans* (head-to-tail) dimers appear to be the most stable. They found that the preferred angle of the bases to the cyclobutane ring was 120 degrees for all dimer conformations. Finally Jordan and Pullman calculated the dipole moments for the ground state dimers, which after correction, compared favorably to the experimentally measured values.

Nagata et al. [13] have adopted a different approach in evaluating the interaction of thymine monomers to form an excited state dimer. The perturbation treatment given by Nagata et al. somewhat resembles that which we will employ, although their procedure arises from the "frontier" π-electron theory. Their approach, however, is defective in that neither the ground state interactions are explicitly included, nor is the overlap or distance of separation specifically included. The charge interactions have not been explicitly accounted for either. Further they have dropped all terms, second order and higher, in overlap.

Nagata et al. have found for a series of aromatic molecules that uracil and thymine have the largest energy of delocalization of π-electrons and have a high ability to form dimers. Regarding the ability to form the isomers of thymine dimers, they report that the *cis* (head-to-tail) and *trans* (head-to-tail) isomers have the greatest energies of π-electron delocalization, and therefore these isomers should predominate.

In addition to his fine studies regarding the role of the triplet state in thymine photodimerization, Lamola [4] has utilized calculations for exciton band splitting to study the mechanism of photo reversal of dimerization of the *cis* (head-to-head) isomer. He calculated from the observed band splitting that the distance of separation for the isolated monomers is 2.8 Å. These results, he viewed as consistent with a multistep model for thymine dimerization that proceeds from monomer to excited state dimer to dimer.

The mechanism proposed for thymine dimerization is a multistep process [4]. Such a mechanism requires that two thymine monomers be in appropriate geometrical relation. If one monomer is raised to an excited state, and interacts with another monomer, a metastable excited state dimer can be formed. There are several pathways available that the excited state dimer can return to the ground state. The excited state dimer, through internal conversion, with appropriate nuclear rearrangement and reorganization of its electronic structure may decay into a ground state photodimer. Such a process is represented schematically in Equations (1-3). The mechanism written in Equations (1-3) involves only a generalized excited state.

$$T \overset{h\nu}{\rightleftarrows} T^* \tag{1}$$

$$T^* + T \rightleftarrows TT^* \tag{2}$$

$$TT^* \rightarrow TT \tag{3}$$

T represents ground state thymine monomer
T* represents excited state thymine monomer
TT* represents excited state thymine dimer
TT represents ground state thymine dimer

Equations (1-3) represent a simplified version of a mechanism of photodimerization. A generalized excited state is represented here; although with only slight modification, it could be a singlet or triplet state. The presence of sensitizers or quenchers complicate the reaction mechanism somewhat; however, one step common to any scheme is that of the formation of an excited state dimer.

It is the purpose of this investigation: 1) to verify the findings regarding the monomer's excited states, 2) to examine quantitively and qualitatively certain possible energetic pathways in the formation of the various isomeric photodimers involving first the formation of an excited state dimer, and 3) to examine a possible mechanism for dimerization to occur in DNA.

The method employed here involves the calculation of all energies of interaction as two ground state thymine molecules approach within bonding distance and comparison with those when one of the two molecules is in an excited state.

II. MONOMER STUDIES

In order to verify the conclusions regarding the findings in previous studies of the characteristics of the ground and excited state monomers, a total valence calculation using Iterative Extended Hückel Theory (IEHT, [14]) was performed to obtain eigenvalues and eigenvectors applicable to thymine. From these total valence electron calculations, all contributions to the π-electron structure were separated and used to calculate the π-electron bond orders, the free valence, and the π-electron density. These values could then be compared directly to those reported by investigators using only π-electron calculations. The π-electron bond orders in ground and excited state are given by the following equations:

$$BO_{ij} = 2\sum_{u=1}^{occ} C_{ui}C_{uj} \qquad \text{ground state} \qquad (4)$$

$$BO_{ij}^{\ell\rightarrow\ell+1} = 2\sum_{u=1}^{\ell-1} C_{ui}C_{uj} + \sum_{u=\ell}^{\ell+1} C_{ui}C_{uj} \qquad \text{excited state} \qquad (5)$$

BO_{ij} represents the π-electron bond order between ith and the jth atoms.
The excitation is from the ℓth to the $(\ell + 1)$ orbitals.
C_{ui} are the molecular orbital coefficients.

$$F_i = 1.732 - BO_{i,i+1} - BO_{i,i-1} \tag{6}$$

The π-electron density was calculated using the following equations for the ground and excited states:

$$q_i = 2\sum_{u=1}^{occ} C_{ui}^2 \qquad \text{ground state} \tag{7}$$

$$q_i^{\ell\rightarrow\ell+1} = 2\sum_{u=1}^{\ell-1} C_{ui}^2 + \sum_{u=\ell}^{\ell+1} C_{ui}^2 \qquad \text{excited state} \tag{8}$$

These calculated indices were then compared with those of the investigators reporting changes in these indices on excitation.

Table 1 gives a comparison of the π-bond orders calculated from the wave functions generated by the IEHT procedure with those of other investigators who have argued that, because of the decrease in the 5-6 double bond in the excited state, this is the site that can dimerize. Our results indicate the same trend. Two other π-electron quantities are also compared with those of other investigators. A calculation of the free valence, indicated that the π components of the IEHT procedure also show the free valences of atom 5 and 6 increasing upon excitation. Finally the π-electron density and total electron densities from the IEHT calculations are compared with the ground and excited state electron densities in the excited state are somewhat varient with both those of Pullman [11] and Danilov [8]. These results tend to support the idea that this bond (the 5-6 double bond) is weakened and particularly vulnerable to attack in the excited state.

TABLE 1. COMPARISON THYMINE MONOMER PROPERTIES

π-Bond Order

BOND	GS^a	GS^b	GS^c	$n\to\pi^a$	$\pi\to\pi^{*a}$	$G\to S^{1b}$	$G\to S^{3b}$	$G\to S^{1c}$	$G\to T^{3c}$
5-6	0.598	0.811	0.903	0.394	0.260	0.411	0.451	0.425	0.205

Free Valence 5-6 Double Bond

ATOM	GS^a	GS^b	GS^c	$n\to\pi^a$	$\pi\to\pi^{*a}$	$G\to S^{1b}$	$G\to T^{3b}$	$G\to S^{1c}$	$G\to T^{3c}$
5	0.859	0.455	0.496	0.958	1.270	0.588	0.561	0.898	1.078
6	0.861	0.544	0.536	1.284	1.254	0.860	0.891	0.878	1.217

π- Electron Density Atoms 5 and 6

ATOM	GS^a	GS^d	GS^c	$n\to\pi^{*a}$	$\pi\to\pi^{*a}$	$G\to S^{1d}$	$G\to S^{1c}$
5	0.805	1.043	0.967	0.906	0.732	0.972	0.778
6	0.919	1.020	1.019	1.328	1.225	1.231	0.934

a π Contribution from IEHT Procedure.

b Pullman, Reference [11].

c Danilov, Reference [8].

d Denis & Pullman, Reference [9].

GS- Stands for ground state.

III. EXCITED STATE DIMER STUDIES

Methods

The procedure used in this study is to examine the total energy of interaction in the formation of the excited state dimer (one molecule in the ground state and one in a generalized excited state). For this present study, we will consider the formation of the excited state dimer as a two step process: that is an excited monomer interacts with another in the ground state where the wave function is only perturbed slightly by the presence of the other molecules. The second substep is the electronic and nuclear reorganization necessary to form the excited state dimer. At the present time we will consider only the first substep in this excited state dimer formation. Simultaneously, we will consider the interactions for both molecules being in their ground states to confirm the absence of a thermal dimerization product. We have decomposed the total energy of interaction into four component terms: 1) a contribution due to the interaction of π-electrons as the molecules approach one another (This will herewith be called the overlap interaction.), 2) a term representing the interaction of the electrostatic charges on both molecules, 3) a term representing the polarization interaction of the σ-electrons, and 4) a term representing the dispersion interaction of the σ of core electrons remaining on the molecular framework.

The Overlap Interaction

$$E_{int} = -\sum_{rr'} (q_r + q_{r'})\eta_{rr'}S_{rr'} - 2\sum_{j}^{occ}\sum_{k'}^{unocc}\Big[\frac{(\sum_{rr'} c_{jr}c_{k'r'}\eta_{rr'})^2}{E_{k'} - E_j} + \frac{1}{4}(E_{k'} - E_j)(\sum_{rr'} c_{jr}c_{k'r'}S_{rr'})^2\Big] - 2\sum_{j'}^{occ}\sum_{k}^{unocc}$$

$$\Big[\frac{(\sum_{rr'} c_{kr}c_{j'r'}\eta_{rr'})^2}{E_k - E_{j'}} + \frac{1}{4}(E_k - E_{j'})(\sum_{rr'} c_{kr}c_{j'r'}S_{rr'})^2\Big] \qquad (9)$$

r and r' refer to atoms in different thymine monomers.

q_r and $q_{r'}$ refer to π-electron charges densities on atomic centers.

E_j and E_k are Hückel molecular orbital energies.

C are associated molecular orbital coefficients in the LCAO expansion.

$S_{rr'}$ is the atomic overlap between the two molecules.

$\eta_{rr'}$ is an interaction energy that is parameterized in this approximation as being proportional to the interatomic overlaps. This constant of proportionality is taken as -9 eV.

The overlap interactions were calculated using a method developed by Salem for π-electron systems [15,16]. However, these calculations, unlike those of Salem, involve the explicit calculation of interatomic overlaps. Equation (9) gives the ground-ground state overlap interaction energy between the two molecules. As can be seen the resultant interaction energy comprises two main terms. The first is a repulsive term, $-(q_r + q_{r'})\eta_{rr'}S_{rr'}$, proportional to the π-electron charge density and roughly proportional to the overlap squared (since $\eta_{rr'}$ is proportional to the overlap). The repulsion arises due to the closed shell configuration of the ground state molecules in which all bonding orbitals are filled. The second is an attractive term due to the mixing of all π shells on one molecule with unoccupied shells on the other.

For the interaction energy, when one molecule has been excited the new interaction energy is the ground state interaction energy plus a small perturbation term, given approximately by Equations (10) and (11):

where
$$\Delta E^*_{int} = E_{int} + \Delta E_{int} \quad (10)$$

$$\Delta E^{(i\to j)}_{int} = -\left(\left|\sum_{rr'} c_{ir}c_{i'r'}\eta_{rr'}\right| + \left|\sum_{rr'} c_{jr}c_{j'r'}\eta_{rr'}\right|\right) + \sum_{rr'} (c_{ir}^2 - c_{jr}^2)\eta_{rr'}S_{rr'} + \sum_{\substack{\text{all } i' \\ (\neq i)}} \left[\frac{(\sum_{rr'} c_{ir}c_{i'r'}\eta_{rr'})^2}{E_{i'} - E_i} + \frac{1}{4}(E_{i'} - E_i)\left(\sum_{rr'} c_{ir}c_{i'r'}S_{rr'}\right)^2\right] - \sum_{\text{all } i' \neq j} \left[\frac{(\sum_{rr'} c_j c_{i'r'}\eta_{rr'})^2}{E_{i'} - E_j} + \frac{1}{4}(E_{i'} - E_j)\left(\sum_{rr'} c_{jr}c_{i'r'}S_{rr'}\right)^2\right] . \quad (11)$$

c_{jr} and $c_{j'r'}$ are the Hückel LCAO coefficients.

$\eta_{rr'}$ is a parameterized constant.

$S_{rr'}$ is the intermolecular atomic overlap.

E is the correspondent molecular orbital energy.

When the molecules are identical, the linear term usually is significant, but when they are different, it disappears and the second order terms in overlap (the remainder), become the lead terms. For our calculations, even though both molecules are identical, we have retained all terms.

To calculate the Hückel energies and molecular orbital coefficients, a Hückel secular determinant was set up utilizing the α and β parameters suggested by Streitweiser [6] and diagonalized. The obtained energies were then converted into electron volts using $\beta = 3.0$ eV.

Electrostatic Interactions

The electrostatic interactions are explicitly included in these calculations, since the molecules of interest have a dipole moment in the ground state and involve heteroatoms. The electrostatic interactions are calculated as a coulombic interaction between net atom charges on one molecule with all net atom charges on the other. The net atom charges used (for ground and excited states) were calculated using the IEHT computer program [14].

$$E_{el} = \sum_{r}\sum_{r'} \frac{q_r q_{r'}}{d_{rr'}} \qquad (12)$$

E refers to the electrostatic energy of interaction.
rr' refers to atomic centers on the unprimed and primed molecules.
$d_{rr'}$ refers to the distance between the rth atoms on the unprimed molecule and the r'th atom on the primed molecule.
q_r is the net atomic charge on the rth atom of the unprimed molecule.
$q_{r'}$ is the net atomic charge on the r'^{th} atom of the primed molecule.

Polarization Interaction

The $\underline{\sigma}$ polarization interaction was included inasmuch as the influence of the core σ-electrons were not explicitly included in the initial overlap interaction. It has been shown that, to the second order approximations used elsewhere, that the contribution of σ-electrons need be included [17-19]*. In this study the monopole bond polarizability approximation was used to investigate the σ polarization energy of interaction. The following equation, due to Rein, Claverie, and Pollak, was used in determining this interaction:

$$E_{pol} = -\frac{1}{2}\left[\alpha^{t}(\xi \cdot \xi) + \delta(\xi \cdot \alpha^{\ell})\right]$$

$$\xi = \sum_{\beta} \frac{\rho(\beta)}{R_{\beta}^{3}} R_{\beta} \qquad (13)$$

$\rho_{(\beta)}$ is the net charge on the βth atom.

α^{t} is the transverse polarizability.

$\delta = \alpha^{\ell} - \alpha^{t}$.

$R_{(\beta)}$ is the distance from the βth atom to the midpoint of the bond being considered.

The calculations are first the net changes on one molecule and the bonds and polarizabilities on the other; then they are repeated reversing the molecules. The polarizabilities used were obtained from Hirshfeld, Curtis and Bird [20], with the exception that the σ polarizability for carbon-carbon single bond was recommended by Claverie. All σ polarizabilities used were for single bonds irrespective of molecular environment. The net charges for ground and excited state configurations were obtained from the IEHT program. In both the polarization on σ dispersion calculations all atoms and bonds were included.

Dispersion Interaction

For the σ-σ dispersion energy, a bond polarizability approximation was used, represented by Equation (14) [17-19]. The molecular ionization potentials used in the case of an excited molecule were obtained by application of Koopman's theorem to the first excited state. The summations in the dispersion interactions evaluation were overall bonds in both molecules.

---

* Rein, Claverie and Pollak have shown that the σ-electrons contributed 60 to 70% of the total interaction in their investigation of the stacking of base pairs in DNA. See [17].

$$E_{dispersion} = -\frac{1}{4}\frac{I_1 I_2}{I_1 + I_2} \sum_{i=1}^{b_1} \sum_{j=1}^{b_2} \frac{1}{r_{ij}^6}\Big[6\alpha_1^T\alpha_2^T + \alpha_1^T\delta_2(3(\alpha_2^L \cdot r) + 1)$$

$$+ \alpha_2^T\delta_1(3(\alpha_1^L \cdot r)^2 + 1) + \delta_1\delta_2[3(\alpha_1^L \cdot r)(\alpha_2^L \cdot r)$$

$$- (\alpha_1^L \cdot \alpha_2^L)]^2\Big] \quad .$$

$\delta = \alpha^\ell - \alpha^t$

I_1, I_2 are molecular ionization potentials.

b_1, b_2 are number of bonds in molecule 1 and 2.

α^t is the transverse sigma polarizability.

α^ℓ is the longitudinal sigma polarizability.

α^L vector is a unit vector directed along the bond.

r_{ij} is the distance between midpoint of the ith bond on molecule 1 to midpoint of jth bond in molecule 2.

r is the vector joining the midpoints of bonds in molecule 1 and 2.

IV. CONFIGURATIONS STUDIED

The geometrical configurations studied were idealized to the extent that both monomers were parallel with the z axis being taken perpendicular to their planes. The four configurations examined were shown in Figure 2.

For the calculation of the perturbation overlap interaction, the configurations of the individual thymines were idealized still further. Firstly, both the real geometry of the six membered thymine ring and that of benzene were compared. No significant change in interaction was found between real and idealized geometries for the overlap interactions. Secondly, the three methyl hydrogens, which together contribute a component to the pi electron system, were replaced with a single pseudo-hydrogen, located 0.5 Å from the methyl carbon and in the plane of the thymine. The pseudo-hydrogen was then given an appropriate component which contributed to the pi electron system in both the näive Hückel and, hence, in the overlap interaction calculations.

For all other interactions, all atoms including all hydrogens were used, the positions of which were determined from the crystallography literature.

Finally all calculations were repeated in increments of 0.2 Å from 1.0 to 4.8 Å separation.

Results

Overlap Interactions

Figure 3 shows the results for the ground state overlap interaction for each of the four isomers studied. Note that at all distances (2.0 to 5.0 Å separation) the ground state overlap interaction is repulsive. It should also be noted that at molecular separation of less than 1.6 Å the perturbation theory used no

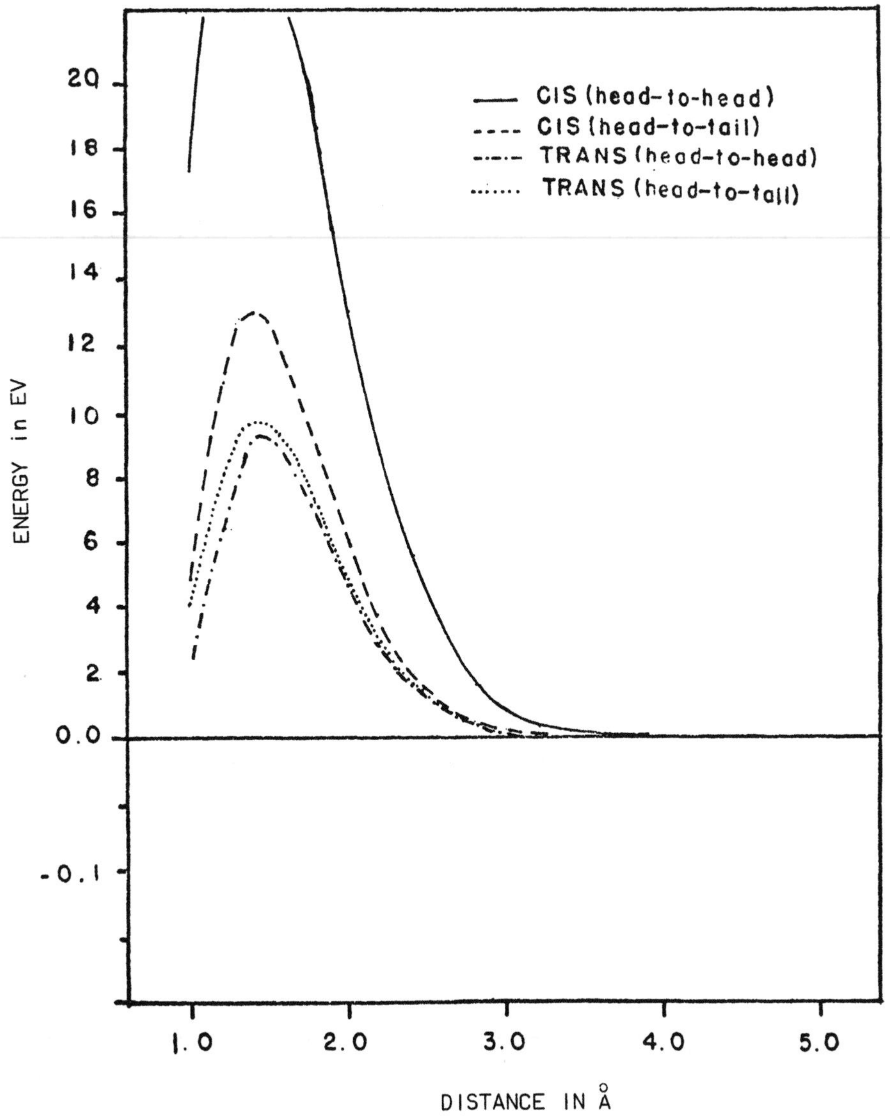

FIGURE 3. Ground state overlap interactions.

longer applies. This breakdown in the theory occurs, because all terms second order and higher in overlap have been neglected. If the overlap becomes larger than 0.2 Å or so, this approximation is no longer appropriate. Also, if the molecules used were to approach so closely, one would need to account for nuclear and electronic rearrangements, which also invalidates the simple perturbation methods used.

Figure 4 gives the results obtained for the excited state overlap interactions for each of the four isomers. In contrast to the previous ground-ground

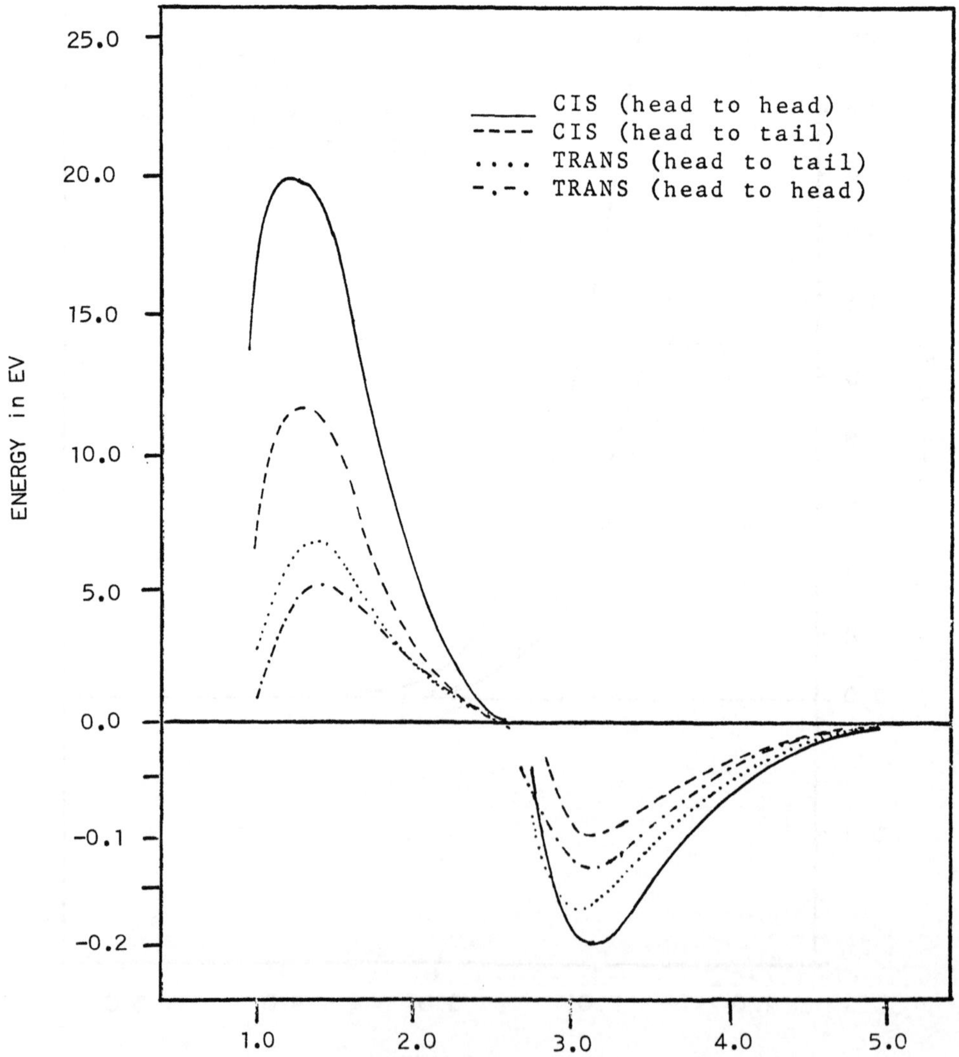

FIGURE 4. Excited state overlap interactions.

state interactions, the results indicate that when an excited state monomer interacts with one in the ground state a net stabilization occurs. An examination of these results indicates that the net stabilization is approximately 0.2 eV or 4.6 kcal/mole.

One additional configuration was tested, which results in a "rare" type of thymine dimer. This is a *trans* type dimer in which the 5-6 double bond on one molecule was interacted with the 3-2 single bond on the other. Initially, when this conformation was tested, it was felt that the presence of a single bond and a nitrogen in position 3 would lead to a situation in which no dimer could be formed, but recently this dimer, too, was found in irradiated DNA [7]. In the ground state the repulsive barrier is observed as in all other conformations studied. However, in the excited state a substantially weaker attraction was found. The interaction reached a maximum that was three times smaller than that for either of the normal *trans* (head-to-head) or *trans* (head-to-tail) isomers, and this occurred when the monomers were 0.2 to 0.4 Å farther apart. This indicates that a less stable excited state dimer was formed.

Electrostatic Interaction

Figures 5 and 6 show the results for both the ground state and excited state electrostatic interactions. The ground state-ground state electrostatic interactions for the *cis* (head-to-head) are always repulsive, while that for the other isomers may contribute a small electrostatic stabilization. In all cases the ground state-excited state electrostatic interactions offer a larger contribution to the possible stabilization of the product.

Polarization Interaction

In Figure 7, the ground and excited state sigma electron polarization interactions are given. The polarization interactions for both ground and excited state interactions (Figure 8) always contribute an attractive interaction. While the polarization interaction is small, it does contribute to a ground state

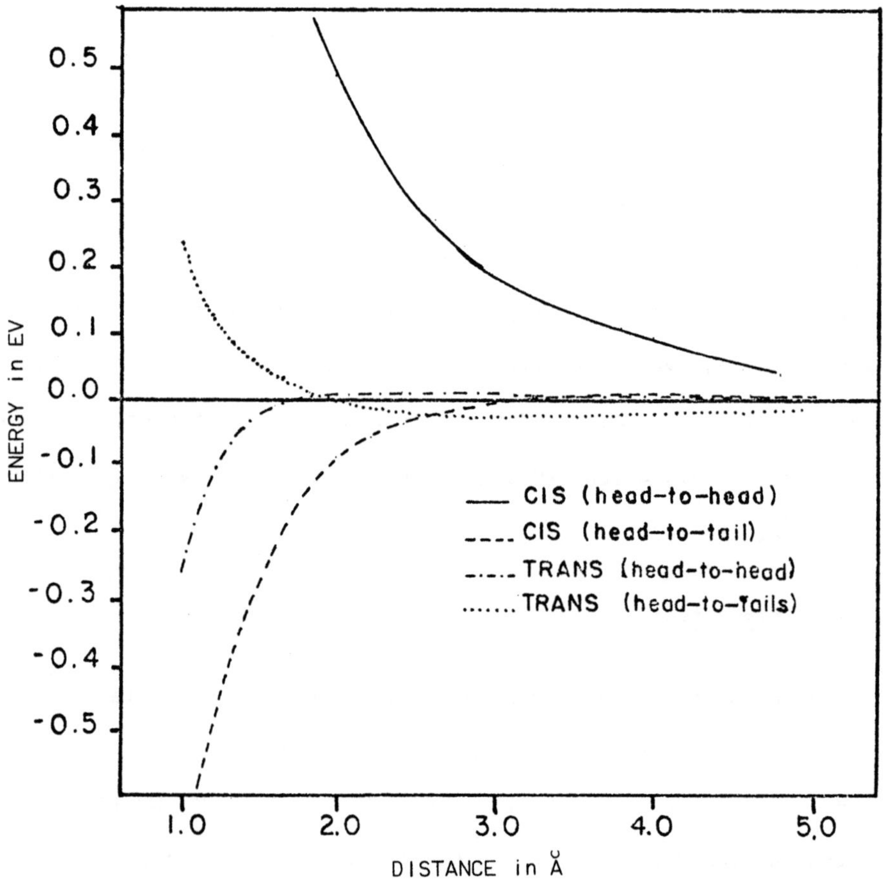

FIGURE 5. Ground state electrostatic interactions.

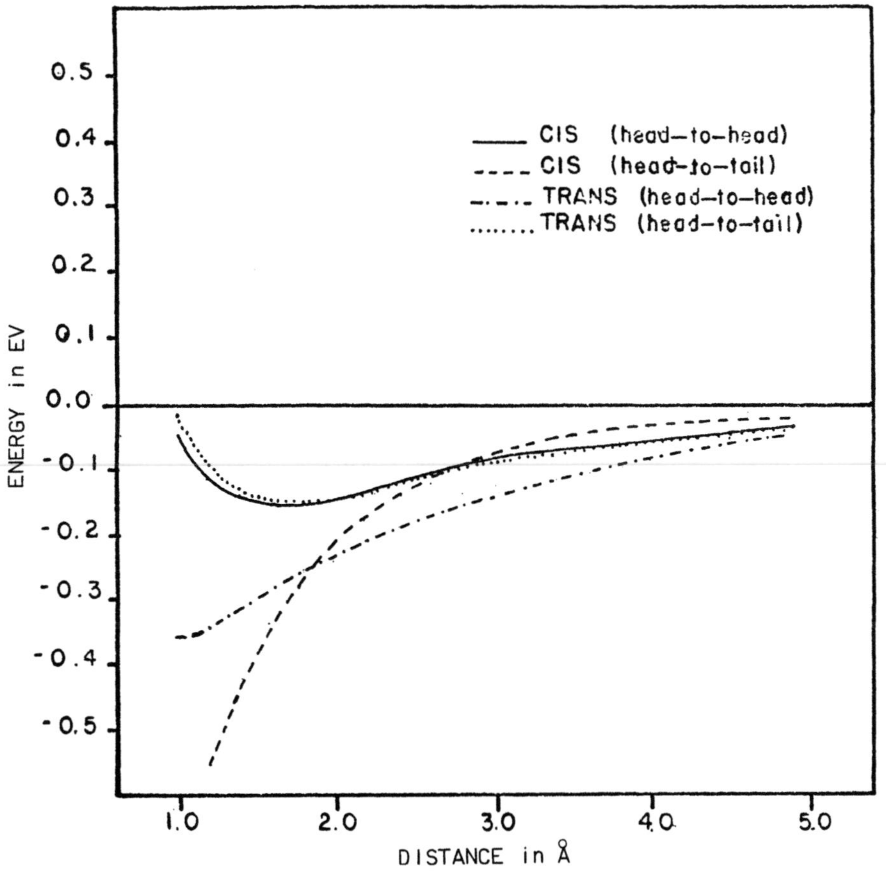

FIGURE 6. Excited state electrostatic interactions.

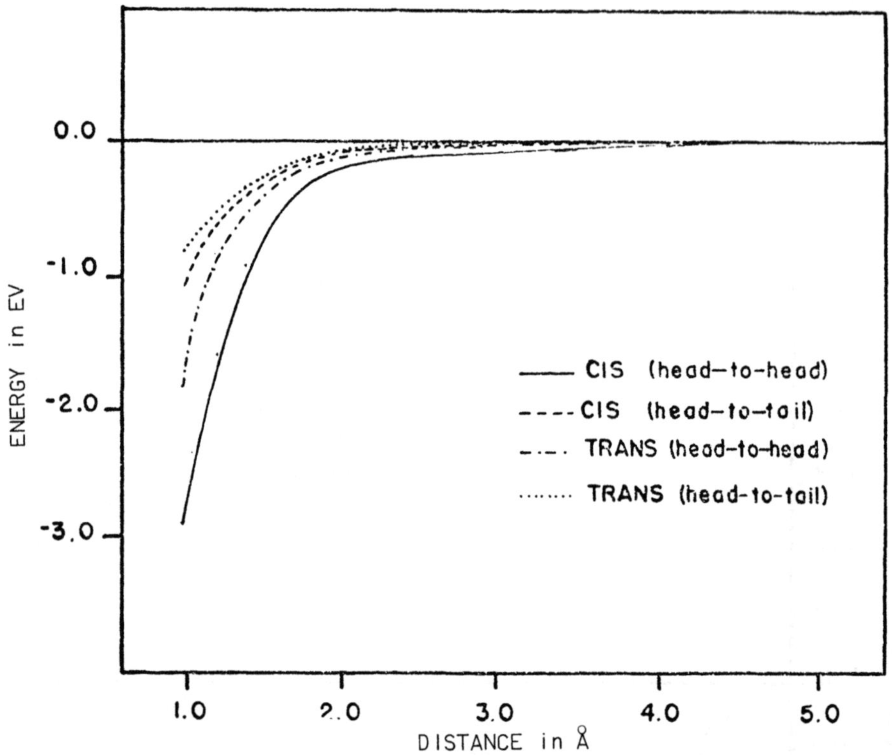

FIGURE 7. Ground state polarization interactions.

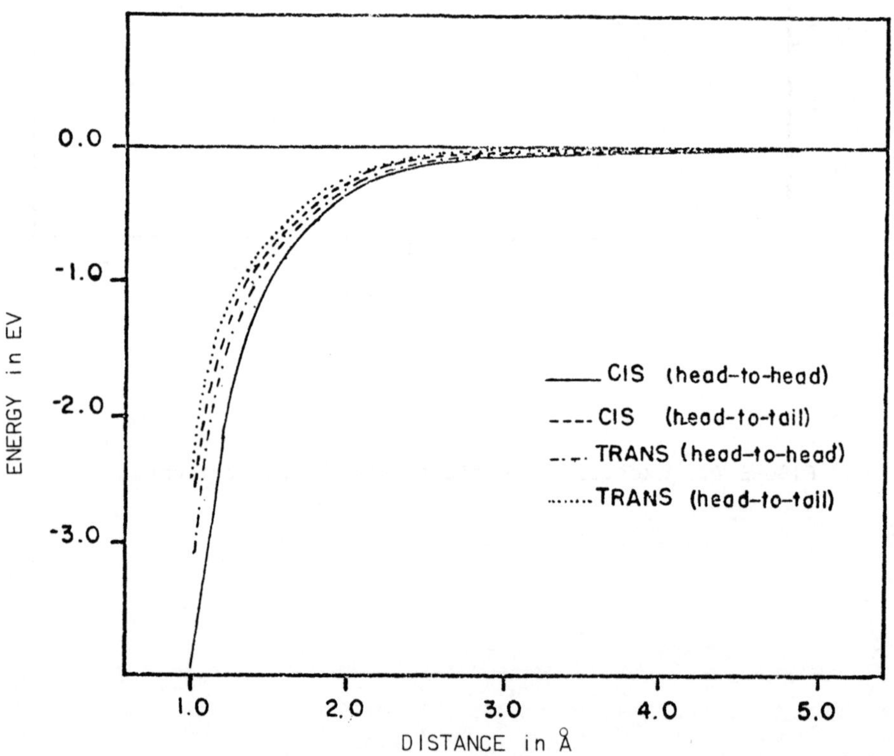

FIGURE 8. Excited state polarization interactions.

stabilization. However, the contribution toward stability for the configurations studied is greater when one molecule is excited, as shown in Figure 8.

Dispersion Interaction

The dispersion interaction, ground-ground state, for the sigma core electrons is shown in Figure 9. Again the ground-ground state interaction tends to

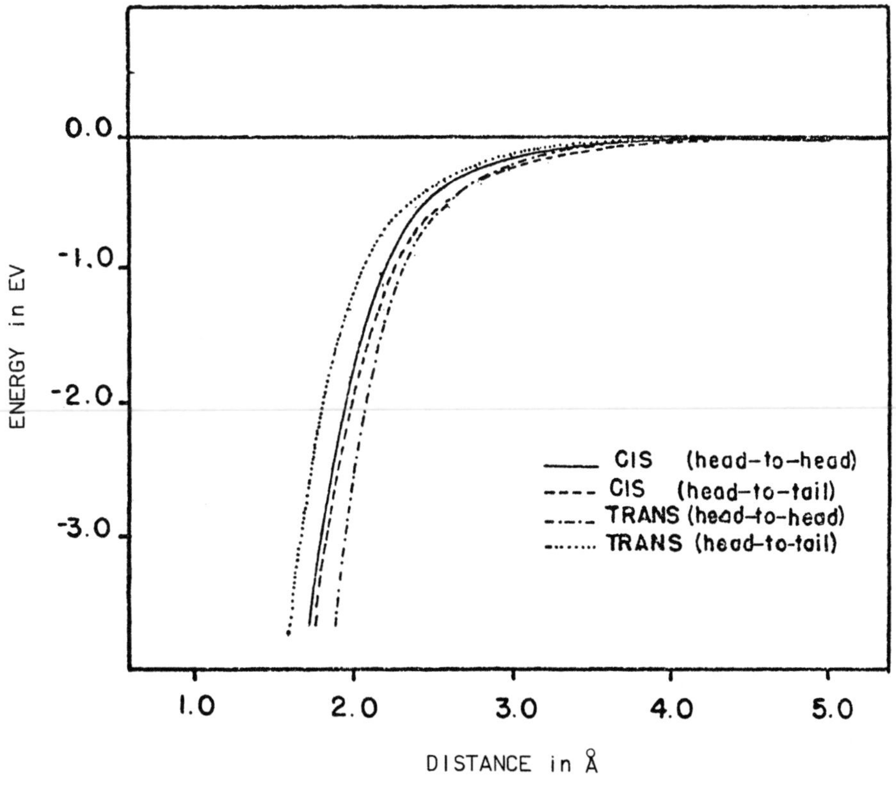

FIGURE 9. Ground state dispersion interactions.

slightly stabilize the two monomers. The results of the ground state-excited state sigma dispersion interactions for the four configurations are shown in Figure 10. In general this interaction, while still small, contributes a larger stabilization to the excited state dimer that occurred in the ground-ground state interaction (Compare Figures 9 and 10). At 2.8 to 3.0 Å this interaction may be two to three times larger (more stable) than that contributed either by the electrostatic or by the sigma polarization interactions.

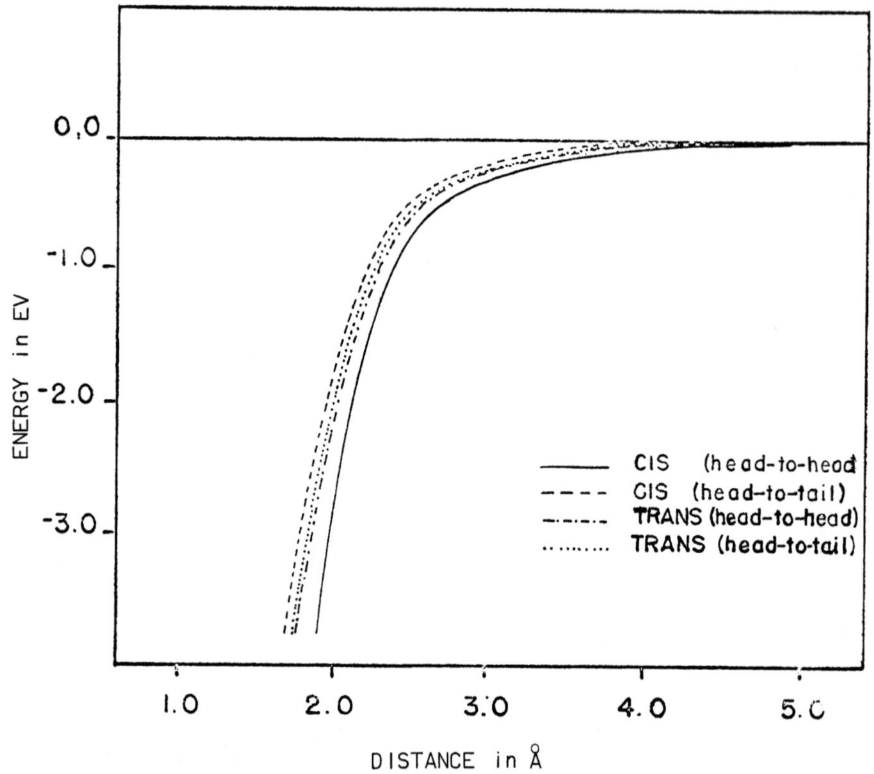

FIGURE 10. Excited state dispersion interactions.

Total Interaction

When all the contributions to the ground-ground state interactions are totalled, one finds for the *cis* (head-to-head) configuration that in the ground state at all distances the monomers repel one another (see Figure 11). While, when one monomer is excited and the other in its ground state, a new stabilization occurs (Figure 12). This stabilization is maximum at about 2.8 Å separation, with the net stabilization energy of about −0.7 eV.

For all other geometrical isomers examined, the total ground-ground state interactions indicate that both ground state molecules are repulsive; however, for configurations, other than *cis* (head-to-head), one may observe a very weakly attractive interaction −0.1 eV or less. The possible significance of these weakly attractive ground state interactions will be discussed later. There is always a

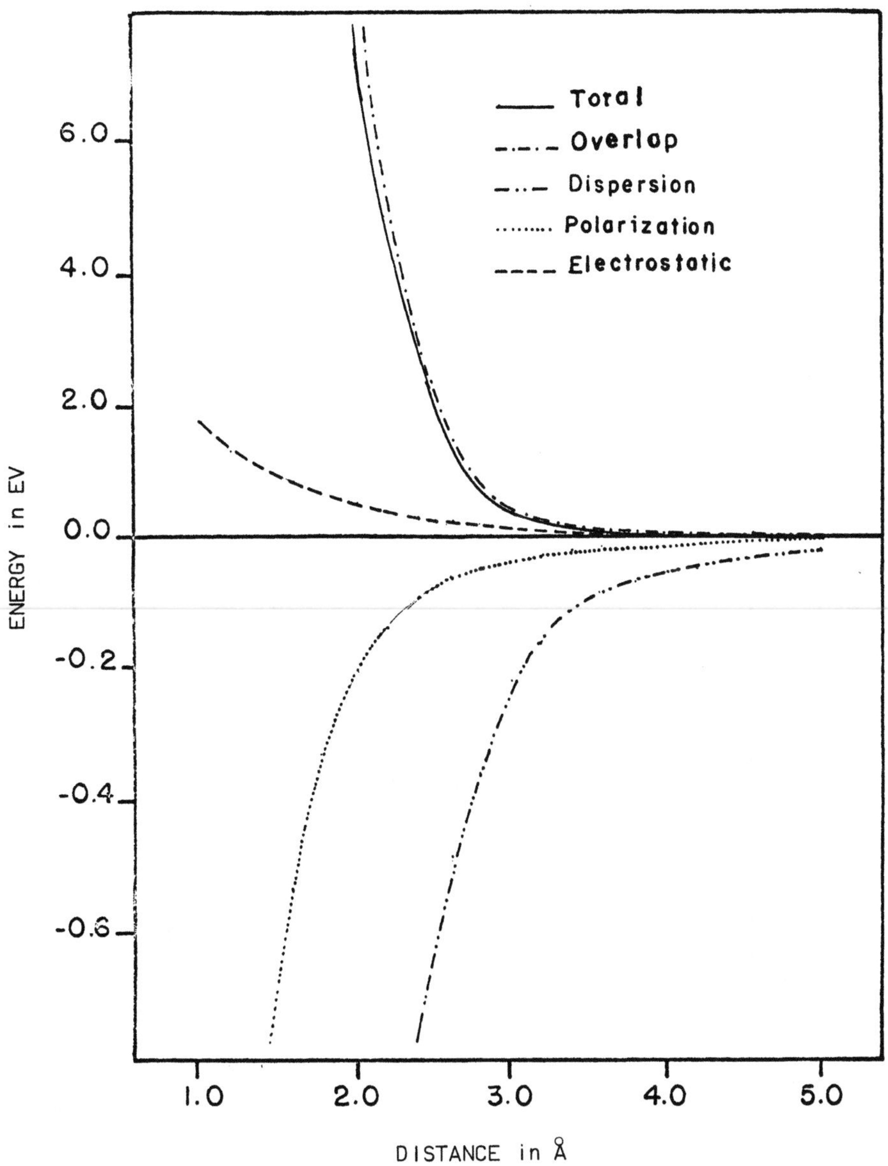

FIGURE 11. Total ground state interaction for *cis* (head-to-head) isomer.

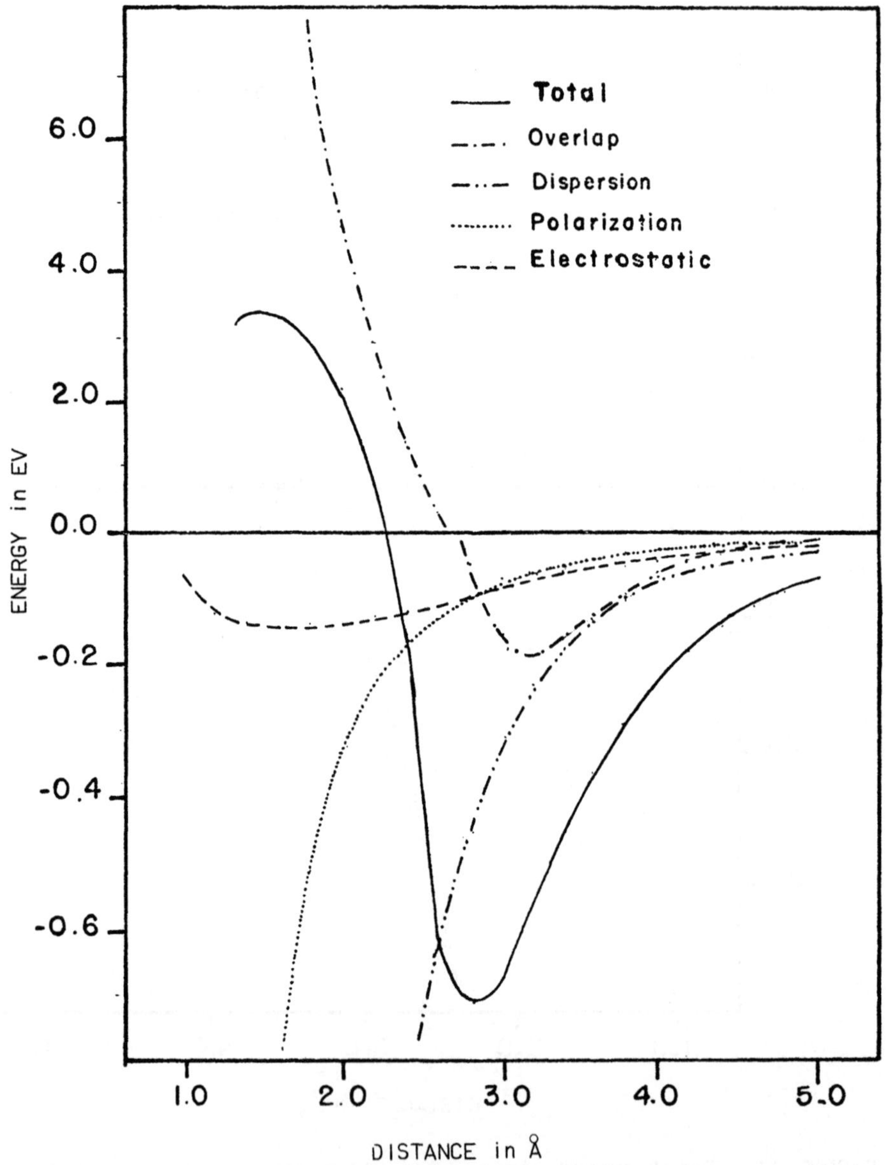

FIGURE 12. Total excited state interaction for *cis* (head-to-head) isomer.

significant energy of stabilization when one molecule is in an excited state. The energy of stabilization is maximum at about 2.8 to 3.0 Å separation.

Discussion of Excited State Dimer Studies

The results shown in Figure 11 for the *cis* (head-to-head) isomer are similar, for all ground-ground state interactions. These results indicate for each isomer studied, that at distances closer than 3.5 Å, the monomers tend to repel one another. This net repulsive interaction constitutes a barrier that would prevent thermal stabilization and subsequent thermal dimerization. In every case examined, this is not the result if one monomer has been excited. There occurs, for each of the four configurations examined, a net attraction if one monomer is excited. This attraction occurs at about 2.8 to 3.0 Å and may lead to the formation of the excited state dimer. If the net excited state overlap interactions for each of the four geometrical configurations are compared (see Figure 4), one observes that the *cis* (head-to-head) produces the greatest degree of stabilization followed in order by the *trans* (head-to-tail), *trans* (head-to-head) and the *cis* (head-to-tail) being the least stable configuration.

When all interactions have been included, the order of stability is identical with that of the overlap interaction alone for the isomers of thymine dimers. However, the total interaction is indeed more stable than the overlap by itself. The order of stability in excited state dimer formation, from most stable to least stable is shown in Table 2. The total maximum interaction occurs at 2.6 to 2.8 Å for the configurations studied.

Jordan and Pullman [12] using an extended Hückel approach calculate the total electronic energies for the ground state of the isomeric dimers. They report that the *cis* (head-to-tail) and *trans* (head-to-tail) thymine dimers appear most stable, while the *cis* (head-to-head) dimer is the least stable. While these results are of interest they are not at variance to those obtained in this study as it would first appear. Their results pertain to the final products; ours to the intermediates. The total energy may or may not be the limiting step that determines yield.

TABLE 2. TOTAL EXCITED STATE INTERACTION ENERGY

Isomer	Maximum Interaction in eV	Separation in Å
Cis (head-to-tail)	-0.702	2.8
Trans (head-to-tail)	-0.685	2.6
Trans (head-to-head)	-0.631	2.8
Cis (head-to-tail)	-0.527	2.8

A comparison could be made between the theoretical stabilities with experimental yields of the various isomers; however, the relevance of this may be questionable - first because the yields are not necessarily controlled either by final product or by the excited dimer stability; and second, because the explicit distinction between yields and isomers is not easily performed experimentally. Many investigators do agree that the *cis* (head-to-head) is the most prevalent. Frozen aqueous solutions of thymine yield only one dimer - the *cis* (head-to-head) isomer [21]. Further the *cis* (head-to-head) isomer is the only isomer isolated from irradiated DNA [4,22]. There is some discussion that the techniques used to isolate the dimer may destroy other isomers. It is significant that the strong attraction to 2.8 to 3.4 Å is the distance the bases are separated in DNA. The *cis* (head-to-head) dimer has been shown by Johns et al. [2] to remain stable under diverse physical and chemical conditions, while the other isomers decompose with similar treatment. This is consistent with this study. Furthermore, only the *cis* (head-to-head) dimer has been obtained in adequate quantity for an X-ray crystallographic determination of its structure [5]. Two considerations should be reiterated: firstly the *cis* (head-to-head) configuration studied here is idealized, compared to that identified by crystallography analysis. Secondly, it is precisely this isomer of the dimer that has been identified in irradiated DNA.

Rotated *Cis* (Head-to-Head) Conformations

The configurations considered thus far are quite idealized. Indeed, the only thymine dimer actually crystallized and studied using X-ray diffraction techniques [5] is the *cis* (head-to-head) thymine dimer. The findings indicate that the planes of the two molecules are inclined at about 28.5°. In addition, the molecules are rotated with respect to each other by about 28°. This configuration specifically requires that the cyclobutane ring is no longer square, but rather a puckered or strained parallelogram, which is no longer planar. However, one must observe caution in speculating that the final geometry of the ground state dimer has any relation whatsoever to the geometrical arrangements through which the excited state dimer formation may pass.

The overlap perturbation calculations were performed to ascertain if the excited state dimer is sensitive to rotations around the 5-6 double bond in the *cis* (head-to-head) conformation. The results for a 28° rotation in the ground and excited state interactions are compared with those for the idealized dimer in Figure 13. As can be seen, in the ground state the repulsive barrier still exists; however, in the excited state the attractive maximum not only is deeper but its maximum is shifted so that both molecules are closer together. The observed 30% increase in interaction appears significant.

Another series of calculations were performed testing the correspondence of 28° rotation to the maximum interaction. The ground and excited state interactions were determined for every 7° rotation. All the ground state calculations exhibited the same sort of repulsive barrier as shown in all earlier overlap perturbation calculations. In Figure 14 where the angle of rotation versus the energy of interaction has been plotted for only the separations of 2.8 and 3.0 Å in the excited state, the maximum interaction occurs at 28° rotation. Such a result may have serious implications concerning possible pathways of dimerization. This is significant in that the most attractive interaction for the excited state dimer, i.e. most stable, occurs when the nuclear geometry most nearly approximates that of the final state dimer. This implies that perhaps only slight nuclear rearrangement may

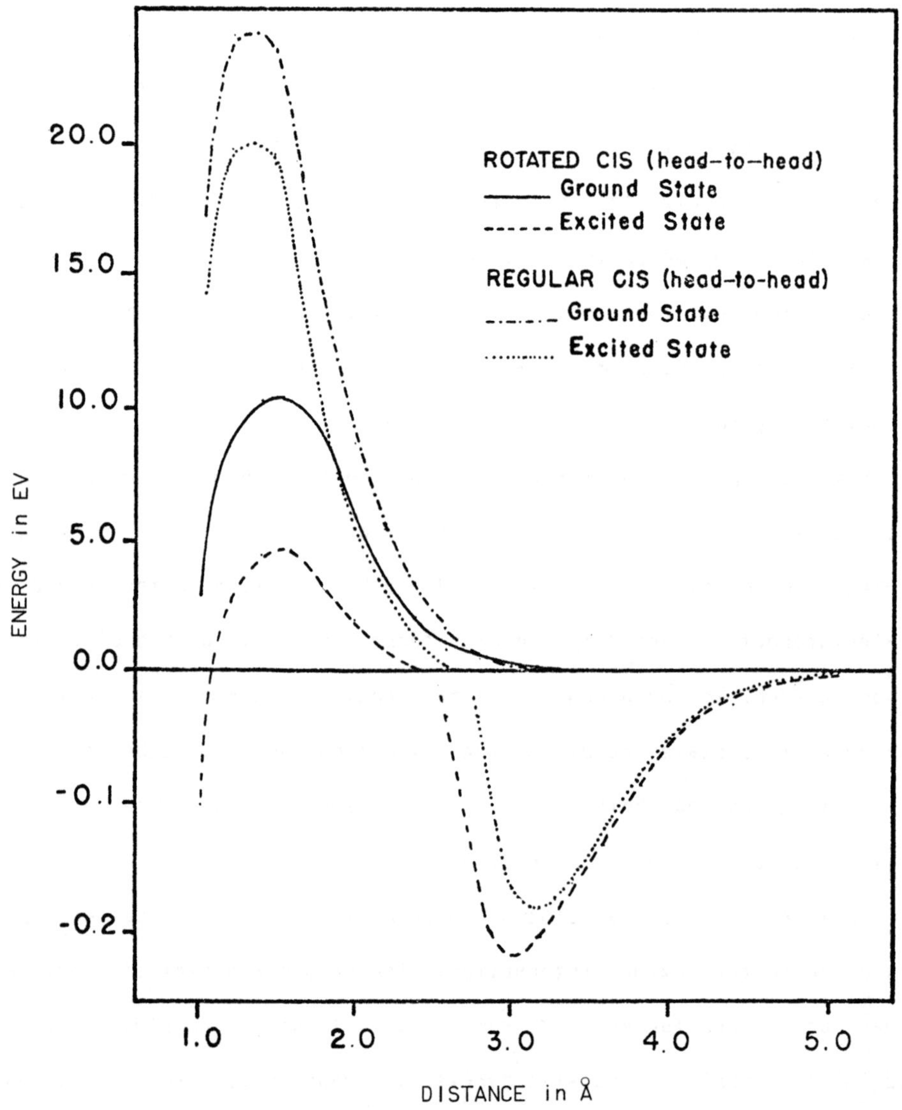

FIGURE 13. Comparison of idealized *cis* (head-to-head) isomer to that rotated 28° around the midpoint of the 5-6 double bond.

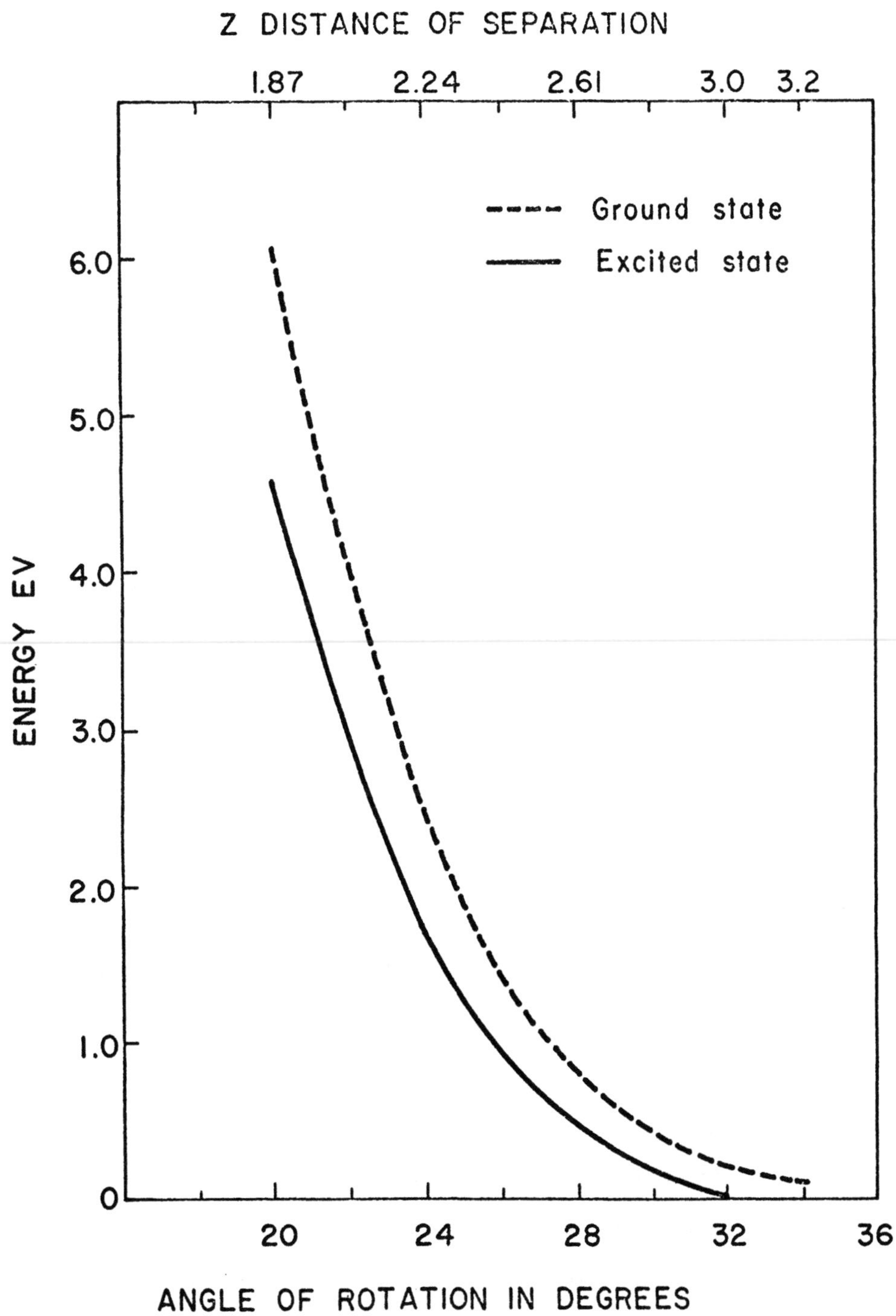

FIGURE 14. Comparison of excited state interaction vs. angle of rotation for *cis* (head-to-head) isomer.

be necessary as the excited state dimer decays into the stable ground state configuration.

V. A POSSIBLE PATHWAY OF PHOTODIMERIZATION IN DNA

One pathway that can be envisaged for the dimerization of thymine in DNA is for the adjacent stacked thymine bases to collapse around the helical axis, that is to translate closer toward one another as they twist around the helical axis. While such a mechanism would put considerable strain and compression on the sugar backbone, the strands of DNA would still resemble a double helix and would have similar configuration that must occur after the dimer is formed.

This possibility was tested utilizing the overlap interaction program. The results are shown in Figure 15. In the ground state, as both molecules rotate and translate into position, the repulsive barrier increases. The same type of repulsive barrier is observed, only slightly smaller, when one molecule has been excited. The presence of the increasing repulsive barrier in both ground and excited state interactions must be taken to mean rotation and compression of the adjacent thymines into a position favorable to dimerization in DNA, results in an unfavorable pathway for dimerization. This would suggest that some other means must be proposed by the *cis* (head-to-head) dimer can be formed as found in DNA.

If one examines the positioning of adjacent stacked thymines using space filling CPK models, one finds that the 5-6 double bonds are quite far apart. An alternative reaction pathway is for at least one of the thymines to break away from the sugar backbone in order to be able to obtain the proper position to dimerize with the adjacent thymine on the same strand. In fact, if the bond with the sugar backbone were to break, it has been shown that the hydrogen bonding with the opposite strand is broken, or at least greatly weakened, when one thymine is excited. Now the thymine could more freely twist and rotate into a geometrically favorable position for dimerization.

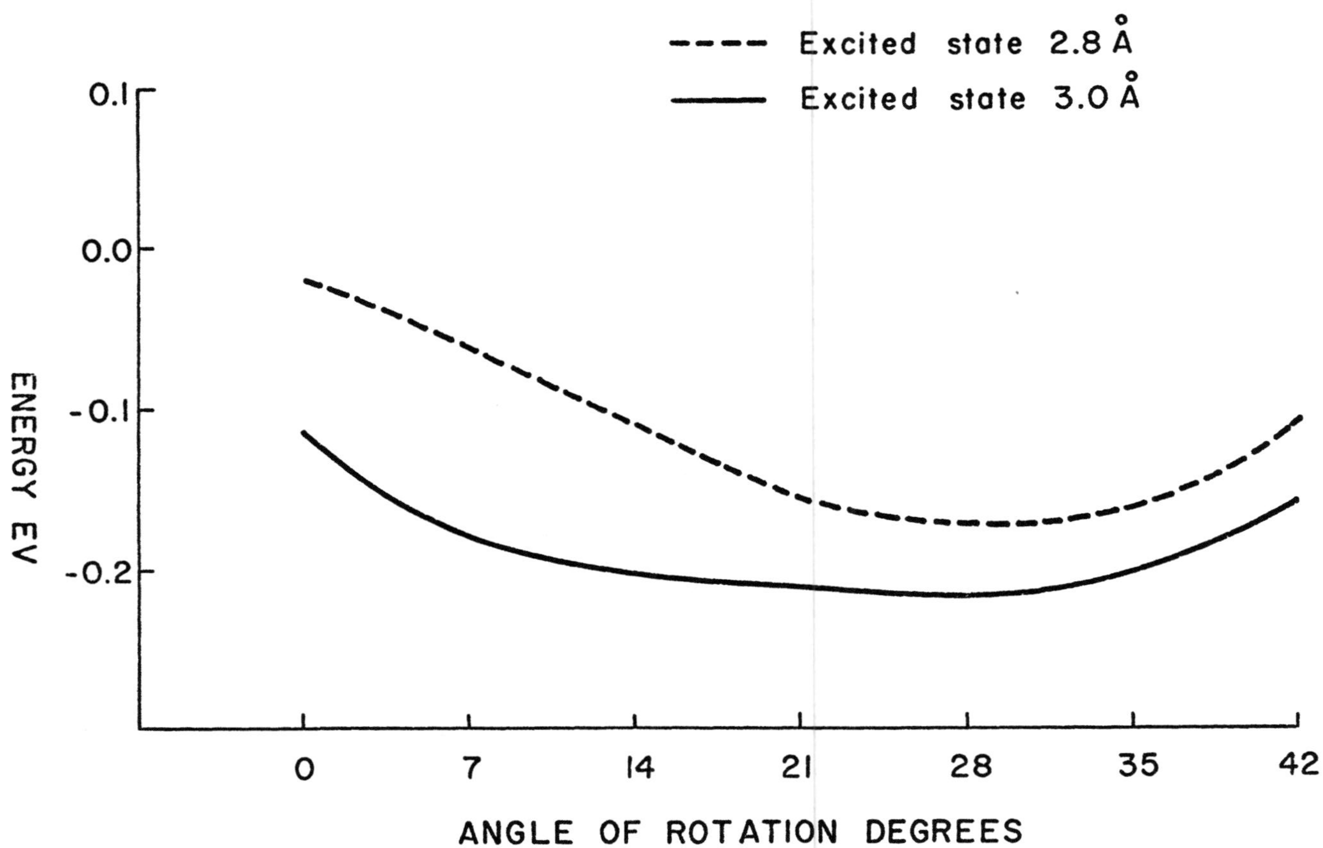

FIGURE 15. Comparison of angle of rotation and distance of separation vs. energy of interaction for thymine stacked and constrained to move around a helical axis.

VI. SUMMARY

Thus in summary we can say that our results support the following view of the reaction mechanism for thymine dimerization. Because of the obvious dependence of the excited state interactions on the nuclear arrangements, it is significant to find that small stabilizations have already occurred between ground state monomers. These stabilizing reactions, although small 0.1 eV and requiring increasing molecular separations 3.2 to 3.4 Å, tend already in the ground state to begin aligning the molecules. Thus once excited, dimerization may proceed.

It is yet significant to reiterate that once the excited dimer has been formed, the maximum interaction tends to position the nuclear centers still closer into the position of the final dimer ground state. This is supported by finding that for the *cis* (head-to-head) conformation that a rotation of 28° around the midpoint of the 5-6 double bond produces the most stable excited state dimer. This rotation corresponds to that found in the crystallized ground state dimer. Thus once formed the excited state dimer may after a simple internal conversion process return to the ground state.

Finally the question of how thymine is able to dimerize in DNA is still open. Our results indicate that one simple pathway is energetically forbidden. Without allowing an excited thymine to break away from its sugar backbone and to be able to freely translate and rotate, dimerization in DNA that produces the *cis* (head-to-head) dimer must be both stearically and energetically a difficult question.

VII. ACKNOWLEDGMENT

We gratefully acknowledge support for this investigation from NASA Grant NGR 33-015-016 and NIH Predoctorial Training Grant (RMS) 5T01GM00718-10. Further we appreciate support given these studies by the Computer Center of the State University of New York at Buffalo.

VIII. REFERENCES

[1] Brueckers, R. and Berends, W., *Biochem. Biophys. Acta.*, 41, 550, (1960).

[2] Johns, H. E. et al., *J. Mol. Biol.* 9, 503, (1964).

[3] Johns, H. E., Rapaport, S. A., and Delbrück, M., *J. Mol.Biol.*, 4, 104, (1962).

[4] Lamola, A. A., *Photochem. Photobiol.*, 7, 619, (1968).

[5] Camerman, N. and Camerman, A., *Science*, 160, 1451, (1968).

[6] Streitweiser, A. J. Jr., *Molecular Orbital Theory for Organic Chemists*, John Wiley, New York, (1966).

[7] Smith, K. C. and Hanawalt, P. C., *Molecular Photobiology: Inactivation and Recovery*, Academic Press, New York, (1969).

[8] Danilov, V. I., *Photochem. Photobiol.*, 6, 233, (1967).

[9] Denis, A. and Pullman, A., *Theoret. Chim. Acta.*, 7, 110, (1967).

[10] Kuprievich, V. A., *Int. J. Quantum Chem.*, 1, 561, (1967).

[11] Pullman, B., *Photochem. Photobiol.*, 7, 525, (1968).

[12] Jordan, F. and Pullman, B., *Theoret. Chim. Acta.*, 10, 423, (1968).

[13] Nagata, C. et al., *J. Theoret. Biol.*, 9, 357, (1965).

[14] Rein, R. et al., *J. Chem. Phys.*, 45, 4743, (1966).

[15] Salem, L., *J. Amer. Chem. Soc.*, 90, 543, (1968).

[16] *Ibid.*, *J. Amer. Chem. Soc.*, 90, 553, (1968).

[17] Rein, R., Claverie, P., and Pollak, M., *Intern. J. Quantum Chem.*, 2, 129, (1968).

[18] Rein, R. and Pollak, M., *J. Chem. Phys.*, 47, 2039, (1967).

[19] *Ibid.*, *J. Chem. Phys.*, 47, 2045, (1967).

[20] Hirschfelder, J. O., Curtis, C. F., and Bird, R. B., *Molecular Theory of Gases and Liquids*, John Wiley, New York, (1954).

[21] Buckers, R., Ylstra, J., and Berends, W., *Rec. Trav. Chim.*, 77, 883, (1959).

[22] Varghese, A. J. and Wang, S. K., *Science*, 160, 186, (1968).

PSYCHEDELIC DRUG ACTIVITY: ELECTRONIC, STERIC AND BIOCHEMICAL CORRELATES*

by

Solomon H. Snyder**

I. INTRODUCTION

Discerning the interaction of any drug and its receptors is difficult. Before a direct attack on a molecular system that mediates a drug's action is possible, indirect approaches are important. One of the most fruitful is to correlate the varying pharmacological potencies of different analogues with varying activities on a test system. As a model of drug-receptor interactions, psychedelic agents present some tempting possibilities as well as almost insuperable difficulties. For instance, d-Lysergic acid diethylamide (d-LSD) is so extraordinarily potent, producing effects in man at doses as little as 20 micrograms per 70 kg, that one can readily postulate a high degree of affinity for its receptor. Also, there are fairly extensive series of psychedelic drugs which, although apparently differing in structure, produce closely similar effects and seem to be acting on the same receptor site--which raises the question of just what psychotropic effects should be labeled "psychedelic".

Psychedelic activity is shared by a series of compounds including representatives of phenylethylamines, amphetamines, tryptamines, and multiringed structures such as d-LSD and its variants. Each of them produces profound subjective experiences most prominent of which is an intense self awareness

---

* Supported by NIH Grants 1-Ro1-NB-07275 and 1-P01-GM-16492. The author is a recipient of NIMH Research Career Development Award K3-MH-33128.

** Departments of Pharmacology and Experimental Therapeutics and Psychiatry and the Behavioral Sciences, The Johns Hopkins University School of Medicine, Baltimore, Maryland.

coupled with a feeling of heightened sensory, cognitive and emotional perception. Best known are the distortions of visual processes which have earned the appellation "hallucinogenic", although frank hallucinations are rare. It is striking that compounds so different chemically as d-LSD and mescaline should produce effects so similar that naive subjects judge them the same, while amphetamine, chemically similar to mescaline produces very different effects. Although a large number of drugs including amphetamines and anticholinergic agents can provoke "psychotic" reactions in humans, only the psychedelic agents produce the unique syndrome described above. Psychedelic drugs have been variously labeled "psychotomimetic", "psychosomimetic", "psychodysleptic", and "hallucinogenic".

What is the best way to assess their relative activities? The simplest approach is to determine minimal active doses. But this is a crude approximation since apparent activity may be related not to "receptor" potency but to variations in metabolic degradation or in ability to penetrate the blood brain barrier. Even if metabolic and transport factors are equal, there are other more subtle complications. As described above, the total spectrum of psychedelic effects embraces several components. Which of these should be the criterion for drug activity? For example, among the methoxyamphetamines, DOM(2,5-dimethoxy-4-methylamphetamine) (Figures 1 and 2) informally designated "STP", produces perceptual and cognitive changes in humans closely resembling in quality, intensity and duration the hallucinogenic-psychotomimetic syndrome of LSD [1,2].

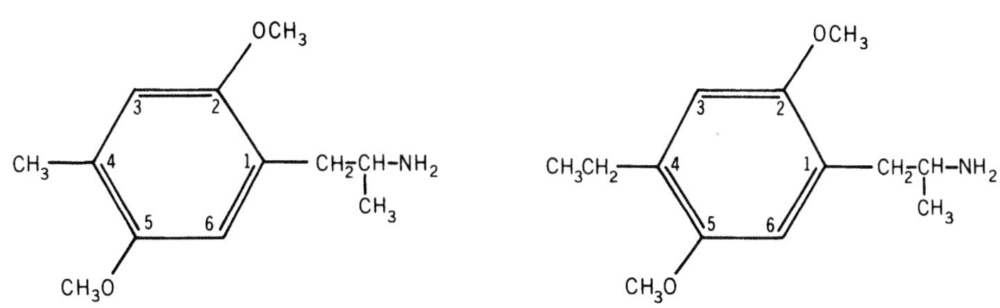

2,5-DIMETHOXY-4-METHYLAMPHETAMINE (DOM) 2,5-DIMETHOXY-4-ETHYLAMPHETAMINE (DOET)

Figure 1

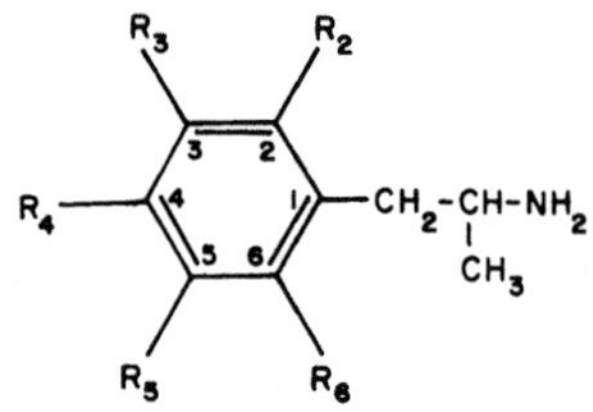

AMPHETAMINE DERIVATIVES

COMPOUND	R_2	R_3	R_4	R_5	R_6
TMA	H	CH_3O	CH_3O	CH_3O	H
TMA-2	CH_3O	H	CH_3O	CH_3O	H
TMA-3	CH_3O	CH_3O	CH_3O	H	H
TMA-4	CH_3O	CH_3O	H	CH_3O	H
TMA-5	CH_3O	CH_3O	H	H	CH_3O
TMA-6	CH_3O	H	CH_3O	H	CH_3O
DOM	CH_3O	H	CH_3	CH_3O	H
DOET	CH_3O	H	CH_3CH_2	CH_3O	H
DMMDA	CH_3O	$O-CH_2-O$		CH_3O	H
DMMDA-2	CH_3O	CH_3O	$O-CH_2-O$		H
MMDA	H	$O-CH_2-O$		CH_3O	H
MMDA-2	H	$O-CH_2-O$		H	CH_3O
MMDA-3a	CH_3O	$O-CH_2-O$		H	H
MDA	H	$O-CH_2-O$		H	H
DMA	CH_3O	H	H	CH_3O	H

Figure 2.

DOET (2,5-dimethoxy-4-ethylamphetamine) (Figures 1 and 2) differs from DOM only in the presence of an ethyl rather than a methyl group at the four position yet shows a markedly different dose-response spectrum. The minimal dose required to produce subjective effects with DOET is half that of DOM [3,4]. At these low doses DOET causes heightened self awareness and a mild euphoria [3,4]. At five times the minimal detectable dose DOET continues to enhance self-awareness but fails to provoke cognitive or perceptual distortions. Thus for certain psychological actions DOET is twice as potent as DOM, yet it is much weaker, perhaps impotent, in inducing psychotomimetic-hallucinogenic changes.

Besides the definition of "psychedelic" effects, important concerns are whether relative potency is the same in humans and animals and whether different types of animal tests provide comparable information about drug potencies. In rats psychedelic drugs have been compared in tests of rope climbing [5], bar pressing [6], and Sidman avoidance procedures [7]. Although such techniques yield similar rank-order potencies for different drugs, the observed effects are by no means specific for psychedelic drugs, since amphetamine also impairs performance. In a general way, relative potencies in rats parallel relative activity in humans. For instance, in bar pressing by rats with a fixed ratio schedule for food reinforcement [8] d-LSD is almost an order of magnitude more potent than 1-LSD, 2-brom-LSD and psilocybin which in turn are an order of magnitude more potent than mescaline.

Careful studies, however, reveal significant species differences. In an extensive series of psychotomimetic methoxyamphetamines (Table 1, Figure 2) activities were similar in two different test procedures in rats and showed some rank-order similarities to squirrel monkeys and man. But while there was a very

TABLE 1. PSYCHEDELIC DRUGS - STRUCTURE: ACTIVITY TRIMETHOXYAMPHETAMINES

Efficacy	Steric Model	Man	Monkey	Rat
Potent	2,4,5-TMA (TMA-2)	2,4,5-TMA (17)	2,4,5-TMA (5.4)	2,4,5-TMA(7.2_u)(4.0_s)
	2,4,6-TMA (TMA-6)	2,3,6-TMA (13)	2,4,6-TMA (3.2)	3,4,5-TMA(4.0_u)(1.5_s)
	2,3,6-TMA (TMA-5)	2,4,6-TMA (10)		
Weak	2,3,5-TMA (TMA-4)	2,3,5-TMA (4)	3,4,5-TMA (1.8)	2,4,6-TMA(1.7_u)(1.0_s)
	3,4,5-TMA (TMA)	3,4,5-TMA (2.2)	2,3,5-TMA (1.1)	2,3,4-TMA(1.6_u)($<1.0_s$)
	2,3,4-TMA (TMA-3)	2,3,4-TMA (<2)	2,3,4-TMA (0.7)	

TMA refers to trimethoxyamphetamine, and the preceding numbers refer to the location of methoxy substituents. The TMA designations in parentheses are the code names assigned to these compounds by Shulgin [43]. Numbers in parentheses refer to potency in mescaline units as explained in the text. Subscripts u and s refer to data of Uyeno [11] and Smythies et al. [7], respectively. Monkey and human data were obtained by Uyeno et al. [9] and Shulgin et al. [10], respectively.

close correlation between man and monkey, there were marked discrepancies between these two species and rats. For instance, 3,4,5-trimethoxyamphetamine (3,4,5-TMA) which is one of the weaker trimethoxyamphetamines in man and monkey, is one of the most potent agents in the rat; and 2,4,6-TMA, one of the most active analogues in man and monkey, is one of the weakest in rats.

Factors accounting for these differences are not readily apparent. The studies in squirrel monkeys measured impairment of visual discrimination [9], those in man reflect the minimum dose required to produce subjective psychological effects [1,4,10] while those in rats involved a Sidman avoidance procedure [7] or a test of orientation in an underwater swimming test [11]. Metabolic differences could account for the variations in potencies. Man and monkey metabolize amphetamine primarily by N-demethylation, while hydroxylation followed by conjugation at the four position is the predominant route in rats [12]. In any event, the investigator attempting to explain structure-activity relationships of psychedelic drugs must decide which species is most relevant.

In summary, studies of structure-activity relationships among psychedelic drugs are confounded by numerous difficulties, including 1) practical difficulties of evaluating compounds in man, 2) the question of which are the most relevant human psychological effects, 3) species differences in potency, and 4) variations among drugs of metabolism and penetration to active sites in the brain.

II. BIOCHEMICAL STUDIES

These limitations of *in vivo* studies tell us loudly and clearly that structure-activity relations of psychedelic drugs will be clarified only when a meaningful *in vitro* system for assessment of drug activity is developed. Biogenic amines, such as serotonin (5-hydroxytryptamine) and norepinephrine, are localized to neuronal systems in the brain mediating emotional behavior. Their structural similarity to psychedelic drugs suggests fruitful models. LSD and other psychedelic drugs increase brain serotonin [13], a phenomenon that seems to be related to a slowing of serotonin turnover in the brain [14]. To determine a neuronal basis for the effects, Aghajanian et al. [15] administered psychedelic drugs to rats and

and measured the firing rates of individual serotonergic neurons. The serotonin containing neurons have their cell bodies in the raphe nuclei of the brain stem with axons and terminals ramifying throughout the rest of the brain [16]. Aghajanian found that as little as 0.025 mg/kg of d-LSD, considerably less than the minimal dose for gross behavioral effects, would slow the firing rate of serotonin neurons. Of a number of neuronal systems evaluated, only the serotonin neurons were affected in this way by psychedelic agents. This effect was shared by all psychedelic drugs examined and was not produced by amphetamine. Thus in Aghajanian's system mescaline behaved like d-LSD and unlike its chemically close relative d-amphetamine, indicating greater specificity for psychedelic drugs than is provided by tests of animal behavior. At least two mechanisms could explain Aghajanian's results. Psychedelic drugs might slow directly the firing rate of these neurons resulting in less discharge of serotonin at their terminals. If this were the case, depletion of brain serotonin should attenuate the behavioral actions of psychedelic drugs. To the contrary, reserpine and p-chloro-phenylalanine, drugs which deplete brain serotonin , accentuate the behavioral effects of d-LSD. A more probable explanation is that psychedelic drugs mimic serotonin at its post-synaptic receptors and a neuronal feedback mechanism "turns off" the serotonin neurons. This explanation is supported by Aghajanian's finding in rats that vigorous stimulation of the serotonin cell bodies, which should produce a high rate of serotonin discharge onto its post-synaptic receptors, mimics the behavioral actions of d-LSD [17].

Some evidence suggests a role for central norepinephrine in psychedelic drug action. Cerletti [18] showed that the psychotropic activity in man of 18 LSD derivatives correlated closely with their ability to provoke a central sympathetic excitatory syndrome in animals consisting of mydriasis, hyperglycemia and hyperthermia. Since psychedelic drugs do not affect the presynaptic dispositions of norepinephrine (such as its release or reuptake), they probably interact with post-synaptic norepinephrine receptors. As with most pharmacological receptors, the identity of the norepinephrine "receptor" is a mystery and its "tagging" an awesome task. When radiolabeled norepinephrine is administered *in vivo* or *in vitro* to peripheral tissues or the brain it is accumulated avidly by noradrenergic nerve terminals. This uptake system probably is responsible for terminating the actions of synaptically released norepinephrine in the periphery [19] and in the brain [20]. However, if this neuronal uptake system is blocked by a drug such as cocaine [21,22] or at high amine concentrations [23] an extraneuronal system for norepinephrine accumulation is unmasked. This "extraneuronal" uptake of norepinephrine is inhibited by adrenergic blocking agents and therefore seems to be associated with norepinephrine receptors. One of the most potent blockers of "extraneuronal-receptor" norepinephrine uptake is normetanephrine, the methoxylated metabolite of norepinephrine, which appears to have more affinity for this uptake than does norepinephrine. The high affinity of normetanephrine for this system suggests that normetanephrine uptake may be a good model for the norepinephrine receptor. Accordingly we studied the uptake of ^{3}H-normetanephrine in rat brain slices [24]. Normetanephrine uptake differed considerably from the neuronal uptake of norepinephrine. While norepinephrine was accumulated to the greatest extent in the corpus striatum, highest normetanephrine levels occurred in the cerebral cortex. Normetanephrine accumulation was much less sensitive to omission of glucose and sodium from the medium, to lowered temperatures and to reserpine (Table 2). Accumulated norepinephrine was highly localized in nerve terminals, but there was very little particulate localization of normetanephrine. Normetanephrine was taken up more rapidly than norepinephrine and accumulation was linear only for one minute, while norepinephrine was accumulated linearly for up to 10 minutes (Figure 3). Normetanephrine uptake was blocked very efficiently by adrenergic blocking agents of which the β-blocker propranolol, was the most potent. Our most striking finding evolved from a study of the actions of the psychotropic methoxyamphetamines. Their ability to inhibit normetanephrine uptake correlated closely with their psychotropic potency in man (Table 3). 2,4,5-Trimethoxyamphetamine (2,4,5-TMA), 2,4,6-TMA, DOM and DOET which are potent psychotropic agents, were considerably more effective in inhibiting normetanephrine uptake than were the less psychoactive compounds 3,4,5-TMA, 2,3,5-TMA and 2,3,4-TMA. DOM and DOET are analogues of 2,4,5-TMA in which the 4-methoxy is replaced by methyl or ethyl respectively. Their very great psychotropic potency is related most likely to resistance to metabolic degradation by

TABLE 2. CHARACTERISTICS OF ^{3}H-NORMETANEPHRINE AND ^{3}H-NOREPINEPHRINE UPTAKES IN CEREBRAL CORTICAL SLICES

Standard Incubation Medium[(a)]	^{3}H-Normetanephrine, 30 Sec Accumulation		^{3}H-Norepinephrine 5 Min Accumulation	
	% Inhibition[(b)]	P[(c)]	% Inhibition[(b)]	P[(c)]
Less Oxygen	11	>0.05	0	---
Less Glucose	22	<0.02	86	<0.001
Na Replaced with Li	20	>0.05	81	<0.01
Plus Ouabain, 10^{-4}M	44	<0.05	81	<0.001
27°	37	<0.05	74	<0.01
	(Q_{10} = 1.6)		(Q_{10} = 3.8)	
Reserpinized Tissue (5 mg/kg ip. 18 hr prev.)	0	---	72	<0.01

(a) Standard incubation medium contained modified Krebs-Henseleit bicarbonate buffer, at 37°C, a gas phase of 95% O_2-5% CO_2, nialamide and 0.1 μM ^{3}H-amines.

(b) % Inhibition was determined as % decrease in tissue: medium ratios as a result of altering the incubation medium, and after the subtraction of 0° tissue: medium uptake ratios as blanks (0.2 for ^{3}H-normetanephrine and 0.8 for ^{3}H-norepinephrine).

(c) P values were determined by t test and were based on data from at least four determinations.

TABLE 3. RELATIVE POTENCIES OF TRIMETHOXYAPHETAMINES AND RELATED COMPOUNDS AS INHIBITORS OF ^{3}H-NORMETANEPHRINE UPTAKE IN CEREBRAL CORTEX.

Inhibitor	^{3}H-Normetanephrine, 30 Sec Uptake		Psychotropic Potency in Man
	ID-50[a]	Relative Potency[b]	Mescaline Units
d-Amphetamine	4.4×10^{-4}M	4.8	---
2,5-Dimethoxy-4-Methyl-amphetamine (DOM)	4.8×10^{-4}M	4.4	50 - 100[d]
2,4,6-Trimethoxyamphet-amine (TMA-6)	5.3×10^{-4}M	4.0	13[c]
2,4,5-Trimethoxyamphet-amine (TMA-2)	5.9×10^{-4}M	3.6	17.7[c]
2,5-Dimethoxy-4-Ethyl-amphetamine (DOET)	7×10^{-4}M	3.0	80 - 130[d]
3,4,5-Trimethoxyamphet-amine (TMA)	1.9×10^{-3}M	1.1	2.2[c]
2,3,5-Trimethoxyamphet-amine (TMA-4)	2.5×10^{-3}M	0.8	4.0[c]
2,3,4-Trimethoxyamphet-amine (TMA-3)	$>5 \times 10^{-3}$M	< 0.4	<2.0[c]

(a) ID-50 values were determined from log probit plots of % inhibition at 3 or 4 concentrations of inhibitor, in quadruplicate, after subtracting 0° uptakes as blank. ^{3}H-amine concentration was 0.1 µM. Data presented are the means of 2-4 independent determinations in which values did not differ by more than 25%.

(b) $\frac{\text{ID-50 dl-Normetanephrine}}{\text{ID-50 Inhibitor}}$

(c) Data are those of Shulgin et al. [10].

(d) Data from Snyder et al. [1,2,4].

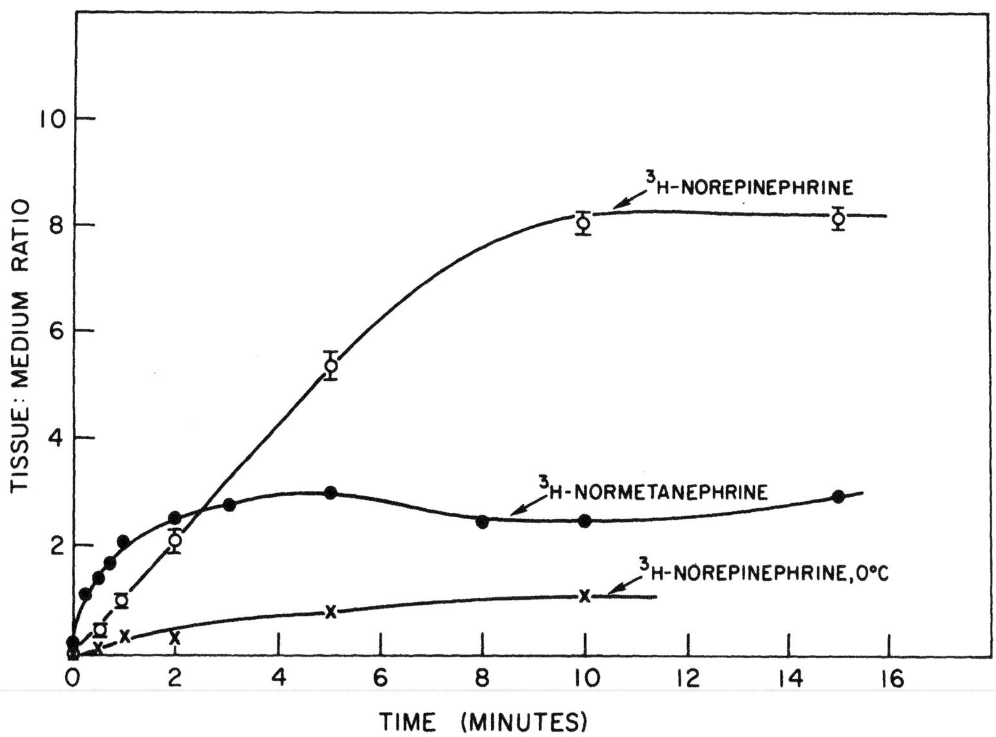

Figure 3

demethylation at C-4 [25,26] rather than to enhanced receptor activity. The correlation of psychotropic activity with inhibition of normetanephrine uptake suggests that its uptake site, which may be a reflection of the noradrenergic receptor, is related in some way to the locus of action of these drugs.

Interestingly, although our normetanephrine studies were performed with rat tissues, methoxyamphetamine activity in this system correlated with relative psychotropic potency in man and monkey but not with psychotropic potency in rat. This suggests that relative activities of these drugs in man are closely related to their "receptor" affinity, while behavioral potency in rats is a less valid model of receptor activity, possibly confounded by more extensive or varied metabolism in rats than in man and monkeys. Thus, in spite of all the limitations discussed above, it appears possible that psychotropic activity in man may be as good a criterion of psychedelic receptor activity as any others available at the present time.

III. ELECTRONIC FACTORS

Several years ago Carl Merril and myself began studies of possible chemical correlates of the human psychotropic potency of psychedelic drugs. We were impressed by the strikingly energetic highest occupied molecular orbital (HOMO) calculated by Karreman, et al. [27] for LSD and their suggestion that psychotropic activity could be related to this measure of the ability of an electron in the highest occupied molecular orbital to be transferred to an acceptor molecular. In reviewing known structure-activity relationships of LSD derivatives, we noticed that changes in the LSD molecule that would decrease HOMO energy would also decrease psychotropic activity. Thus it is likely that reduction of the doublebond at C_9-C_{10} would markedly decrease HOMO energy. Loss of this doublebond by hydrogenation or hydration (as in dihydro-LSD and lumi-LSD respectively) abolishes psychotropic activity [18]. It is thought that charge transfer reactions may involve electron donations from localized portions of a molecule, the region of highest "frontier electron density" [28]. One of the positions of highest frontier electron density in tryptamines and presumably in LSD is at the number 2 carbon atom. Thus if a charge transfer action were involved in the psychotropic activity of LSD, C-2 should be critical for activity. In reviewing the literature we noted that substitution at C-2 with sterically obstructing substituents as in brom-LSD [18] and 2-oxy-LSD [29] resulted in molecules that are devoid of psychedelic activity even though they readily entered the brain. These observations prompted our performing semi-empirical Hückel molecular orbital calculations [30] on a series of psychedelic compounds [31,32]. These were performed using a Honeywell 800 digital computer with a program designed by Dr. Howard deVoe. Of the tryptamine psychedelic drugs and their analogues (Figure 4) the most energetic HOMO was observed with the most potent agent, the 4-hydroxylated N,N-dimethyltryptamine, psilocin. Bufotenine, which differs from psilocin only in the position of its hydroxyl group which is at C-5 as opposed to C-4 in psilocin, is much less active psychotropically than psilocin [33]. Bufotenine has a considerably lower HOMO energy (0.5147 β-units; see legend to

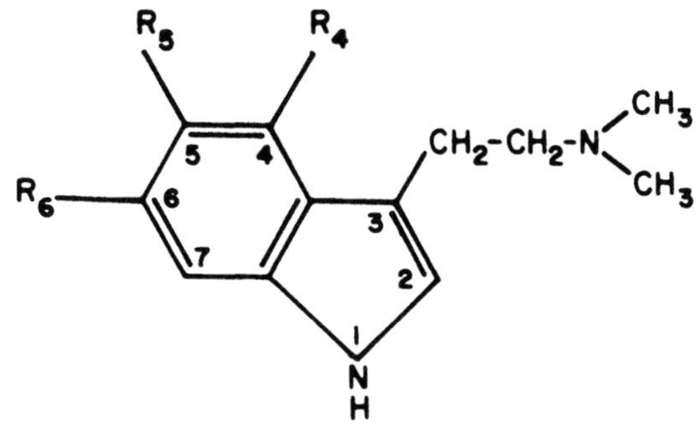

N,N-DIMETHYLATED TRYPTAMINE DERIVATIVES

COMPOUND	R_4	R_5	R_6
Dimethyltryptamine	H	H	H
Bufotenine	H	OH	H
6-Hydroxy-N,N-Dimethyltryptamine	H	H	OH
Psilocin (4-Hydroxy-N,N-Dimethyltryptamine)	OH	H	H

Figure 4

Table 4 for definition) than psilocin (0.4603 β-units). 6-Hydroxydimethyltryptamine has a HOMO energy (0.4700 β-units) intermediate between psilocin and bufotenine. There is some controversy over whether this compound is psychedelic in man. Alkylated tryptamines are hydroxylated at the 6 position in the liver [34] and their psychotropic activity is closely related to the extent of 6-hydroxylation [35]. Moreover, introducing a fluorine atom at position 6 to prevent 6-hydroxylation results in a molecule devoid of psychedelic activity [36]. In preliminary experiments, Szara and Hearst [35] found 6-hydroxydiethyltryptamine highly active in humans. More recently, however, Rosenberg et al. [37] were unable to produce psychotropic effects in man with 6-hydroxdimethyltryptamine.

At the time of our initial calculations, the psychotropic activity of only three trimethoxyamphetamines had been reported in the literature. If their potency is expressed relative to the activity of mescaline, hence in mescaline units (M.U.), 2,4,5-TMA and 3,4,5-TMA have potencies of 17 and 2.2 M.U. respectively. 2,3,4-TMA appeared to be devoid of psychotropic activity in doses examined and was certainly less than 2 M.U. The HOMO energies for these compounds correlated closely with their psychotropic activity (Table 4). This is especially striking since there is no apparent difference in lipid solubility or susceptibility to metabolic degradation among these three isomers. Mitoma (personal communication) found that C^{14}-labeled 2,4,5-TMA and 2,3,4-TMA, the most and least potent agents respectively showed no differences in metabolic degradation or in penetration into the brain in rats. When new data on the human activity of the 6 isomers of trimethoxyamphetamine became available [10] the correlation of psychotropic potency in man and HOMO energy broke down (Table 4). Interestingly, however, these HOMO energies still correlate with behavioral effects in rats.

TABLE 4. TRIMETHOXYAMPHETAMINES: ELECTRONIC CONFIGURATION AND PSYCHOTROPIC POTENCY

Compound	Homo[(a)]	Psychotropic Activity (M.U.) Man	Monkey	Rat
2,4,5-TMA (TMA-2)	.4810	17	5.4	7.2_u 4.0_s
2,3,5-TMA (TMA-4)	.5134	4	1.1	---
2,3,6-TMA (TMA-5)	.5250	13	---	---
3,4,5-TMA (TMA)	.5356	2.2	1.8	4.0_u 1.5_s
2,3,4-TMA (TMA-3)	.5696	<2	0.7	1.6_u $<1.0_s$
2,4,6-TMA (TMA-6)	.5740	10	3.2	1.7_u 1.0_s

(a) Expressed in β units which are related inversely to capacity for electron donation so that 2,4,5-TMA is a better electron donor and poorer acceptor than 2,4,6-TMA.

TMA refers to trimethoxyamphetamine, and the preceding numbers refer to the location of methoxy substituents. The TMA designations in parentheses are the code names assigned to these compounds by Shulgin [43]. Numbers in parentheses refer to potency in mescaline units as explained in the test. Subscripts u and s refer to the data of Uyeno [11] and Smythies et al. [7] respectively. Monkey and human data were obtained by Uyeno et al. [9] and Shulgin et al. [10] respectively.

IV. STERIC CORRELATES

Even with elegant correlations, molecular orbital calculations failed to account for the most dramatic feature of psychedelic drug structure-activity, the similar psychotropic activity produced by compounds of very different chemical classes such as mescaline and LSD. To examine this question, we made molecular models (Dreiding-Stereo Models [Swissco]) of psychedelic tryptamines and methoxy-amphetamines and observed that they can all approximate a conformation simulating in part the indole ring system of LSD (Figure 5) which we will refer to as rings A

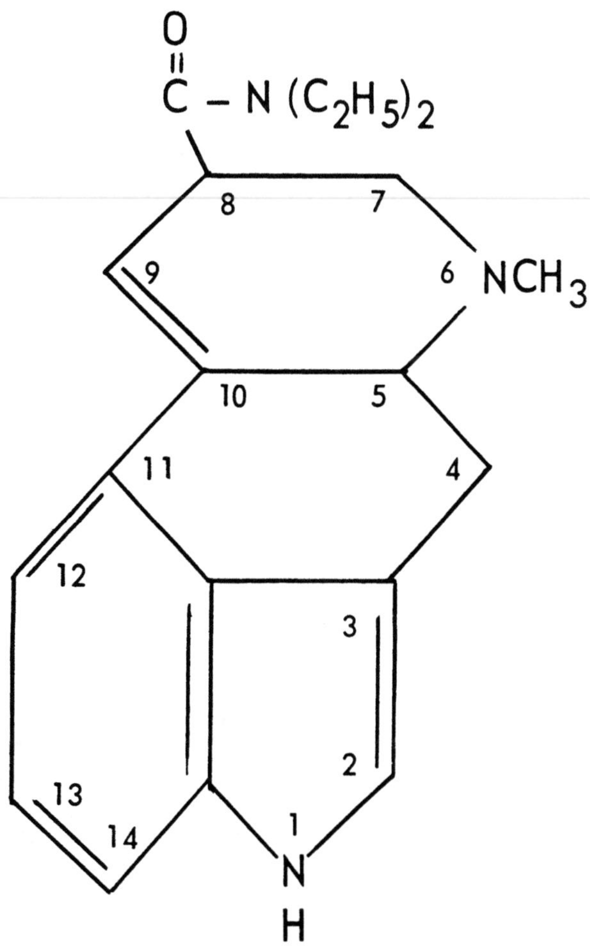

LYSERGIC ACID DIETHYLAMIDE

Figure 5

and B, as well as the saturated ring surmounting the indole nucleus, which will be referred to as ring C [38-40]. The more potent derivatives contain structural features that might permit the stabilization of the hypothetical "active" conformation enabling the preduction of the psychotropic activities of a number of psychedelic drugs.

In this formulation psychedelic drug potency will refer to the minimally detectable dose in humans or ED-50 in animals, expressed as mescaline units (M.U.) and defined as the effective dose of mescaline divided by the effective dose of the compound evaluated.

Tryptamine derivatives. As mentioned above, with these drugs there are marked differences in activity with small variations in structure. Psilocin (4-hydroxydimethyltryptamine) (Figures 4,6) is the most potent one, about 31 M.U. while bufotenine (5-hydroxydimethyltryptamine) appears to be inactive. N,N-dimethyltryptamine is an effective drug but only 1/8 as potent as psilocin [41]; its activities may or may not be mediated by a 6-hydroxylated intermediate. All of the tryptamines possess the indole moiety of LSD (rings A and B). The side chain of

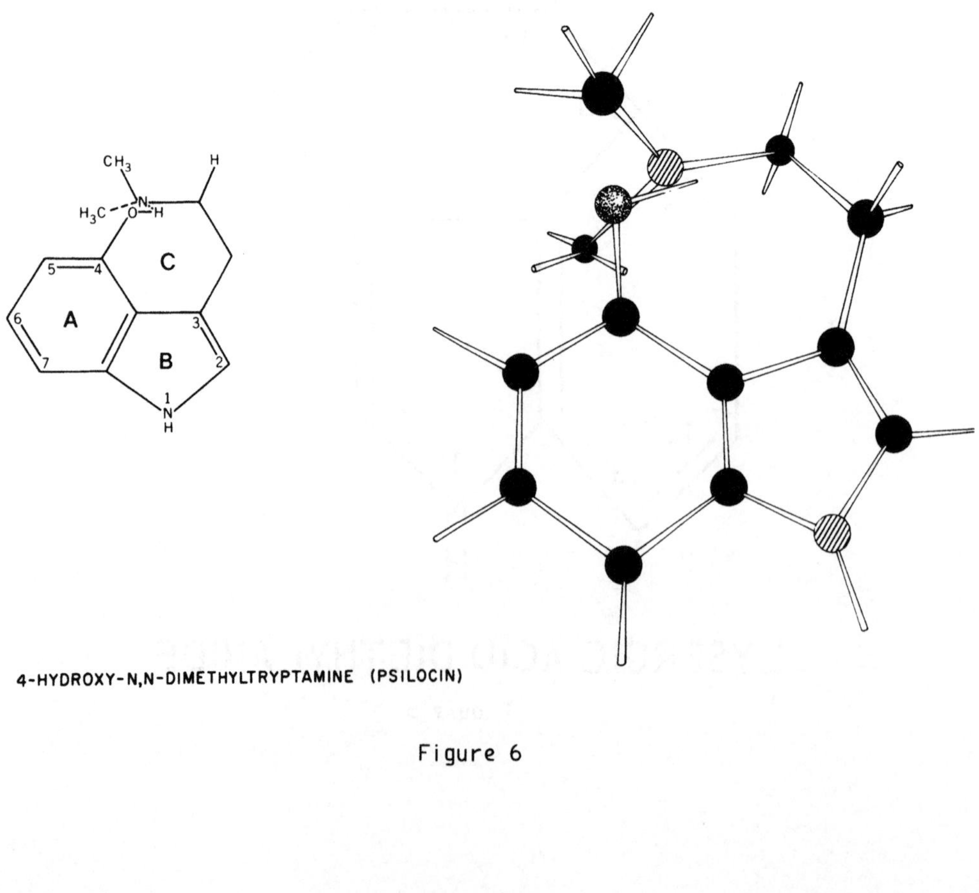

4-HYDROXY-N,N-DIMETHYLTRYPTAMINE (PSILOCIN)

Figure 6

these compounds can fold back on the indole ring to approximate the C ring of LSD. However, since the side chain is freely rotating, it may assume a great number of other conformations. The C ring conformation would occur more frequently if there were some means of its stabilization. In the molecular model of psilocin (Figure 6) the amine moiety of the side chain approaches the hydroxyl group of the benzene ring and physically permits hydrogen bonding between the two groups. Such hydrogen bonding with the hydrogen of the 4-hydroxyl and the tertiary amine nitrogen would stabilize an 8 membered ring which, in three dimensions, would resemble ring C of LSD. The distance separating groups forming the bond would be 1.7 angstrom units which is in the range of values seen for strong hydrogen bonds, although in Figure 6 they appear closer. Such intramolecular hydrogen bonding could not take place for bufotenine or dimethyltryptamine. Thus the structure of psilocin, the most potent psychedelic tryptamine, favors the LSD conformation more than the less potent tryptamines. Stabilization of psilocin's ring C in this way requires that the amine grouping be nonprotonated which would be the case if the hypothetical receptor site were lipid like. If at the receptor psilocin's amine group were protonated, as might occur at physiological pH in aqueous solution, this type of hydrogen bonding would not be feasible. In this case, the protonated amine could interact with the oxygen of the 4-hydroxyl group stabilizing the C ring. In addition to fostering the resemblance to ring C of LSD, the conformation described here for psilocin would also make it more lipid soluble. Indeed Gessner et al. [42] has found that psilocin is much more lipid soluble than bufotenine.

Methyoxyamphetamines. A large number of trimethoxyamphetamines, dimethoxyamphetamines, and methoxymethylenedioxyamphetamines have been synthesized and evaluated in man (Figure 2) [10]. As already discussed there are marked differences in psychotropic activity of the trimethoxyamphetamines. With these compounds as has been suggested for mescaline by numerous other investigators, the side chain might fold down toward the ring resembling an indole nucleus (rings A and B of LSD). Such a conformation might conceivably be stabilized by hydrogen bonding between the hydrogen of the amine side chain and pi electrons of the benzene ring at C-2 or C-6. However, in order for the amine side chain to interact with the pi electrons of the ring it would have to assume a position above the plane of the ring and accordingly would not be coplaner with the benzene ring as in a true indole structure. Moreover, this type of interaction would probably be fairly weak and has therefore not been utilized for prediction of psychotropic activity in the present model.

A more interesting possibility is that for isomers with methoxy substituents at C-2 or C-6 an interaction could take place between the hydrogen of the amine side chain and the oxygen of the methoxy group at C-2 or C-6 to form a seven membered ring that, sterically, closely resembles ring C of LSD (Figures 7,8). In approximating this C-ring conformation, the methoxy group at C-2 must fulfill a relatively rigid spatial arrangement. Molecular models show that if there is a methoxy group at C-3 ortho to the methoxy at C-2, the free rotation of the methoxy at C-3 sterically would hinder the ability of the C-2 methoxy to assume its required arrangement. This steric hindrance would interfere with formation of ring C in compounds possessing the group at both C-2 and C-3, i.e., 2,3,5-TMA and 2,3,4-TMA. Compounds with methoxy groups at C-2 or C-6 whose ability to approximate the side chain amine is not hampered by methoxy substituents at C-3 or C-5 respectively should be quite potent. These predictions (Table 1) correspond closely to the potencies of these compounds in man and in squirrel monkeys.

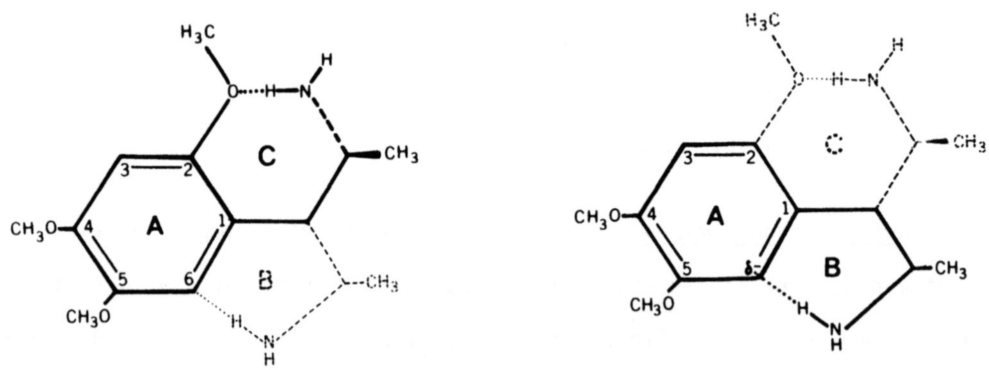

2,4,5-TRIMETHOXYAMPHETAMINE (TMA-2)

Figure 7

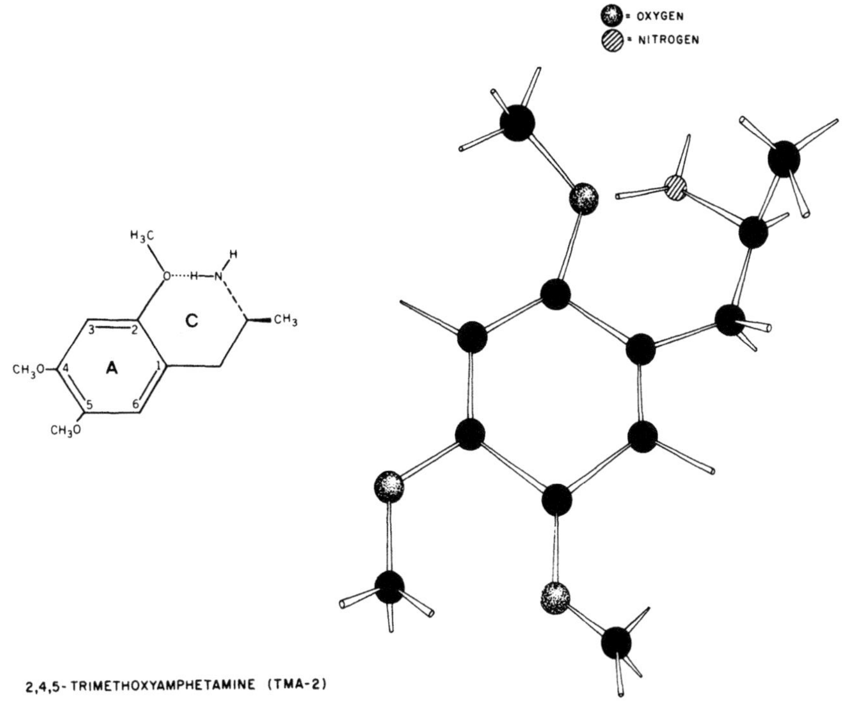

Figure 8

<u>Methoxymethylenedioxyamphetamines</u>. These compounds are analogues of the trimethoxyamphetamines in which methylenedioxy bridges replace two adjacent methoxys (Figure 2). In naming these compounds, a hyphen between position numbers will be used to designate a methylenedioxy linkage. 3-Methoxy-4,5-methylenedioxyamphetamine (3,4-5-MMDA) the analogue of 3,4,5-TMA has a potency of 3 M.U. similar to 3,4,5-TMA [10]. 2-Methoxy-4,5-methylenedioxyamphetamine (2,4-5-MMDA), the analogue of 2,4,5-TMA has a potency of 12-20 M.U. similar to 2,4,5-TMA. 2-Methoxy-3,4-methylenedioxyamphetamine (2,3-4-MMDA) (Figures 2,9) is the analogue of 2,3,4-TMA. Although 2,3,4-TMA is inactive as a psychedelic agent, 2,3-4-MMDA is a very potent psychedelic agent (12-20 M.U.). The striking difference in activity between 2,3,4-TMA and 2,3-4-MMDA can be explained by their relative capacities to approximate ring C of LSD. As mentioned above, the formation of ring C in 2,3,4-TMA is hindered sterically by the freely rotating methoxy at C-3. In 2,3,-4-MMDA the methylenedioxy substituent constitutes a fixed linkage between C-3 and C-4 removing the steric hindrance to the formation of ring C.

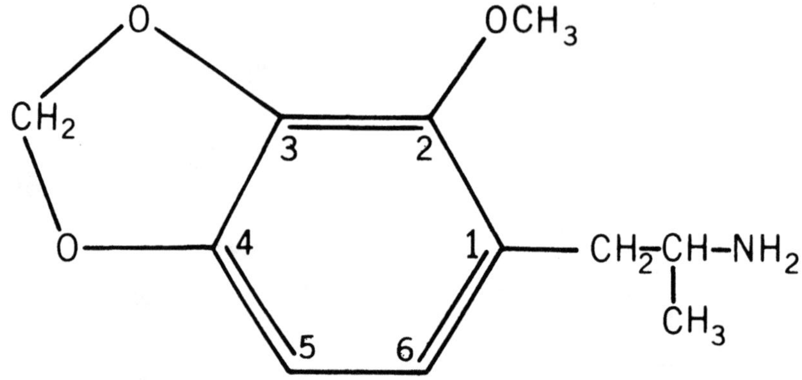

2-METHOXY-3,4 METHYLENEDIOXY-AMPHETAMINE (MMDA-3a)

Figure 9

Two dimethoxymethylenedioxyamphetamines have been synthesized and tested in humans. 2,5-dimethoxy-3,4-methylenedioxyamphetamine (DMMDA) (Figure 10) is equivalent to 2,3-4-MMDA with an additional methoxy grouping at C-5. As with 2,3-4-MMDA, ring C can be readily formed. DMMDA is an active psychedelic agent, with a potency of 12 M.U. (10). 2,3-Dimethoxy-4,5-methylenedioxyamphetamine (DMMDA-2)

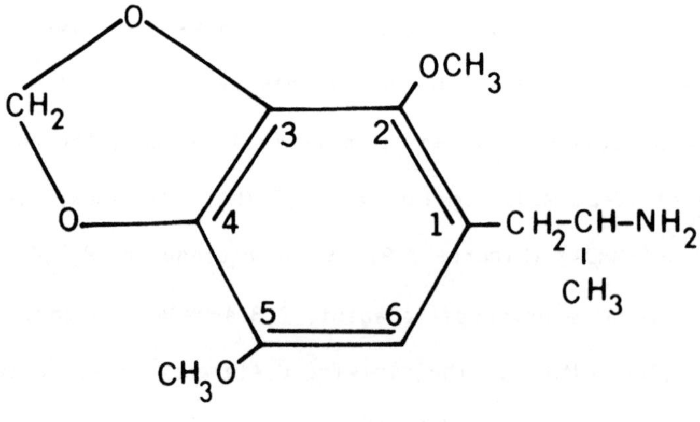

DMMDA

(2,5-DIMETHOXY-3,4-METHYLENEDIOXYAMPHETAMINE)

Figure 10

(Figure 11) differs from DMMDA only in the position of the methylenedioxy bridge. However, it is less than half as potent (5 M.U.) as DMMDA [10]. The decreased potency is readily explicable in terms of the relative capacity of the methoxy at C-2 to form ring C with the side chain amine. In DMMDA-2 just as in 2,3,4-TMA there is a freely rotating methoxy group at C-3 that sterically would hinder interactions between the methoxy at C-2 and the side chain.

The three methoxymethylenedioxyamphetamines which our model predicts to be active are indeed potent in man (Table 5) while the two which our model predicts to be relatively weak, are considerably less potent.

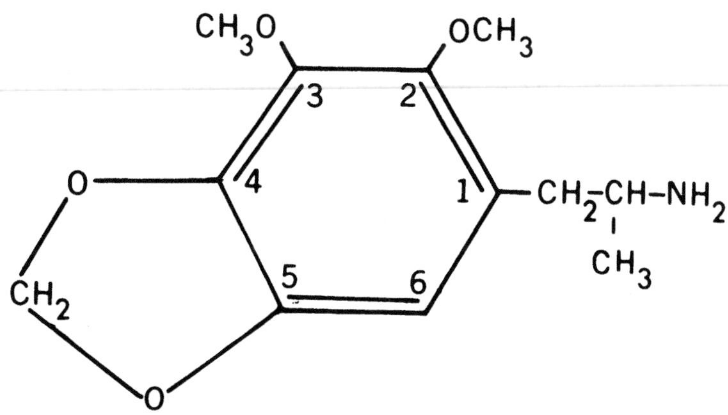

DMMDA-2

(2,3-DIMETHOXY-4,5-METHYLENEDIOXYAMPHETAMINE)

Figure 11

TABLE 5 . PSYCHEDELIC DRUGS - STRUCTURE: ACTIVITY
METHOXYMETHYLENEDIOXYAMPHETAMINES

Efficacy	Steric Model	Man
Potent	2,4-5-MMDA (MMDA-2)	2,4-5-MMDA (12)
Potent	2,3-4,5-DMMDA (DMMDA)	2,3-4,5-DMMDA (12)
Potent	2,3-4-MMDA (MMDA-3a)	2,3-4-MMDA (10)
Weak	2,3,4-5-DMMDA (DMMDA-2)	2,3,4-5-DMMDA (5)
Weak	2-3,4-MMDA (MMDA-3)	2-3,4-MMDA (3)

MMDA and DMMDA refer to methoxymethylenedioxyamphetamine and dimethoxymethylenedioxyamphetamine respectively. Hyphens between numbers preceding compounds indicate methylenedioxy bridges. Lettered designations in parentheses refer to code names assigned [43]. Numbers in parentheses are psychotropic potency in mescaline units as reported by Shulgin et al. [10].

Dimethoxyamphetamines. When this model was first proposed [38] only one of the dimethoxyamphetamines had, to our knowledge, been evaluated in man for psychotropic potency. As with the other amphetamine analogues, our model would predict that the potent isomers would be those containing a methoxy grouping at C-2 whose interaction with the side chain would not be hindered by a methoxy group at C-3. Thus, we would predict that 2,5-dimethoxyamphetamine and 2,4-dimethoxyamphetamine should be relatively potent while 3,5-dimethoxyamphetamine, 3,4-dimethoxyamphetamine and 2,3-dimethoxyamphetamine would be relatively weak (Table 6). Recently Shulgin et al. [10] have shown than in man, 2,5-dimethoxyamphetamine and 2,4-dimethoxyamphetamine are relatively potent (8 M.U. and 5 M.U., respectively) while 3,4-dimethoxyamphetamine is inactive. There is at least one methoxyamphetamine whose activity is not explained by the above model. Thus 4-methoxyamphetamine, which could not readily form ring C is moderately active in man [10] and quite potent in disrupting rat behavior [7].

It would be interesting to mesh the electronic and steric models of psychedelic drug activity. One would expect that electronic considerations would determine drug activity only after a compound had first fulfilled whatever steric considerations were required for interaction with the receptor. For instance, 4-methoxypsilocin possess a more energetic HOMO than Psilocin [31,32] and, if steric considerations are insignificant, it should be a more potent psychedelic agent than psilocin. However, introduction of a methyl group at the number 4 position (assuming that the nitrogen of the amine side chain is not protonated), according to the steric model, would yield a psychedelic agent less active than psilocin. We are unaware of any studies in humans of 4-methoxypsilocin, but in behavioral tests in rats and monkeys, 4-methoxypsilocin is less potent than psilocin (Uyeno, personal communication).

TABLE 6. PSYCHEDELIC DRUGS - STRUCTURE ACTIVITY DIMETHOXYAMPHETAMINES

Efficacy	Steric Model	Man
Potent	2,5-DMA	2,5-DMA (8)
Potent	2,4-DMA	2,4-DMA (5)
Weak	3,4-DMA	3,4-DMA (<1)
	3,5-DMA	
	2,3-DMA	

DMA refers to dimethoxyamphetamine. Numbers in parentheses are psychotropic potency in mescaline units reported by Shulgin et al. [10].

V. REFERENCES

[1] Snyder, S. H., Faillace, L., and Hollister, L., *Science*, 158, 669, (1967).

[2] Snyder, S. H., Faillace, L. A., and Weingartner, H., *Amer. J. Psychiat.*, 125, 357, (1968).

[3] Snyder, S. H., Faillace, L. A., and Weingartner, H., *Arch. Gen. Psychiat.*, 21, 95, (1969).

[4] Snyder, S. H., Weingartner, H., and Faillace, L. A., in *Psychotomimetic Drugs*, (ed. by D. H. Efron), Raven Press, New York, (1969, in press).

[5] Smythies, J. R. and Levy, C. K., *J. Mental Sci.*, 106, 531, (1960).

[6] Freedman, D. X., Appel, J. B., Hartman, F. R., and Molliver, M. E., *J. Pharmacol. Exp. Therap.*, 143, 309, (1964).

[7] Smythies, J. R., et al., *Nature*, 216, 128, (1967).

[8] Appel, J. B. and Freedman, D. X., *Life Sci.*, 4, 2181, (1967).

[9] Uyeno, E. T., Otis, L. S., and Mitoma, C., *Comm. Behav. Biol.*, A1, 83, (1968).

[10] Shulgin, A. T., Sargent, T., and Naranjo, C., *Nature*, 221, 537, (1969).

[11] Uyeno, E. T., *J. Pharmacol. Exp. Therap.*, 159, 216, (1968).

[12] Ellison, T., Gutziat, L., and Van Loon, E. J., *J. Pharmacol, Exp. Therap.* 152, 383, (1966).

[13] Freedman, D. X., *Amer. J. Physchiat.*, 119, 843, (1963).

[14] Diaz, P., Ngai, S. H., and Costa, E., *Pharmacologist*, 9, 372, (1967).

[15] Aghajanian, G. K., Foote, W. E., and Sheard, M. H., *Science*, 161, 707, (1969).

[16] Hillarp, N. A., Fixe, K., and Dahlstrom, A., *Pharmacol. Rev.*, 18, 727, (1966).

[17] Aghajanian, G. K. and Sheard, M. H., *Comm. Behav. Biol.*, 1, 37, (1968).

[18] Cerletti, A., p. 117 in *Neuropharmacology*, (ed. by P. B. Bradley, et al.), Elsevier, Amsterdam, (1959).

[19] Iversen, L. L., *The Uptake and Storage of Noradrenaline in Sympathetic Nerves*, Cambridge University Press, New York, (1967).

[20] Glowinski, J. and Baldessarini, R. J., *Pharmacol. Rev.*, 18, 1201, (1966).

[21] Eisenfeld, A. J., Axelrod, J., and Krakoff, L., *J. Pharmacol. Exp. Therap.*, 156, 107, (1967).

[22] Eisenfeld, A. J., Landsberg, L., and Axelrod, J., *J. Pharmacol. Exp. Therap.* 158, 378, (1967).

[23] Iversen, L. L., *British J. Pharmacol.*, 25, 18, (1965).

[24] Hendley, E. D. and Snyder, S. H., *Federation Proc.*, 28, 674, (1969).

[25] Schweitzer, J. W. and Friedhoff, A. J., *Biochem. Pharmacol.*, 15, 2097, (1966).

[26] Sargent, T. W., et al., *Biochem. Biophys. Res. Commun.*, 29, 126, (1967).

[27] Karreman, G., Isenberg, I., and Szent-Gyorgyi, A., *Science*, 130, 1191, (1959).

[28] Fukui, K., Yonezawa, T., and Nagata, C., *J. Chem. Phys.*, 27, 1247, (1957).

[29] Axelrod, J., Brady, R. O., Witkop, B., and Evarts, E. V., *Ann. N.Y. Acad. Sci.*, 66, 435, (1957).

[30] Streitweiser, A., *Molecular Orbital Theory for Organic Chemists*, Academic Press, New York, (1961).

[31] Snyder, S. H. and Merril, C. R., *Proc. Nat. Acad. Sci., U.S.*, 54, 258, (1965).

[32] Snyder, S. H. and Merril, C. R., p. 229 in *Amine Metabolism in Schizophrenia*, (ed. by H. Himwich and Smythies), Pergamon Press, New York, (1966).

[33] Turner, W. J. and Merles, S., *A.M.A. Arch. Neurol. Psychiat.*, 81, 121, (1959).

[34] Szara, S. and Axelrod, J., *Experientia*, 15, 216, (1959).

[35] Szara, S. and Hearst, E., *Ann. N.Y. Acad. Sci.*, 96, 134, (1962).

[36] Kalir, A. and Szara, S., *J. Med. Chem.*, 6, 716, (1963).

[37] Rosenberg, D. E., Isbell, H., and Miner, E. J., *Psychopharmacologia*, 4, 39, (1963).

[38] Snyder, S. H. and Richelson, E., *Proc. Nat. Acad. Sci., U.S.*, 60, 206, (1968).

[39] Snyder, S. H. and Richelson, E., p. 1199 in *Psychotomimetic: A Review of Progress*, (ed. by D. H. Efron), Public Health Service, Washington, D.C., (1968).

[40] Snyder, S. H. and Richelson, E., in *Psychotomimetic Drugs*, (ed. by D. H. Efron), Raven Press, New York, (1969, in press).

[41] Szara, S., p. 460 in *Psychotropic Drugs*, (ed. by S. Garattini and V.Ghetti), Elsevier, Amsterdam, (1957).

[42] Gessner, P. K., Godse, D. D., Krull, A. H., and McMullan, J. M., *Life Sci.*, 7, 267, (1968).

[43] Shulgin, A. T., *Experientia*, 20, 366, (1964).

MOLECULAR ORBITAL THEORY AND PHARMACOLOGIC RECEPTOR THEORY AS INTEGRATED EXPERIMENTAL TOOLS

by

Arnold J. Wohl*

I. INTRODUCTION

A. Fundamental Assumptions

It has only been within the past decade that high-speed computers and all-valence-electron quantum chemical methods have become available. These techniques are an absolute necessity to provide quantitative information about Szent-Györgyi's "clouds" [1] in molecules of biological interest. Despite this current faculty, however, quantitative structure-activity studies using the information provided by quantum chemistry have been surprisingly few in number. Those studies which have appeared [2,3] have not led to new insights into drug design or subsequent studies on submolecular mechanisms of drug action, and this fact remains the case despite the valuable information which Kier's conformational studies [4-7] and the theoretical work of Cammarata [8,9] have made available.

There are, presumably, two reasons for this lack of results. Preeminently, there has been, until the very recent general acceptance of the mechanics of receptor theory, [10,11] a misunderstanding among chemists as to the meaning of the pharmacologists' "mechanism of action". Most of the pharmacological literature which deals with what is called "mechanisms of action" is misnamed, since drug effects and their physiological localization is the topic actually treated. Mechanism of action, in a quantum-biological sense, is meant to imply a dissection of the intermolecular forces at the electronic level which are presumed responsible for receptor involvement, in turn thought to always result in a given response of the

* Department of Pharmacology, Schering Corporation, Bloomfield, New Jersey.

biological system under study. In concrete terms, the electronic interactions of a series of compounds which have all been shown to have the same "mechanism of action", in molecular pharmacological terms, at a presumed constant receptor, is as close as modern pharmacology can now approach to the "ultimate" mechanism of action. This mechanism of action, however, is many levels of integration removed from the current terminology.

The second difficulty is conceptual and technical as well. It is unrealistic to expect singularity of drug-receptor attachment, and little, generally, is done in structure-activity studies to protect against random "sites of loss". The flexibility of drug-receptor interactions virtually excludes one-point attachment, meaning that, even using quantum chemical data, simple regression analyses are unlikely to provide predictive or even intuitively useful data. Multiple regression techniques are necessary, and these are notable for their absence in all but a few such studies.[2,3]

The approaches implicitly outlined above, that is, uniformity of molecular mechanism of action as described by receptor theory, and multiple regression analyses, have been followed in this study of the quantum-biological mechanism of action of a series of antihypertensive agents.

B. Molecular Mechanism of Action

The benzothiadiazine antihypertensive drug, diazoxide, has been shown [12, 13] to compete with barium or calcium for activation of a receptor responsible for contraction of vascular smooth muscle. The compound is, therefore, a "partial biostere" [10] for calcium, and a number of representatives of the class were evaluated as competitive antagonists of barium by techniques described by Ariëns [10] and van Rossum [14] and employed in the studies on diazoxide referred to above.

The structure-activity relationships of a series of compounds can only be rationally discussed after the constancy of the activity is assured. In these studies, all compounds were evaluated by study of dose-response curves, in addition to quantification of competitive blocking potency, to assure an equivalence of mechanism in all cases.

While analytical techniques have been discussed, a brief review is indicated. By a current theory, a competitive blocking agent is one able to occupy a receptor in such a way that a response is not effected (either because the compound is unable to produce the chemical stimulus or because there is a conflicting and negative stimulus which results in a cancellation), hence the receptor is made temporarily unavailable to the agonist. When sufficient receptors are occupied by a competitive antagonist, the minimum concentration of agonist required to cause a response is increased. That is, plots of dose-response curves in the presence and absence of antagonists show a shift to the right as in Figure 1, where curve (1) is in the absence of and curve (2) in the presence of a competitive antagonist.

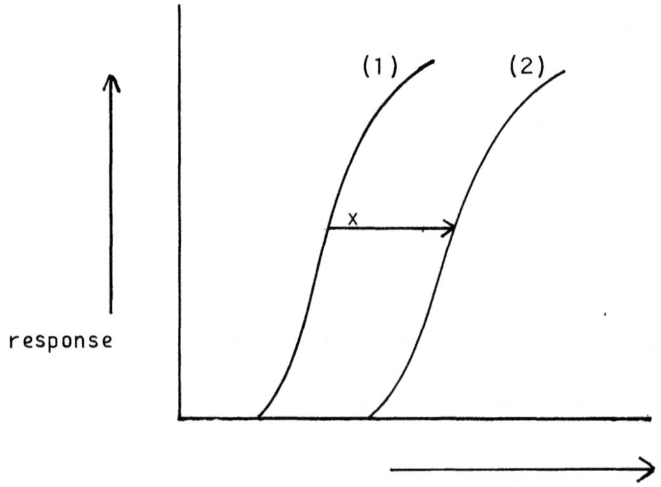

FIGURE 1. Log concentration of agonist

The parallelism of the curves is a consequence of the ability of ever-increasing agonist concentrations to displace antagonist molecules by simple mass-action relationships, the situation being one of random "hits". This parallelism allows the measurement of the displacement, the shift x, at any point on the curves. In practice this shift is measured at the midpoint of the response and used as in (1).

$$\log(x - 1) = -\log K + pA_x \; . \qquad (1)$$

In this equation, x is the dose ratio required for equivalent effect, pA_x is the negative log of the molar antagonist concentration at which the shift was produced. When $X = 2$, the left-hand side of the equation disappears and the $pA_{x=2} = \log K$ is the antagonist-receptor dissociation constant.

This value, the pA_2, is as good a measure as is presently available of the chemical (i.e., electronic and steric) interaction of drug and receptor. It is also a measure of an action (receptor site function) rather than an effect.

In any such study, it is absolutely vital that the biological activity being used as the dependent variable in the regression analysis be measured in a simple medium, at least for preliminary study, and that this medium have relevance to the possible therapeutic utility of the compound series. The drug-receptor interaction should be uncomplicated by membrane transports, metabolism, distribution and so on. These preconditions to accurate data practically restrict consideration to *in vitro* biological systems.

The benzothiadiazine-1,1-dioxides [15,16] treated in this paper were studied as described for diazoxide [12], and appear to act as the neutral molecule (personal communication: Dr. J. G. Topliss, Schering Corporation).

II. METHODOLOGY

A. Biological

The techniques applied to study the locus of action of the benzothiadiazine antihypertensive agents have been discussed above and in an earlier publication in some detail. [12] Since these agents act on vascular smooth muscle, the use of the rat aorta *in vitro* was considered a relevant testing system which permitted accurate pA_2 determinations for all compounds involved in this study. These values, and the structures of the compounds under discussion, are tabulated (Table 1).

B. Quantum Chemical

Extended Hückel Theory

Hoffmann's formulation of the Hückel molecular orbital approach, known as Extended Hückel Theory (EHT) [17] has been described in numerous recent publications and will not be discussed *per se* in the present paper. The use of EHT for this work follows that of Kier [4]. A compilation of parameter values, all taken

TABLE 1. STRUCTURE AND NUMBERING OF BENZOTHIADIAZINES AND SIMILAR COMPOUNDS

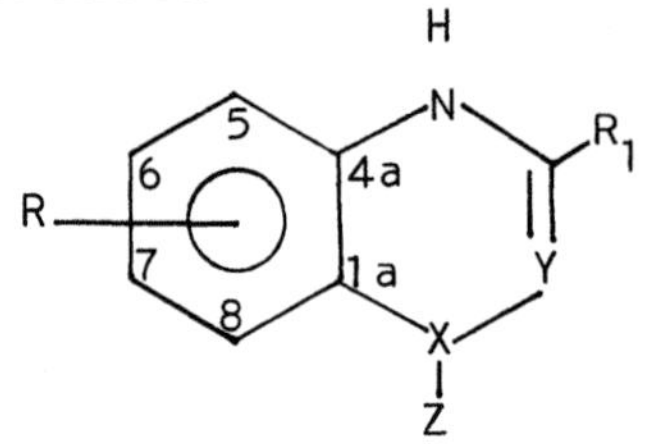

Compound Number	R	R_1	X	Y	Z	pA_2 ± S.E.M.
1	7-AZA	H	S	N	O_2	3.76 ± 0.17
2	H	CH_3	S	N	O_2	3.76 ± 0.14
3	6-Cl	H	S	N	O_2	4.92 ± 0.15
4	H	H	S	N	O_2	3.62 ± 0.04
5	7-Cl	CH_3	S	N	O_2	5.11 ± 0.01
6	6-Cl	CH_3	S	N	O_2	5.40 ± 0.13
7	8-Cl	CH_3	S	N	O_2	4.39 ± 0.10
8	5-Cl	CH_3	S	N	O_2	3.94 ± 0.17
9	6,8-Cl_2	CH_3	S	N	O_2	4.63 ± 0.19
10	5,7-Cl_2	CH_3	S	N	O_2	4.68 ± 0.09
11	6,7-Cl_2	CH_3	S	N	O_2	6.12 ± 0.21
12	6-CH_3	CH_3	S	N	O_2	4.34 ± 0.16
13	7-CH_3	CH_3	S	N	O_2	4.26 ± 0.21
14	6-Cl-7-CH_3	CH_3	S	N	O_2	5.82 ± 0.13
15	5-CH_3-7-Cl	CH_3	S	N	O_2	4.63 ± 0.09
16	6,7,8-Cl_3	CH_3	S	N	O_2	5.85 ± 0.18
17	7-F	CH_3	S	N	O_2	4.68 ± 0.13
18	6-NO_2-7-Cl	CH_3	S	N	O_2	5.54 ± 0.13
19	7-Cl	CH_3	S	N	O	4.44 ± 0.17
20	6-Cl		S	N	O_2	5.41 ± 0.21
21	6-Cl		S	N	O_2	4.16 ± 0.20
22(a)	5-THIA-6-Cl	CH_3	S	N	O_2	3.60 ± 0.23
23(b)	6,7-Cl_2	C_5H_9	S	N	O_2	7.73 ± 0.13
24	6,7-Cl_2	Δ^1-C_5H_7	S	N	O_2	4.59 ± 0.11
25	6,7-Cl_2	Δ^2-C_5H_7	S	N	O_2	7.00 ± 0.17
26	6,7-Cl_2	Δ^3-C_5H_7	S	N	O_2	7.84 ± 0.21
27(c)	6,7-Cl_2	C_7H_7	S	N	O_2	6.64 ± 0.27
28	6-CH_3-7-Cl	H	S	N	O_2	5.46 ± 0.12
29	7-Cl	H	S	N	O_2	4.12 ± 0.25
30	7,8-Cl_2	CH_3	S	N	O_2	5.34 ± 0.08
31	6-CH_3-7-Cl	CH_3	S	N	O_2	5.70 ± 0.15
32	5-CH_3	CH_3	S	N	O_2	3.86 ± 0.14
33	6-Cl-7-SH	Δ^3-C_5H_7	S	N	O_2	7.27 ± 0.18
34	6,7-Cl_2	CH_3	C	N	O	5.19 ± 0.07
35	6-Cl	CH_3	S	C	O_2	4.85 ± 0.23
36	6-OCH_3	CH_3	S	N	O_2	4.78 ± 0.16

(a) Thieno ring fused
(b) This and following three compounds are cyclopentyl and pentenyl
(c) 1-Cycloheptatrienyl

from the work of Hinze and Jaffé [18], is presented in Table 2. The version of EHT used in this study is that offered by the Quantum Chemical Program Exchange of Indiana University (QCPE) and is available from this organization as QCPE 64. It is able to accommodate up to 140 orbitals and to handle third row atoms.

TABLE 2. EHT PARAMETERS

Atom Type	Slater Orbital Exponent	Ionization Potential (Orbital)[(a)]	
H	1.000	-13.60 (1s)	
C	1.625	-21.40 (2s)	-11.40 (2p)
N	1.950	-26.00 (2s)	-13.40 (2p)
O	2.275	-35.30 (2s)	-17.76 (2p)
F	2.600	-38.24 (2s)	-20.86 (2p)
S	1.818	-20.08 (3s)	-13.32 (3p)
Cl	2.033	-25.23 (3s)	-13.34 (3p)

(a) Ionization potential given in eV.

Although no provision is made for other than s- and p-orbitals in QCPE 64, sulfur 3d-orbitals could have been considered through the use of a similar program graciously supplied to the author by Hoffmann. Several authors [19,20,21] have proposed that the sulfur atom, when attached to electronegative ligands (as is the case in the benzothiadiazines), may undergo a contraction of the diffuse 3d radial functions compatible with chemical bonding. Sulfur 3d-orbitals were not considered in this study because the results of several calculations with inclusion did not change either the charge distribution of the molecule (except for the sulfur charge) or the order or energy of the bonding orbitals. Furthermore, since the SO_2 grouping is a very consistent feature of the compounds under study, it was felt that the absence of 3d-orbital inclusion could be related to a similar series of calculations with such inclusion by a simple scaling factor.

It is also recognized that EHT calculations produce exaggerated charge distributions. Self-consistency within the series of molecules was felt to obviate consideration of this problem as well, bearing in mind that the typical difference in results between EHT and the more theoretically complete CNDO/2 calculations may not be the sign but only the magnitude of charge, equivalent to introduction of another simple scaling factor.

The geometry of the molecule is required as input to the EHT computation. This was provided by a program to calculate Cartesian coordinates (PRØXYZ; QCPE 94) using bond length and bond angle information from the compilations of Sutton [22, 23] and from Alléaume and Decap [24].

Tautomerism and Conformation

The molecules treated in this study may assume either of two tautomeric forms (Figure 2). This tautomerism was initially assumed to possess an equilibrium constant of 1.0 for interconversion of 2-H and 4-H tautomers. Calculations were therefore conducted at equivalent $N_2 - C_3$ and $C_3 - N_4$ bond distances and valency angles (1.35 Å - 120°).

Further observations were made with varying bond lengths and angles but the conclusions were found not to differ from those found when the calculations were conducted assuming true interconvertibility unless unrealistic single- and double-bond values were used for the tautomeric atoms (for numbering of atoms see Figure 2).

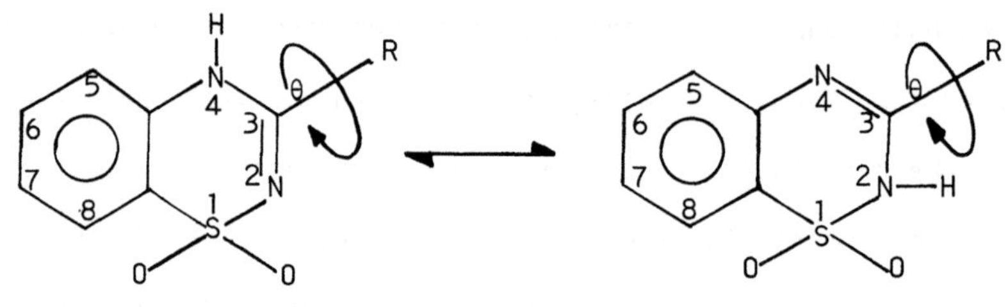

4 - H   2 - H

FIGURE 2. Tautomers and numbering of benzothiadiazine-1,1-dioxide.

Rotation about the plane of the benzothiadiazine nucleus may occur for all substituent groups. The angle of rotation, θ (Figure 2) was varied through the complete range of nonequivalence for all substituents.

Where applicable, that is with molecules capable of changes in conformation by virtue of substituent rotation, the preferred tautomer was determined at the preferred rotational conformer for each of the tautomers.

Since no information is available regarding the electronic nature of the benzothiadiazine-"Ca^{++}-receptor" interaction, a variety of quantum chemical indices obtained from Extended Hückel Theory (EHT) calculations performed as in the preceding paper were considered as independent variables (see C. below). The molecular orbital calculations performed by EHT yield net atomic charges for each atom in the molecule which is further partitioned into σ and π electronic charges ($q(N)^{\sigma}$, $q(N)^{\pi}$). Summed regional π- and σ-charges were calculated for 3-substituents as Streitweiser [33] has recently done for a reaction problem in organic chemistry. This is symbolized $q(3R)^{\sigma \text{ or } \pi}$.

The energy levels of the molecular orbitals are also part of the computer print-out. The highest (most energetic) molecular orbital (HOMO) which contains a full electron complement (of 2 electrons) frequently participates in chemical reactions [25,26] and has been found of biological significance [27,28] along with the least energetic (lowest) unoccupied orbital (LEMO). These numbers are negative quantities. As multiplied by −1 they are symbolized E_{HOMO} and E_{LEMO}, respectively. It should be pointed out, however, that the negative sign of E_{LEMO} is an artifact of EHT since non-empirical calculations yield a positive value for this quantity.

Additional quantities are the approximate nucleophilic and electrophilic superdelocalizabilities ($S'_{(N)}E$, $S'_{(N)}N$) where the subscript refers to the atom in question. These indices appear to be a measure of the tendency [29,30] for incoming (interacting) electron-rich or electron-poor centers to be localized at an atom and have found chemical as well as biological use [2,29]. These superdelocalizabilities refer to π-electron orbitals, and thus likely relate to $\pi - \pi$ drug-receptor interaction at specific atoms in the drug molecule.

An additional set of MO quantities are the atomic and bond polarizabilities [29]. These quantities roughly measure the electric moment induced at an atom by itself, self-atom polarizability, and at one atom by another adjacent one, atom-atom polarizability. These are also reaction indices and have found chemical use [25]. The frontier approximation employed in calculating superdelocalizability, which restricts attention to the HOMO and LEMO as the reaction-determining orbitals was also used to calculate polarizabilities ($\pi'_{N,N}$, $\pi'_{N,N+1}$).

Although mis-ordering of orbitals has on occasion been noted with EHT, a σ-orbital occasionally appearing as the HOMO rather than a π-orbital, calculations on the benzothiadiazines invariably showed there to be a π-orbital at a very similar energy whenever this mis-ordering of energy levels occurred. For the polarizabilities, as well as the superdelocalizabilities discussed above, the computations were done on the frontier π-orbital.

Preliminary results were obtained by utilizing the above information which selected the particular atoms in the molecule which, based on the results of the regression analyses, might be involved in the interaction with the receptor. Attempts were then made to refine the work by introducing several additional quantities.

Coulomb's Law gives the direct electrostatic (charge-charge) interaction between two points centers of charge as

$$F = q_d q_r / \epsilon R_{dr} \tag{2}$$

where q_d is a charge on a drug atom d and q_r is the corresponding charge on receptor atom r, with ϵ as the dielectric constant of the medium and R_{dr} is the separation between atoms d and r. For all atoms in drug and all atoms in the receptor

$$F = \sum_d \sum_r \frac{q_d q_r}{\epsilon R_{dr}} . \tag{3}$$

But we may consider the receptor as constant, and the dielectric constant as unchanged by drug. The preliminary results to be discussed implicated certain atoms in the drugs as participants in the interaction, so unit positive charges symbolizing q_r were located at points in space topographically corresponding to the drug atoms at reasonable distances, and denoted by [A] as one of 7 such points (Figure 3), and Coulombic interactions between drug atoms and points [A] through [G] were calculated by

$$F^{[A]} = \sum_d \frac{q_d}{R_{d\,[A]}} . \tag{4}$$

A second type of drug atom-receptor atom intermolecular energy may be simplified, for a series of molecules, as the field created by a series of charges upon the midpoint of a bond located a given distance away. [31,32] The midpoints

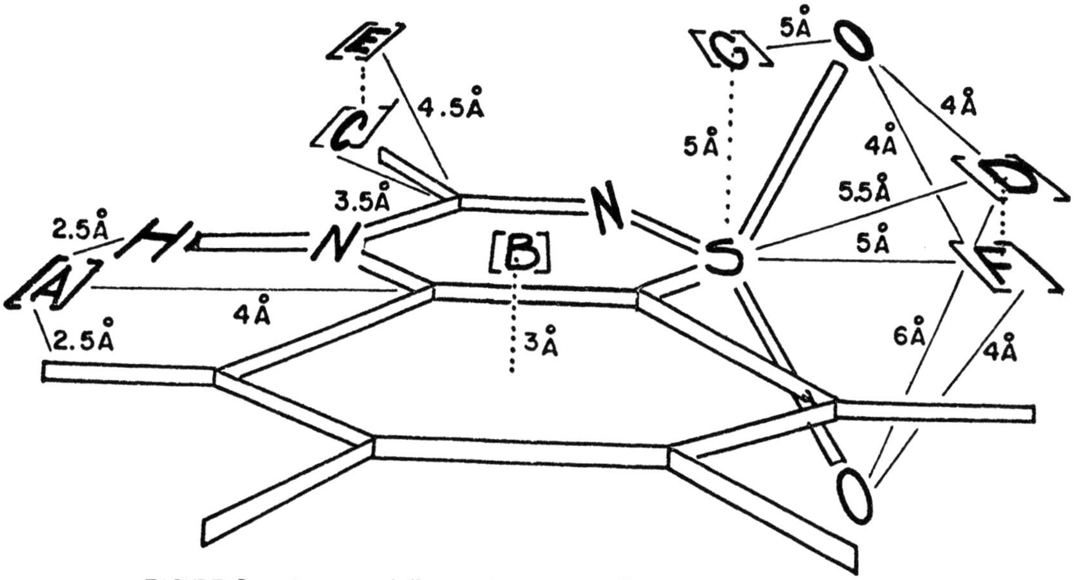

FIGURE 3. Proposed "receptor points" and relationship to benzothiadiazine molecule .

of receptor intramolecular bonds were also considered to be located at points [A] to [G] and the electric field calculated by

$$E^{[A]} = \sum_d \frac{q_d}{R^3_{d[A]}} \cdot r_{d[A]} \tag{5}$$

where $r_{d[A]}$ is the vector distance.

These two calculations were performed for all molecules in the series.

The list of variables employed in the preliminary and in the final regression analyses follows:

q^{σ}_{N} = net σ-charge on atom N

q^{π}_{N} = net π-charge on atom N

Q_N = net total ($\sigma + \pi$) charge on atom N

$q(3R)^{\sigma,\pi}$ = summed net regional charge over all atoms in 3-R group (σ or π)

E_{HOMO} = energy $\cdot$ (-1) in eV of HOMO

E_{LEMO} = energy $\cdot$ (-1) in eV of LEMO

$S'_{(N)}N$ = approximate (frontier) nucleophilic superdelocalizability on atom N

$S'_{(N)}E$ = approximate (frontier) electrophilic superdelocalizability on atom N

$\pi'_{N,N}$ = frontier self-atom polarizability of atom N

$\pi'_{N,N+1}$ = frontier atom-atom polarizability between atom N and atom N + 1

$F^{[A]}$ = intermolecular Coulombic interaction energy for a molecule and point [A]

$E^{[A]}$ = electric field created at point [A] by set of charges on a molecule .

C. Statistical

The compounds studied were treated as individual "observations" in which the dependent variable, pA_2, was assumed to correlate with one or more of the numerous EHT-MO quantities treated as independent variables. The assumption implicit in this treatment is that receptor structure and mechanism of action hold constant, while pA_2 varies throughout the series presumably with one or more of the independent variables.

The standard multiple regression techniques used to treat these data can be evaluated by all of three criteria; the multiple correlation coefficient, r, the standard error of the estimates, $Sy \cdot \Sigma_x$, and the F-statistic. Of the three, r is the least reliable as an estimate of "goodness of fit" of the derived equation to the Y values, for r may increase to very high values (→ 1.0), while $Sy \cdot x$ increases. This circumstance indicates multicolinearity, that is, high correlations among the MO variables treated, which mathematically results in a high r. There are often significant intercorrelations between the MO variables; only when inclusion of intercorrelated variables decreases the $Sy \cdot x$ are such variables important.

The F-statistic measures the significance of the coefficient of a variable as it contributes to the overall regression, and only highly significant contributions are considered.

The assumption is made that a high r, coupled with a low $Sy \cdot x$ for a regression equation, the coefficients of the variables of which are highly significant, indicates something of real biological import. It is, strictly speaking, improper and invalid to imply causality to a correlation, however high it may be. Appeal is made here, however, to the pragmatic, the experimental: if such a regression equation, applied to compounds other than those treated, yields a prediction of the pA_2 within the statistical limits of experimental data, it is felt that the equation in question is, if not a real, then at least a working description of the electronic factors which determine the receptor attack of a molecule and its consequent biological effects.

III. RESULTS AND DISCUSSION

A. Chemical

Tautomerism

Calculations were carried out on the 2-H and 4-H tautomers of a number of variously substituted benzothiadiazines. The tautomer possessing the lowest (most negative) total molecular energy was considered, as is usual in such studies, the more stable species, whereas the difference between the two was taken to represent the energy barrier for tautomer interconversion. The energy barrier and the equilibrium constant for 2-H $\longleftrightarrow$ 4-H tautomerism are given for 21 compounds in Table 3.

The selection of compounds given here comprise six different 3-position substituents, three different types of nuclei, and a large number of positional and substituent variations in the benzenoid nucleus. Although the degree of 4-H tautomer preference varies widely over the series, the consistency as well as the magnitude of the preferences calculated is convincing demonstration that the benzothiadiazines are likely, in general, to exist as the 4-H tautomer.

Additional calculations were carried out on a few compounds for which the N_2-C_3 and C_3-N_4 distances were reduced to 1.31 Å when double-bonded, and 1.39 Å when single-bonded. Even with this large separation, tantamount to assuming a considerable energy barrier for $\Delta^{2,3} \rightleftharpoons \Delta^{3,4}$ tautomerization, the $\Delta^{2,3}$ or 4-H tautomer was consistently favored, although the energy difference had decreased to values centering about 2.4 kcal/mole, for which $\log K^{37^\circ} = 1.0$. It must be borne in mind that EHT is too crude for detailed analyses of energetics.

Independent chemical evidence for these results is provided by the UV spectroscopic work of Novello, et al. [34] This confirmation of the present work obviates, in part, a frequent objection to the applicability of MO methods (which

TABLE 3. TAUTOMERIC STABILITY IN BENZOTHIADIAZINES

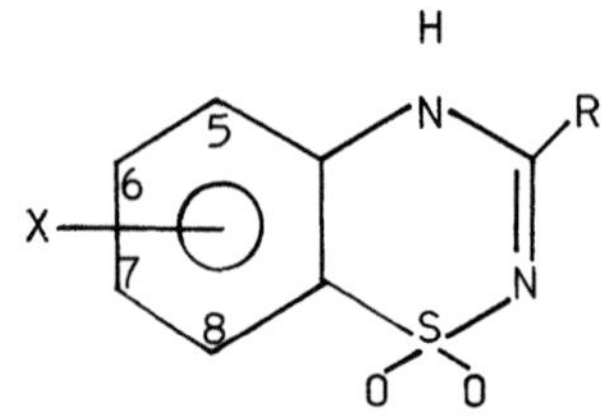

R	X	ΔF (4-H — 2-H)[(a)]	Log $K^{37°}$[(b)]
H	H	6.508	4.588
CH_3	H	6.485	4.572
CH_3	5-Cl	6.491	4.576
CH_3	6-Cl	6.448	4.546
CH_3	7-Cl	6.473	4.564
CH_3	8-Cl	6.508	4.588
CH_3	6,7-Cl_2	6.450	4.547
CH_3	7-F	6.476	4.566
CH_3	7-CH_3	6.537	4.609
CH_3	6-Cl-7-CH_3	6.517	4.595
CH_3	6-NO_2-7-Cl	6.476	4.566
H	6-Cl-7-SO_2NH_2	6.615	4.664
CF_3	6-Cl	6.450	4.547
CH_3	5-CH_3-7-Cl	0.424	0.299
H	5-AZA	4.985	3.514
H	7-AZA	6.705	4.727
CH_3 (sulfoxy)	7-Cl	6.090	4.294
CH_3	6-Cl-THIENO	3.927	2.769
Phenyl	6-Cl	5.995	4.227
Δ'-Cyclopentyl	6,7-Cl_2	6.224	4.388
2-Furyl	6-Cl	5.444	3.838

(a) Free energy difference in kcal/mole.

(b) Equilibrium constant for 2-H ⟶ 4-H conversion at 37°C.

treat molecules in total isolation) to systems involving solutions or even within crystal structures.

Conformation

The single bond between the 3-carbon of the ring system and attached groups is one about which rotation may occur. The compounds to be discussed below show sizable energy barriers to such rotation.

Figure 4 (A-G) shows the results obtained with seven different types of 3-position substituents. These results are summarized in Table 4.

That these results are likely to represent actual conformations may be inferred from the size of the rotational barriers. Hoffmann [17] calculated the staggered-eclipsed rotational barrier in ethane to be 4 kcal/mole. Microwave determinations of this energy barrier [35,36] yield values of 2.815-3.030 kcal/mole. While EHT probably exaggerates the magnitude of such barrier determinations, the procedure has yielded useful and often quite accurate conformational analyses in a large variety of chemical systems. [37-40]

It is interesting to note the correspondence between biological potency and the preferred rotational isomer, maximum potency being attained when mutual perpendicularity obtains between substituent group and benzothiadiazine nucleus. It is of interest to speculate that a segment of the receptor at which these agents function, a "site of attachment", is situated so as to produce maximum interaction when the plane of the 3-substituent group, rather than one or more of its component atoms, is presented to the receptor surface.

It may even be possible to deduce some information relating to the nature of the proposed site with which the 3-substituent interacts. Figure 5 shows that positive charge and conformation are not unrelated, and that the increased group positivity may be the actual determinant of potency rather than conformation, *per se*. The nature of the interaction would thus seem, at least with regard to this presumed site, to be that of a charge-charge attraction, and so we may tentatively assign anionic character to the proposed site, based on these results.

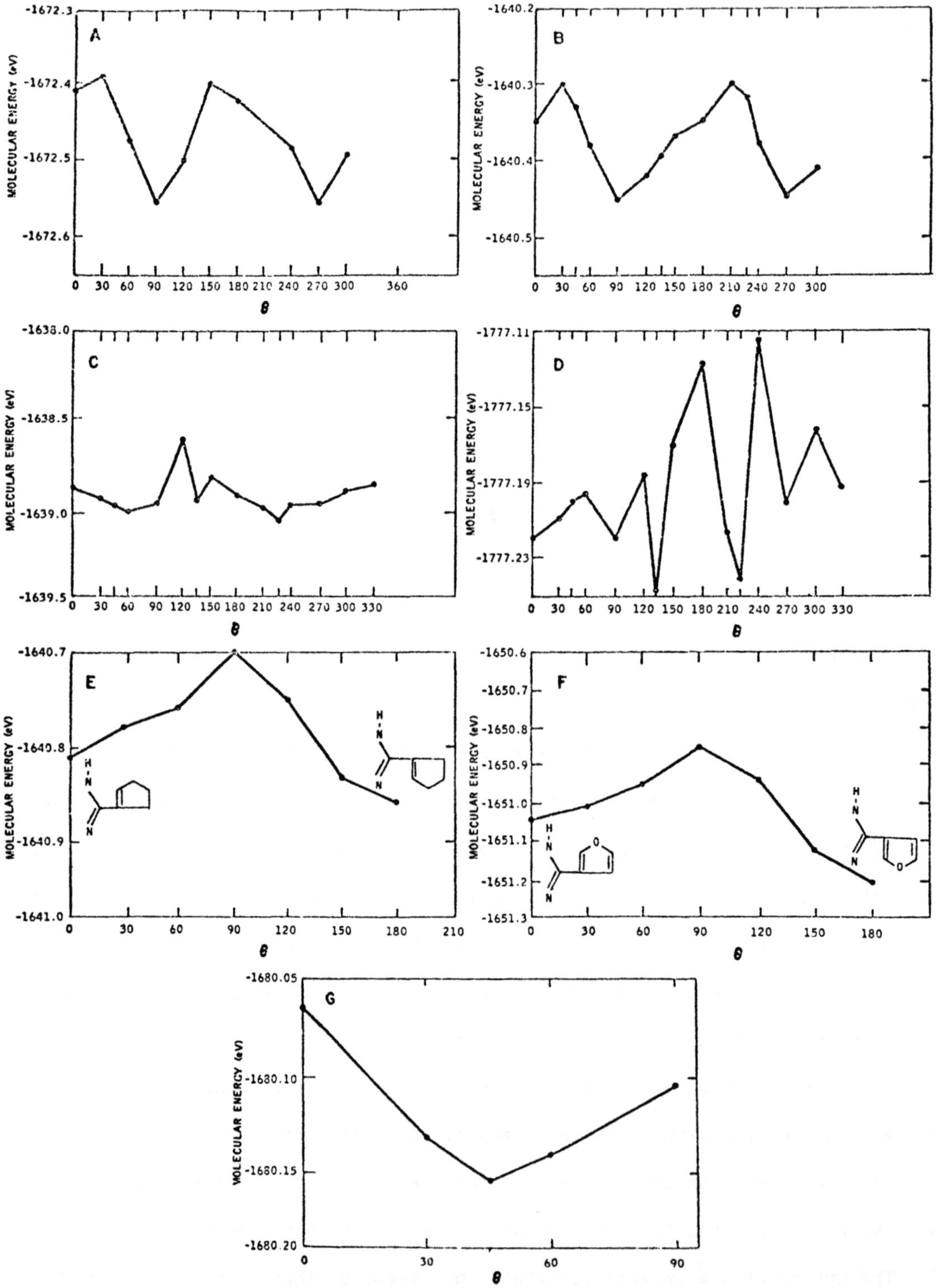

FIGURE 4. Rotational conformation of 3-R group. Ordinate is the molecular energy in eV, abscissa is the angle, θ, of rotation about the plane of the benzothiadiazine nucleus in degrees. A. R = cyclopentyl; B. R = Δ^3-cyclopentenyl; C. R = Δ^2-cyclopentenyl; D. R = 2,4,6-cycloheptatrien-1-yl; E. R = Δ^1-cyclopentenyl; F. R = 2-furyl; G. R = phenyl.

TABLE 4. SUMMARY OF CONFORMATIONAL PREFERENCE

Group	Rotamer Preferred[(a)]	Energy Barrier[(b)]	Antihypertensive Potency[(c)]
2-furyl	0	7.8	1
Δ^1-cyclopentenyl	0	3.6	2
phenyl	45	2.1	3
1-cycloheptatrienyl	45	3.0	4
Δ^2-cyclopentenyl	45	3.9	5
cyclopentyl	90	4.1	6
Δ^3-cyclopentenyl	90	4.1	7

(a) Dihedral angle in degrees between plane of nucleus and that of substituent.

(b) Difference in kcal/mole between rotamer of lowest and highest stability.

(c) Rank of *in vitro* "antihypertensive potency". See following for full discussion.

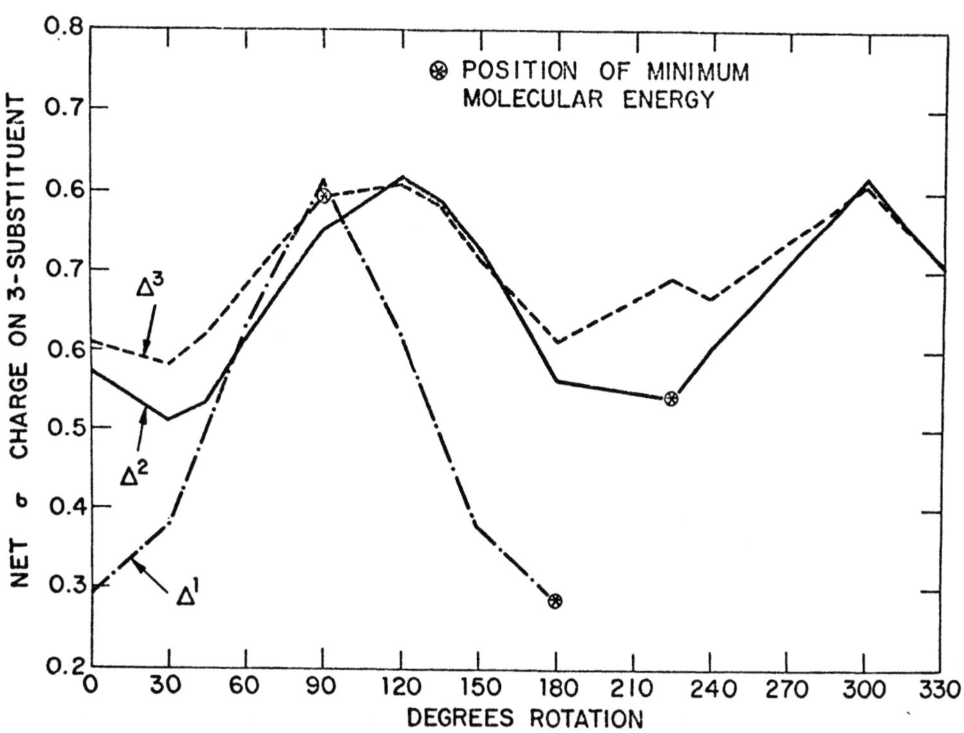

FIGURE 5. Net σ group charge in three isomers of cyclopentenyl-benzothiadiazines as a function of the angle of rotation about the benzothiadiazine ring plane.

B. Biological

Antihypertensive Potency

Preliminary Data. Regression Equation (6) below is the result obtained from stepwise analysis of compounds 1-7, 9, 11-14, and 16-19 in Table 1. The pA_2 range of this set of 16 compounds is 3.76-6.12, a 230-fold potency spread.

$$pA_2(\hat{Y}) = 28.34 - 1.96\, E_{HOMO} - 52.99 S'_{(5)}{}^{E} + 48.38 S'_{(5)}{}^{N} - 56.07 S'_{(4)}{}^{E} + 98.57 S'_{(6)}{}^{N} \quad (6)$$

$r^2 = 0.947 \quad Sy \cdot x = 0.23 \quad F = 48.31\ (p < 0.0005)$

The statistical significance of the regression equation is high, for, in addition to the high correlation coefficient and F-test value, the standard error of the estimate is such that the potential inaccuracy of the equation goes from a low of 3.8 percent to a maximum of 6.1 percent. Predictively, however, the equation is useful only for compounds included within the relatively narrow selection of structural types indicated. Predictions of activity for compounds possessing R groups other than H or CH_3 are uniformly low by an order or two of magnitude, and predictions for 5-substituted compounds such as 8, 10, 15, and 32 are uniformly too high by approximately an order of magnitude. It is clear, then, that Equation (6), while a regression of high statistical significance, covers too narrow a structural type to be useful.

There are salient features of Equation (6), however, which are of interest. No charge terms are included, indicating that the interaction may be frontier-controlled. [41,42] The presence of the E_{HOMO} would imply, since the coefficient for this term is negative, that the more energetic (the smaller this number, the higher the pA_2) is HOMO, the more facile electron donation from the compound would be, and consequently, that electron donation may play some role in the action of these compounds.

The negative coefficients for position 4 and 5 electrophilic superdelocalizabilities and the positive coefficients for the nucleophilic superdelocalizabilities at positions 5 and 6 confirm the above reasoning, and more accurately locate the areas of possible importance for this effect within the drugs' structure.

Equation (7), which considers the 23 compounds 1-7, 9, 11-14, 16-21, and 23-27, and covers the 12,000-fold pA_2 range 3.65-7.84, is a more satisfactory description.

$$pA_2(\hat{Y}) = 64.12 - 5.16\ E_{HOMO} + 55.09S'_{(5)}N + 115.78S'_{(6)}N + 5.16\ q(3R)^{\sigma} \quad (7)$$

$$r^2 = 0.960 \quad Sy \cdot x = 0.28 \quad F = 62.31\ (p < 0.0005)$$

The statistical significance of Equation (7) is roughly equivalent to that of (6), with the standard error going from 3.6-7.7 percent, and the high correlation coefficient and F-value corroborating the accuracy of the regression. Equation (7) however, is a big improvement over (6) by virtue of distinctly adequate predictions over a much wider range of structural prototypes. The form of this equation is similar to that of (6) except for the apparently important inclusion of the regional charge on the 3-substituent, implying, in addition to electron donation from electron-rich areas on the aromatic ring, a charge-charge interaction which may be involved in stabilization of the drug-receptor complex.

The absence of the seemingly important sulfonyl group is, in all probability, an artifact of the basically limited compound selection, for all compounds are quite similar. The involvement of these atoms, however, does become clear when intermolecular forces are considered in the next section of this paper.

The general usefulness of Equation (7) is still limited, however, for it is inadequate to predict (account for) the potency of 5-substituted compounds in that it consistently over-estimates. Since it seemed that the breadth of structural types included in Equation (7) was quite large, it was difficult to account for the inability of the regression equation to successfully deal with 5-substitution unless the assumption was made that the 5-position was so intimately involved in the reaction mechanism that either steric or direct electronic interactions had to be considered in order to establish a generally useful regression equation.

Refined Equations. Equation (8) should be compared with (6) above for it is the result of performing a multiple regression analysis on the same 16-compound set as for that earlier equation but where the list of variables included the intermolecular energy calculations discussed in the methods section.

$$pA_2(\hat{Y}) = 38.34 - 2.99\, E_{HOMO} + 13.78S'_{(5)}N - 0.004\pi'_{6,7} + 0.04\pi'_{1a,8} + 11.03E^{[A]} \quad (8)$$

$$r^2 = 0.996 \qquad Sy \cdot x = 0.07 \qquad F = 202.57\ (p \ll 0.0005)$$

Equation (8) differs from (6) in two salient respects: a far better, almost perfect, fit of the experimental data has been obtained, and it shows the likelihood of a receptor point located at point [A] (Figure 3). The 1a-8 and 6-7 polarizabilities are correlated with the SN of position 6 and consequently represent that term in Equation (6). It is evident from the size of the coefficient in $\pi'_{6,7}$ that this term is of limited importance. The interpretation of (8), therefore, is the same as was given for (6), and the greatly increased goodness-of-fit is likely the result of the inclusion, in the stepwise procedure, of $E^{[A]}$, of an electric field effect upon a presumed receptor site located in the plane of the nucleus and in the area of atoms 4, 4a, and 5.

Despite the adequacy of (8) in predicting the activity of compounds falling within its narrow structural breadth, it fails quite as completely as the much less accurate (6) with regard to 3-substitution, although (8) is the first equation which satisfactorily accounts for the potency of 5-substituted compounds.

Equation (9) includes the 25 compounds represented by 1-9, and 11-15 in Table 1. While the requirements of compound variety have forced the addition of several additional terms, (9) can be seen to be an entirely satisfactory regression equation spanning the 17,000-fold potency range of 3.60-7.84.

$$pA_2(\hat{Y}) = 1.95 + 8.63S'_{(1)}N - 135.08S'_{(4)}E + 78.14E^{[D]} + 54.52S'_{(3)}N - 0.03\pi'_{5,5} - 0.03\pi'_{1a,1a} + 61.60F^{[E]} + 1.49\, q(3R)^{\sigma} \quad (9)$$

$$r^2 = 0.994 \qquad Sy \cdot x = 0.12 \qquad F = 265.34\ (p \ll 0.0005)$$

Several interesting differences are clear between (8) and (9). The E_{HOMO} requirement has disappeared, evidently because, in this much wider structural range, it is now of less determinantal importance for activity than the limit imposed by the statistical significance threshold of the regression analysis. It has, in effect, been diluted in importance by the presence of large numbers of compounds of roughly equal E_{HOMO} but whose potency is primarily determined by other quantities.

The $E^{[A]}$ quantity found in (8) has been replaced by the correlated self-atom polarizability at position 5 (which allows correct predictions for the 5-thia compound (number 22 in Table 1) and $S'_{(4)}E$. The sulfur and oxygen atoms are shown to be important now by the inclusion of $E^{[D]}$ and $S'_{(1)}N$, and permit tentative placement of another receptor site at [D], making three altogether, at [A], [D], and [E], of the seven originally chosen as likely candidates (Figure 6).

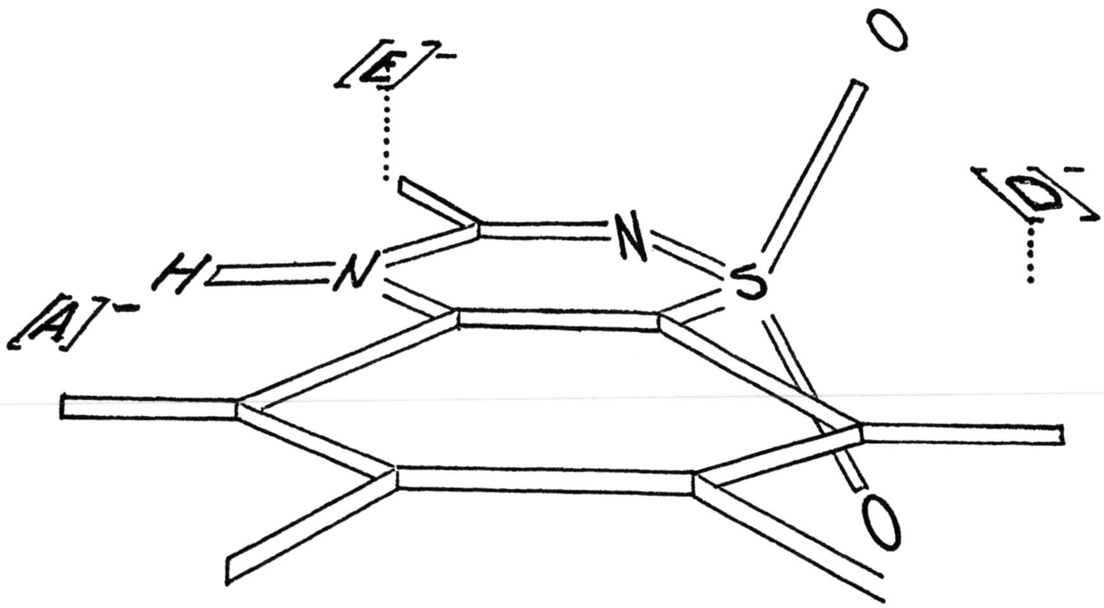

FIGURE 6. Three of the original seven (see Figure 3) proposed "receptor points" which possess apparent physical reality.

An important qualification to multiple regression analyses, even when performed stepwise, is the possible complications induced by multicolinearity, that is significant intercorrelations between supposedly independent variables. Table 5 shows the one such event which appears in Equation (9), a high correlation between $F^{[E]}$ and $q(3R)^{\sigma}$. The statistical significance (F-test) of the equation is, however, markedly reduced by excluding either term, so it must be assumed that, despite intercorrelation, each term says overlappping but different things about the drug-receptor interaction.

Correlations, however, even of high statistical significance, are of only passing interest unless one is able to derive verifiable hypotheses from them and/ or utilize them predictively. Table 6 shows the agreement between predicted and

TABLE 5. CORRELATION MATRIX FOR REGRESSION EQUATION (9)

	Y	$q\sigma^3$	$S'_N{}^{(1)}$	$S'_E{}^{(4)}$	$E^{[D]}$	$S'_N{}^{(3)}$	$\pi'_{5,5}$	$\pi'_{1a,1a}$	$F^{[E]}$
Y	1.0	.795	.375	-.484	.251	.088	-.283	-.306	.600
$q\sigma^3$		1.0	.047	-.336	.084	-.210	-.276	-.126	.702
$S'_N{}^{(1)}$			1.0	.158	.493	.059	.415	-.363	.166
$S'_N{}^{(4)}$				1.0	.462	.065	.493	-.125	-.109
$E^{[D]}$					1.0	.067	.280	-.369	.368
$S'_N{}^{(3)}$						1.0	.123	.003	-.448
$\pi'_{5,5}$							1.0	-.382	-.216
$\pi'_{1a,1a}$								1.0	.013
$F^{[E]}$									1.0

TABLE 6. PREDICTION OF POTENCY BY EQUATION (9)

Compound Number	Observed pA_2 ± S.D.	Predicted pA_2	Deviation
10[a]	4.68 ± 0.16	4.52	0.16
15	4.63 ± 0.14	4.68	-0.05
20[a]	5.41 ± 0.27	5.43	-0.02
21	4.16 ± 0.32	4.27	-0.11
22[a]	3.60 ± 0.27	3.59	0.01
23[a]	7.73 ± 0.31	7.83	-0.10
24	4.59 ± 0.11	4.57	0.02
25	7.00 ± 0.34	7.09	-0.09
26	7.84 ± 0.27	7.64	0.20
27	6.57 ± 0.47	6.83	-0.26
28	5.46 ± 0.12	5.13	0.33
29	4.12 ± 0.37	4.59	0.47
30	5.34 ± 0.13	5.20	0.14
31	5.70 ± 0.19	5.56	0.14
32	3.86 ± 0.13	3.68	0.18
33	7.27 ± 0.31	7.60	-0.33
34	5.19 ± 0.12	4.84	0.35
35	4.85 ± 0.24	4.73	0.12
36	4.78 ± 0.27	4.65	0.13

(a) Included in regression.

experimentally found pA_2 values using regression Equation (9). In 6 of the 19 cases the deviation between predicted and experimental values slightly exceeds one standard deviation of the experimental values themselves. For the other 13 cases tabulated, the estimates of potency are quite close. The pA_2 range covered by these 19 compounds is some 12,000-fold; the range of structural types exceeds the breadth included in the derivation of (9), compound 35 being a 1,4-benzothiazine rather than a 1,2,4-benzothiadiazine and compound 34 being a 4-quinazolinone. It should be clear that (9) is an excellent predictor as well as merely an excellent multiple regressor.

Table 7 shows agreement between experiment and prediction for 3 compounds included in (9) and 6 compounds representing structural types which were not included in the derivation. The largest difference (last column) between experiment and prediction, in micrograms/ml (drug concentration), is only some 30 μg/ml.

From inspection of the data presented below, it seems that the information obtained from the EHT computations has successfully encompassed the salient determinants of potency for this series of compounds. It is of interest to speculate on the electronic mechanism of action of these compounds.

TABLE 7. PREDICTION VS. EXPERIMENT FOR EQUATION (9) (WEIGHT/VOLUME)

Compound Number	Experimental Range	Mean	Predicted Range	Mean	$\overline{X}_E - \overline{X}_P$
5[a]	1.59-2.01 μg/ml	1.79 μg/ml	1.59-2.77 μg/ml	2.19 μg/ml	-0.39 μg/ml
22[a]	18.4-192.2	59.4	45.1-78.3	61.7	-2.3
26[a]	0.001-0.011	0.004_2	0.003-0.006	0.004_5	-0.0003
27	0.034-0.12	0.089	0.037-0.064	0.049	0.04
28	0.43-1.49	0.80	1.30-2.25	1.71	-0.91
30	0.73-2.06	1.22	1.27-2.21	1.68	-0.46
32	21.0-63.4	39.0	52.7-91.7	69.5	-30.5
34[b]	0.87-2.51	1.48	2.51-4.36	3.31	-1.83
35[c]	1.91-5.51	3.24	3.24-5.63	4.27	-1.03

(a) Included in Regression.
(b) Quinazoline-4-one.
(c) 1,4-Benzothiazine.

Electronic Molecular Mechanism of Action

Without invoking any particular conceptualization of drug-induced receptor alteration, we may speculate that the drug molecule moves by diffusion in the biophase into equilibrium position for the formation of three, not necessarily simultaneous, weak molecular bonds at sites [A], [D], and [E] (Figure 6). While it is impossible to decide upon the sequence with which these bonds are formed, and being entirely aware that this hypothesis, is, necessarily, quite speculative, we note the early and continuous appearance in all the regression equations of the apparent importance of the area around the 4-4a-5 bond system in the molecule and say that the bond with site [A] is formed first. The compound is weakly affixed to sites [D] and [E] next, and the molecule now occupies the receptor.

The receptor, however, normally activated by Ca^{++}, may only be composed of sites [A] and [E], or any combination of two such sites for it is difficult to see how the dipositive calcium ion could interact at more than two sites. Sites [A] and [E] are chosen as the likely centers for the Ca^{++}-receptor because the distance between [A] and [E] is 3.5 Å. The diameter of the singly-hydrated Ca^{++} is 3.7 Å.[43] This interesting similarity may, of course, be of no more than coincidental interest. The distance, however, between sites [D] and either [A] or [E] is much greater, and it may be that [D] serves as the accessory site permitting stabilization of the receptor occupation.

With drug molecule in 3-point attachment to receptor, an electron or fraction thereof could possibly be donated to the receptor from the drug. With this event the charge distribution in the drug molecule changes so as to markedly decrease binding at [A]. Binding at [D] and [E] is slightly enhanced, but presumably, not sufficiently so, especially in view of the likelihood that the electron donation occurs from an orbital centered on or near position 5, to overcome the effective lack of binding at [A], and so the molecule is easily disengaged from the receptor either by Ca^{++} or solvent forces, or by changed charge characteristics of the receptor itself.

If this hypothesis is correct, at least in general outline, 4-methylated compounds, which possess very low $E^{[A]}$ values, should be inactive. This has been experimentally verified. Compounds substituted in the 3-position with highly negatively charged substituents such as trifluoromethyl should also be inactive, again in keeping with experimental data. Compounds devoid of oxygen at position 1 should also be inactive, as they are, but this result is open to doubt as a result of the very poor solubility characteristics of such compounds.

The hypothesis does not account satisfactorily for the observation that 3-oxo derivatives do possess respectable activity, but in this case the 2-nitrogen carries a hydrogen atom and this structural difference complicates interpretation of the laboratory finding.

IV. ACKNOWLEDGMENTS

The compounds discussed in this paper were synthesized by J. G. Topliss, Department of Medicinal Chemistry, Schering Corporation, Bloomfield, New Jersey. The pA_2 values were gathered by the painstaking efforts of Miss Lorraine Hausler and Mrs. Emma Eynon of the Department of Pharmacology. The regression analyses and conversion of computer programs were notably aided by Mrs. Margaret Hanks and Mrs. Barbara Uhrmacher of the Department of Statistics and Scientific Programming. Special thanks are due Mr. Robert Meese, of the Singer-General Precision Corporate Data Center, Wayne, New Jersey, for programming help and advice.

V. REFERENCES

[1] Szent-Györgyi, A., *Introduction to a Submolecular Biology*, Academic Press, New York (1960).

[2] Cammarata, A., and Stein, R. L., *J. Med. Chem.*, 11, 829 (1968).

[3] Neely, W. B., White, H. C., and Rudzik, A., *J. Pharm. Sci.*, 57, 1176 (1968).

[4] Kier, L. B., *Mol. Pharmacol.*, 3, 487 (1967).

[5] Kier, L. B., *Mol. Pharmacol.*, 4, 70 (1968).

[6] Kier, L. B., *J. Pharmacol. Exp. Therap.*, 164, 75 (1968).

[7] Kier, L. B., *J. Med. Chem.*, 11, 915 (1968).

[8] Cammarata, A., *J. Med. Chem.*, 11, 1111 (1968).

[9] Cammarata, A., *J. Med. Chem.*, 12, 314 (1969).

[10] Ariëns, E. J., Editor, p. 124 in *Molecular Pharmacology*, Vol. 1, Academic Press, New York (1964).

[11] Arunlakshana, O., and Schild, H. O., *Brit. J. Pharmacol. Chemotherap.*, 14, 48 (1959).

[12] Wohl, A., Hausler, L. M., and Roth, F. E., *J. Pharmacol. Exp. Therap.*, 158, 531 (1967).

[13] Wohl, A., Hausler, L. M., and Roth, F. E., *Life Sci.*, 7, 381 (1968).

[14] Van Rossum, J. M., *Arch. Intern. Pharmacodyn.*, 143, 299 (1963).

[15] Topliss, J. G., et al., *J. Med. Chem.*, 7, 269 (1964).

[16] Rubin, A. A., et al., *J. Pharmacol. Exp. Therap.*, 136, 344 (1962).

[17] Hoffmann, R., *J. Chem. Phys.*, 39, 1397 (1963).

[18] Hinze, J., and Jaffe, H. H., *J. Am. Chem. Soc.*, 84, 540 (1962).

[19] Moffitt, W., *Proc. Roy. Soc. (A)*, 200, 409 (1950).

[20] Clark, D. T., *Tetrahedron*, 24, 2663 (1968).

[21] Price, C. C., and Oae, S., *Sulfur Bonding*, The Ronald Press Co., New York (1962).

[22] Sutton, L. E., Editor, *Interatomic Distances*, (Special Publication No. 11), The Chemical Society, (London) (1958).

[23] Sutton, L. E., Editor, *Interatomic Distances Supplement*, (Special Publication No. 18), The Chemical Society, (London) (1965).

[24] Alleaume, M., and Decap, J., *Acta Cryst.*, 18, 731 (1965).

[25] Streitweiser, A., Jr., *Molecular Orbital Theory for Organic Chemists*, John Wiley and Sons, Inc., New York (1961).

[26] Woodward, R. B., and Hoffmann, R., *J. Am. Chem. Soc.*, 87, 2046 (1963).

[27] Pullman, B., and Pullman, A., *Proc. Natl. Acad. Sci.*, 44, 1197 (1958).

[28] Snyder, S., Merril, C. R., and Bradley, D. F., *Biochim. Biophys. Acta*, 118, 316 (1966).

[29] Fukui, K., Yonezawa, T., Nagata, C., *J. Chem. Phys.*, 27, 1247 (1957).

[30] Fukui, K., Nagata, C., and Imamura, A., *Science* 132, 87 (1960).

[31] DeVoe, H., and Tinoco, I., *J. Mol. Biol.*, 4, 500 (1962).

[32] Rein, R., Claverie, P., and Pollak, M., *Intern. J. Quantum Chem.*, 2, 129 (1968).

[33] Streitweiser, A., Jr., *Quantum Aspects of Heterocyclic Compounds in Chemistry and Biochemistry*, (The Second Jerusalem Symposium, March 30-April 4, 1969), Jerusalem, Israel (In Press).

[34] Novello, F. C., et al., *J. Org. Chem.*, 25, 970 (1960).

[35] Pitzer, K. S., *Discussions Faraday Soc.*, 10, 66 (1951).

[36] Lide, D. R., *J. Chem. Phys.*, 29, 1426 (1958).

[37] Chirgwin, B. H., and Coulson, C. A., *Proc. Roy. Soc. (London)*, A291, 196 (1950).

[38] Henneike, H. F., and Drago, R. S., *J. Am. Chem. Soc.*, 90, 5112 (1968).

[39] Baldwin, J. E., and Foglesong, W. D., *J. Am. Chem. Soc.*, 90, 4311 (1968).

[40] Trahanovsky, W. S., *J. Org. Chem.*, 30, 1666 (1965).

[41] Klopman, G., and Hudson, R. F., *Theoret. Chim. Acta*, 8, 165 (1967).

[42] Klopman, G., *J. Am. Chem. Soc.*, 90, 223 (1968).

[43] Mullins, L. J., *Ann. N.Y. Acad. Sci.*, 94, 390 (1961).

ATTENDEES

QUANTUM BIOLOGY SEMINAR

Battelle Seattle Research Center
Seattle, Washington

Mr. Gordon Amidon
College Pharmacy
University of Michigan
Ann Arbor, Michigan 48104

Dr. Arthur Cammarata
College of Pharmacy
Temple University
Philadelphia, Pennsylvania 19140

Dr. David Chang
Boeing Scientific Research Laboratory
P. O. Box 3981
Seattle, Washington 98124

Dr. B. Vernon Cheney
The Upjohn Company
Kalamazoo, Michigan 49003

Dr. Ralph Christoffersen
Department of Chemistry
University of Kansas
Lawrence, Kansas 50707

Mr. Jim Crow
Department of Pharmacology
School of Medicine
University of Mississippi
Jackson, Mississippi 39216

Prof. David A. Deranleau
Department of Biochemistry
University of Washington
Seattle, Washington 98105

Dr. Harvey Drucker
Pacific Northwest Laboratory
Battelle Memorial Institute
P. O. Box 999
Richland, Washington 99352

Dr. W. Dale Felix
Pacific Northwest Laboratory
Battelle Memorial Institute
P. O. Box 999
Richland, Washington 99352

Dr. Jack P. Green
Mount Sinai School of Medicine
5th Avenue & 100th Street
New York, New York 10029

Dr. Corwin Hansch
Department of Chemistry
Pomona College
Claremont, California 91711

Dr. Robert B. Hermann
Physical Chemistry Research Div.
Eli Lilly and Company
Indianapolis, Indiana

Dr. W. C. Holland
Department of Pharmacology
School of Medicine
University of Mississippi
Jackson, Mississippi 39216

Dr. James Hoyland
Columbus Laboratories
Battelle Memorial Institute
505 King Avenue
Columbus, Ohio 43201

Mr. Carl L. Johnson
Department of Pharmacology
Baylor College of Medicine
Houston, Texas 77025

Dr. Donald Kalkwarf
Pacific Northwest Laboratory
Battelle Memorial Institute
P. O. Box 999
Richland, Washington 99352

Dr. Stewart C. Keeton
Pacific Northwest Laboratory
Battelle Memorial Institute
P. O. Box 999
Richland, Washington 99352

Dr. L. B. Kier (Chairman)
Columbus Laboratories
Battelle Memorial Institute
505 King Avenue
Columbus, Ohio 43201

Dr. Herbert Kollmar
Battelle Institut e.V
Wiesbadenerstrasse, Postfach
900160
6000 Frankfurt, 90
Germany

Dr. Jackson Lynn
Columbus Laboratories
Battelle Memorial Institute
505 King Avenue
Columbus, Ohio 43201

Dr. Ray McCullough
Boeing Scientific Research Laboratory
P. O. Box 3981
Seattle, Washington 98124

Dr. Gerald Maggiora
Department of Chemistry
University of Kansas
Lawrence, Kansas 66044

Dr. Kenneth M. Maloney
Pacific Northwest Laboratory
Battelle Memorial Institute
P. O. Box 999
Richland, Washington 99352

Mr. Victor Marquez
College of Pharmacy
University of Michigan
Ann Arbor, Michigan 48104

Dr. W. H. Matchett
Battelle Seattle Research Center
4000 N. E. 41th Street
Seattle, Washington 98105

Dr. John Morrey
Battelle Seattle Research Center
4000 N. E. 41st Street
Seattle, Washington 98105

Dr. W. Brock Neely
The Biochemical Research Laboratory
Dow Chemical Company
Midland, Michigan 48640

Prof. Hans Neurath
Chairman, Department of Biochemistry
University of Washington,
Seattle, Washington 98105

Prof. Philip Portoghese
Department of Medical Chemistry
College of Pharmacy
University of Minnesota
Minneapolis, Minnesota 55455

Dr. Bernard Pullman
Institut de Biologie Physico-Chimique
Fondation Edmond de Rothschild
13, Rue Pierre et Marie Curie
Paris, France

Dr. William Purcell
College of Pharmacy
University of Tennessee
Memphis, Tennessee 38103

Dr. Robert Rein
School of Pharmacy
State University of New York at Buffalo
Buffalo, New York 14214

Dr. Rudolf Ritter
Institut Battelle
7, route de Drize
1227 Carouge/Genève
Switzerland

Dr. E. B. Roche
College of Pharmacy
University of Nebraska
Lincoln, Nebraska 68505

Dr. Jurgen Schnakenberg
Battelle Institut e.V
Wiesbadenerstrasse, Postfach 900160
6000 Frankfurt, 90
Germany

Dr. M. Sernetz
Battelle Institut e.V
Wiesbadenerstrasse, Postfach 900160
6000 Frankfurt
Germany

Miss Judy Singer
Department of Chemistry
Southwestern College
Memphis, Tennessee 38112

Dr. Soloman Snyder
Johns Hopkins School of Medicine
Baltimore, Maryland 21205

Dr. James Stubbins
Medical College of Virginia
Richmond, Virginia 23219

Dr. Werner Surber
Institut Battelle
7, route de Drize
1227 Carouge/Genève
Switzerland

Dr. David J. Triggle
351 Acheson Hall
State University of New York at Buffalo
Buffalo, New York 14214

Dr. E. B. Truitt
Columbus Laboratories
Battelle Memorial Institute
505 King Avenue
Columbus, Ohio 43201

Dr. William Wiley
Pacific Northwest Laboratory
Battelle Memorial Institute
P. O. Box 999
Richland, Washington 99352

Dr. J. P. G. Williams
Columbus Laboratories
Battelle Memorial Institute
505 King Avenue
Columbus, Ohio 43201

Dr. Arnold J. Wohl
Schering Corporation
Bloomfield, New Jersey 07003

Prof. Allan Young
School of Medicine
Department of Physiology and
Biophysics
University of Washington
Seattle, Washington 98105

GPSR Compliance

The European Union's (EU) General Product Safety Regulation (GPSR) is a set of rules that requires consumer products to be safe and our obligations to ensure this.

If you have any concerns about our products, you can contact us on ProductSafety@springernature.com

In case Publisher is established outside the EU, the EU authorized representative is:

Springer Nature Customer Service Center GmbH
Europaplatz 3
69115 Heidelberg, Germany

Batch number: 10684220

Printed by Printforce, the Netherlands